Essentials of Paediatrics

SECOND EDITION

EDITED BY

NANDU THALANGE
MB BS BSc MRCP MRCPCH

Consultant Paediatrician, Jenny Lind Children's Department,
Norfolk & Norwich University Hospitals NHS Foundation Trust, Norfolk

RICHARD BEACH
MB BS BSc MD FRCP FRCPCH

Consultant Paediatrician (Retired), Jenny Lind Children's Hospital,
Norfolk & Norwich University Hospitals NHS Foundation Trust, Norfolk

DAVID BOOTH
MBChB MRCPCH MMedSci BSc

Consultant Neonatal Paediatrician, Jenny Lind Children's Hospital,
Norfolk & Norwich University Hospitals NHS Foundation Trust, Norfolk

LISA JACKSON
MB BS BSc MRCGP DCH DFFP DipTher

Honorary Senior Lecturer, University of East Anglia, and General
Practitioner, East Norwich Medical Partnership, Norwich, Norfolk

SAUNDERS
ELSEVIER

EDINBURGH LONDON NEW YORK OXFORD PHILADELPHIA ST LOUIS SYDNEY TORONTO 2013

ELSEVIER
SAUNDERS

First edition 2006
Second edition 2013

ISBN 978-0-7020-4359-8

British Library Cataloguing in Publication Data
A catalogue record for this book is available from the British Library

Library of Congress Cataloging in Publication Data
A catalog record for this book is available from the Library of Congress

Series preface

Medical students and doctors in training are expected to travel to different hospitals and community health centres as part of their education. Many books are too large to carry around, but the information they contain is often vital for the basic understanding of disease processes.

The *Pocket Essentials* series is designed to provide portable, pocket-sized companions to larger texts, such as our own *Kumar and Clark's Clinical Medicine*. They are most useful for clinical practice, whether in hospital or the community, and for exam revision.

All the books in the series have the same helpful features:
- succinct text
- simple line drawings
- emergency and other boxes
- tables that summarize causes and clinical features of disease
- examination questions and explanatory answers.

They contain core material for quick revision, easy reference and practical management. The modern format makes them easy to read, providing an indispensable 'pocket essential'.

Parveen Kumar and Michael Clark
Series Editors

Preface

In the first edition of this book, we sought to convey our vision of paediatrics as an exciting and challenging specialty, covering, as it does, the full breadth of modern medicine, from intensive care, to chronic disease and disability; from maximising life potential to safeguarding children from harm at the hands of those who should protect them.

Modern medicine is making progress, and this edition marks many breakthroughs in knowledge and advances in management. Every chapter has been revised. Some needed little change – the basic tenets of paediatric care remain the same – but some chapters have been entirely rewritten. In particular, the advancing role of genetics in modern medicine is marked by a new chapter covering this important topic. The appendices, too, have all been updated, including revised algorithms for resuscitation and emergency management of the sick child. A new addition is the management of unexpected child death – thankfully rare in the modern era, but Britain's child mortality rates are the highest of any Western European country – a reminder that there is still much to be achieved.

As before, we have written this book in the hope that it will appeal to a broad constituency of readers – undergraduates, junior doctors in training, general practitioners, nurses and allied health professionals. The knowledge we share in this book is firmly grounded in the realities of medical practice in primary care, a busy hospital children's department and the wider health community. Those realities are illustrated by the many case histories which we have selected to illuminate each chapter. We hope the cases bring the text to life and make your reading enjoyable, as well as more memorable.

The book has grown a little in revision, but, we hope, still fulfils its purpose as an essential and concise summary of modern paediatric practice in the UK. We apologise in advance for any errors or omissions and gratefully thank the diligent team at Elsevier who have worked so hard behind the scenes to bring the book to fruition. Finally, we thank those who inspire us – the children and families of Norfolk who daily enrich our professional lives.

Nandu Thalange
David Booth
Lisa Jackson
Richard Beach

Contributors

Kate Armon
DM FRCPCH MRCP DCH
DRCOG BMedSci BMBS
Consultant Paediatrician
Jenny Lind Children's Hospital
Norfolk & Norwich University
Hospitals NHS Foundation
Trust
Norfolk

Peter Bale
MB ChB MRCPCH
Paediatric Specialist Trainee
Ipswich Hospital
Suffolk

Richard Beach
MB BS BSc MD FRCP
FRCPCH
Consultant Paediatrician
(Retired)
Jenny Lind Children's Hospital
Norfolk & Norwich University
Hospitals NHS Foundation
Trust
Norfolk

Jane Black
RGN RM HV
Named Nurse for
Safeguarding Children
Norfolk Community
Health & Care
Norfolk

David Booth
MBChB MRCPCH MMedSci
BSc
Consultant Neonatal
Paediatrician
Jenny Lind Children's Hospital
Norfolk & Norwich University
Hospitals NHS Foundation
Trust
Norfolk

Graham Derrick
BM BS BMedSci FRCPCH
MRCP
Consultant Paediatric
Cardiologist
Royal Hospital for Sick Children
Great Ormond Street
London

Rosalind Howe
B Pharm MRPharmS
Paediatric Pharmacist
Norfolk & Norwich University
Hospitals NHS Foundation
Trust
Norfolk

Lisa Jackson
MB BS BSc MRCGP DCH
DFFP DipTher
Honorary Senior Lecturer
University of East Anglia, and
General Practitioner
East Norwich Medical
Partnership
Norwich, Norfolk

George Millington
BSc MB PhD MRCP
Consultant Dermatologist
Norfolk & Norwich University
Hospitals NHS Foundation
Trust
Norfolk

Mary-Anne Morris
MBBS FRCPCH MRCP
BSPGHAN
Consultant Paediatrician
Jenny Lind Children's Hospital
Norfolk & Norwich University
Hospitals NHS Foundation
Trust
Norfolk

Jo Ponnampalam
MBBS MRCP MRCPCH Dip
Pall Med(Paeds)
Consultant Paediatrician
Jenny Lind Children's Hospital
Norfolk & Norwich University
Hospitals NHS Foundation
Trust
Norfolk

Ros Proops
MB ChB FRCP FRCPCH
DCH
Consultant Community
Paediatrician
Norfolk Community
Health & Care
Norfolk

Nishi Puri
MB BS MRCPsych
Consultant Child
Psychiatrist
Child & Family Centre
Mary Chapman House
Norwich, Norfolk

Rahul Roy
MB BS MRCPCH DCH
Consultant Neonatal
Paediatrician
Jenny Lind Children's Hospital
Norfolk & Norwich University
Hospitals NHS Foundation
Trust
Norfolk

Sarah Steel
MB ChB MSc MRCP
MRCPCH
Consultant Community
Paediatrician
Norfolk Community
Health & Care
Norfolk

Nandu Thalange
MB BS BSc MRCP MRCPCH
Consultant Paediatrician
Jenny Lind Children's
Department
Norfolk & Norwich University
Hospitals NHS Foundation
Trust
Norfolk

Chris Upton
MB ChB DM FRCPCH FRCP
DCH
Consultant Paediatrician
Jenny Lind Children's Hospital
Norfolk & Norwich University
Hospitals NHS Foundation
Trust
Norfolk

Contents

Contents

A&E	accident and emergency
ABC	airway, breathing and circulation
ACE	angiotensin-converting enzyme
ACTH	adrenocorticotrophic hormone
ADH	antidiuretic hormone
ADHD	attention deficit hyperactivity disorder
AIDS	acquired immune deficiency syndrome
ALL	acute lymphoblastic leukaemia
AML	acute myeloid leukaemia
APTT	activated partial thromboplastin time
ART	anti-retroviral therapy
ASD	atrial septal defect
ASOT	anti-streptolysin O test
BCG	Bacille Calmette-Guerin
BLS	basic life support
BMT	bone marrow transplantation
CAH	congenital adrenal hyperplasia
CAMHS	Child and Adolescent Mental Health Service
CBT	cognitive behavioural therapy
CF	cystic fibrosis
CFRD	cystic fibrosis related diabetes
CFS	chronic fatigue syndrome
CFTR	cystic fibrosis transmembrane regulator
CK	creatine kinase
CMV	cytomegalovirus
CNS	central nervous system
CP	cerebral palsy
CPAP	continuous positive airway pressure
CPK	creatine phosphokinase
CPR	cardiopulmonary resuscitation
CRP	C-reactive protein
CSF	cerebrospinal fluid
CT	computed tomography
CVS	chorionic villous sampling
DC	direct current
DDAVP	deamino-D-arginine vasopressin (desmopressin)
DDH	developmental dysplasia of the hip
DFP	deferiprone
DFX	deferasirox
DKA	diabetic ketoacidosis

DLA	Disability Living Allowance
DMAC	disseminated *Mycobacterium avium-intracellulare*
DMSA	dimethylsuccinic acid
DNA	deoxyribonuclease
DNase	deoxyribonuclease
DSD	disorders of sexual development
DTaP	diphtheria, tetanus, acellular pertussis (vaccine)
ECG	electrocardiogram
EEG	electroencephalogram
ENT	ear, nose and throat
ESR	erythrocyte sedimentation rate
ET	endotracheal
FB	foreign body
FBC	full blood count
FEV	forced expiratory volume
FHF	fulminant hepatic failure
FII	fabricated or induced illness
FISH	fluorescence in situ hybridization
FSH	follicle-stimulating hormone
FUO	fever of unknown origin
G6PD	glucose-6-phosphate dehydrogenase
GBS	group B *Streptococcus*
GCS	Glasgow Coma Scale
GDM	gestational diabetes mellitus
GnRH	gonadotrophin-releasing hormone
GORD	gastro-oesophageal reflux disease
GP	general practitioner
HCG	human chorionic gonadotrophin
HDU	high-dependency unit
HiB	*Haemophilus influenzae* type B (vaccine)
5-HT	*5-hydroxytryptamine/serotonin*
HIV	human immunodeficiency virus
HSV	herpes simplex virus
HUS	haemolytic-uraemic syndrome
ICP	intracranial pressure
IM	intramuscular
IO	intraosseous
IPV	inactivated poliovirus (vaccine)
ITP	idiopathic thrombocytopenic purpura
IUGR	intrauterine growth restriction
IV	intravenous
JIA	juvenile idiopathic arthritis
LH	luteinizing hormone
MAC	*Mycobacterium avium-intracellulare* complex

MCADD	medium-chain acyl-CoA dehydrogenase deficiency
MCUG	micturating cystogram
Men C	meningococcus C (vaccine)
MMR	measles, mumps and rubella
MODY	maturity-onset diabetes of the young
MRI	magnetic resonance imaging
NF1/NF2	neurofibromatosis type 1/type 2
NICE	National Institute for Health and Clinical Excellence
NSAID	non-steroidal anti-inflammatory drug
NSAP	non-specific abdominal pain
OSA	obstructive sleep apnoea
PCP	*Pneumocystis carinii* pneumonia
PCR	polymerase chain reaction
PCV	pneumococcal conjugate vaccine
PDA	patent ductus arteriosus
PEF	peak expiratory flow
PET-CT	positron emission tomography CT
PICU	paediatric intensive case unit
PIND	progressive intellectual and neurological deterioration
PKD	polycystic kidney disease
PKU	phenylketonuria
PNET	primitive neuro-ectodermal tumour
PPI	proton-pump inhibitor
PPO	police protection order
PSNI	permanent sensorineural hearing impairment
PTH	parathyroid hormone
QDS	four times a day
ROSC	return of spontaneous circulation
RSV	respiratory syncytial virus
SCID	severe combined immunodeficiency
SIADH	syndrome of inappropriate antidiuretic hormone secretion
SLE	systemic lupus erythematosus
SPA	suprapubic aspiration of urine
SUDEP	sudden unexpected death in epilepsy
SUFE	slipped upper femoral epiphysis
SVT	supraventricular tachycardia
TB	tuberculosis
TNF	tumour necrosis factor
ToRCH	toxoplasmosis, rubella, cytomegalovirus, herpes simplex, HIV
TRH	thyrotrophin-releasing hormone
TSH	thyroid-stimulating hormone
U&E	urea and electrolytes

UAC	umbilical arterial catheter
URTI	upper respiratory tract infection
UTI	urinary tract infection
UV	ultraviolet
UVC	umbilical venous catheter
VF	ventricular fibrillation
VSD	ventricular septal defect
VT	ventricular tachycardia
VWD	von Willebrand's disease
WBC	white blood cells

Assessing childhood illness

1

(Lisa Jackson, Nandu Thalange)

CHAPTER CONTENTS

TALKING TO CHILDREN AND THEIR FAMILIES

Talking to children and their families is the key to understanding any child's health. It may be diagnostic. It can be therapeutic. It is extremely rewarding.

Working with sick children is challenging and difficult. A kind, thorough and systematic approach will give the child and parents confidence.

Taking a history is important for the development of the relationship between the doctor and child. It is an opportunity to put the family at ease. The history should naturally flow into, and overlap with, the examination.

What do families want?

Children are taken to see a doctor for many reasons. The parents' concerns might be quite different from those of the doctor:

Parents' thoughts	*Doctor's thoughts*
'Sam coughs at night'	'Sam coughs at night'
'It keeps all of us awake'	'His brother has asthma'
'He's had chest infections before'	'It's probably viral-induced wheeze'
'He needs antibiotics'	'Maybe he needs an inhaler'
'The doctor will give me a prescription'	'I need to make a diagnosis'

It is important to think about the ideas, concerns and expectations that parents have about their child's symptoms. If these are not established early on, they will feel dissatisfied or frustrated. Asking a family about their concerns focuses the consultation and helps to manage the problem.

The paediatric history

The traditional, structured history is important, but the order in which things are done in the consultation should be flexible.

The consultation needs to be interactive – try and involve children so that they feel a part of the process.

Be prepared

- Read the referral letter
- Look at the previous notes

- Where appropriate, speak to other professionals who have had contact with the child
- Record observations – temperature, pulse, respiratory rate
- Plot the height and weight on a growth chart – do not forget to look at the Personal Child Health Record.

Environment

An appropriate environment is needed. Think about:
- The consultation room – position the furniture appropriately
- Safety in the room – are plug sockets, sharps bins and other medical paraphernalia safe?
- Suitable toys – these need not be expensive or numerous; drawing paper and pens have magical properties.

General principles

Greeting

Be friendly – the family and child might be more frightened than you are. An appropriate introduction helps; tell them who you are and what you do. Find out who you are talking to.

Presenting complaint

Break down the history into a set of problems.

History of presenting complaint

Find out what has been happening. Sometimes the way parents describe a problem may be very illuminating:

'Jimmy vomited over my new coat and I was so angry. I told him to tell me if he was going to be sick.'

Make sure you cover the:
- Nature and duration of the symptoms
- Relieving and aggravating factors
- Impact of the illness on the family.

Sometimes you will be seeing a child with a chronic medical problem and then you will need to think about the everyday practical problems the family are facing. For example, how does the child get dressed? How does he go to the toilet? How does he get to and from school? Does the family receive any financial help?

Past medical history

Make sure you find out about:
- Pregnancy
- Birth history – include place of birth
- Illnesses/accidents/operations
- Hospital/A&E visits
- Immunizations (see Box 1.1)
- Growth
- Diet and feeding
- Allergies.

Drug history

Take note of the following:
- Current medication, including dose and route; ask about compliance – is the medication actually taken?
- Relevant recent medication, e.g. courses of steroids for asthma
- Non-prescribed treatment, e.g. vitamins and homeopathic remedies.

Box 1.1 Immunization schedule in the UK

2 months

Diphtheria, tetanus, acellular pertussis, inactivated polio virus, *Haemophilus influenzae* type B vaccine (DTaP/IPV/HiB); pneumococcus (pneumococcal conjugate vaccine, PCV)

3 months

DTaP/IPV/HiB; meningococcus C (Men C)

4 months

DTaP/IPV/HiB; PCV; Men C

12–13 months

HiB/Men C; PCV; measles, mumps, rubella (MMR)

3 years 4 months – 5 years ('preschool booster')

DTaP/IPV; MMR

Girls 12–13 years

Human papilloma virus [course of 3 injections]

13–18 years

TD/IPV

Other immunizations may be indicated in specific 'at risk' groups, e.g. hepatitis B, BCG (Bacille Calmette-Guerin), seasonal influenza, PCV

(From *Immunisation Against Infectious Disease* ('The Green Book'), Department of Health, London, January 2011)

Family and social history

Who lives at home? What is their relationship to the child? Is there any family history of medical problems? Ask about the health of those living at home. Do the parents work? Are there any housing issues? It may be appropriate to ask if the child has a social worker.

This history is about placing a child within a context (see also Figure 1.1).

Developmental history

For a preschool child, ask to see the Personal Child Health Record, which is usually a red book. There is a wealth of information in this book, and parents usually carry it with them. There is no substitute for learning the key milestones. Look for discrepancies in development in the key skills areas of:

● Gross motor skills
● Fine motor skills
● Speech and language
● Vision and hearing
● Social development.

In the older child, ask about school progress and attendance. Ask about any problems with sleeping or continence. Are there concerns about behaviour or mood?

Systems review

Direct questioning related to relevant systems should include:

● **Respiratory:** cough, wheeze, difficulty breathing, night-time symptoms
● **Cardiovascular:** cyanosis, palpitations, exercise tolerance
● **Gastrointestinal:** constipation, diarrhoea, abdominal pain
● **Neurological:** fits, faints, turns, headache

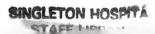

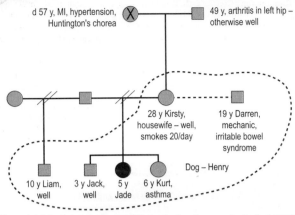

Figure 1.1 A family tree is often useful for understanding complex family dynamics. MI, myocardial infarction.

- **Genitourinary:** dysuria, frequency, haematuria
- **ENT:** sore throat, earache, nasal discharge
- **Skin:** rashes.

Child protection

It is important to recognize that, in some circumstances, we may have concerns about a child's welfare. Some children may be suffering, or at risk of suffering, significant harm, either as a result of a deliberate act, or a failure on the part of a parent or carer to act or to provide proper care, or both. These children need to be made safe from harm, alongside meeting their own needs.

Teaching to assess childhood illness rightly stresses the importance of listening to and believing what parents and carers tell us. Child protection training shows that in order to safeguard this group of children we must also be prepared to think the unthinkable. Any professional in contact with children must receive appropriate child protection training. It is vital to pick up the warning signs from the history or examination.

EXAMINING CHILDREN

First impressions

Does the child look sick or well, and why?

The well child	The sick child
1. Plays	1. Quiet
2. Feeds	2. Still
3. Interacts	3. Pale
4. Smiles	4. Drowsy
5. Responds	5. Unresponsive

Recognizing whether a child is ill or well is the single most important aspect of the examination. These signs correlate very well with the severity of illness. For example, Babycheck™ is a scoring system – devised for infants under 6 months for use by parents and professionals – that uses these principles to help them judge illness.

During the history, observe the interaction of the parents and the child. Look for physical signs such as a limp or cough, which might not be forthcoming during the examination.

Making friends

This is about trust. Children trust friendly doctors. Parents trust friendly, competent doctors. Of course, the practicalities of modern medicine do not always allow the time to develop such a relationship. Other strategies that help:

- Examine the child while the child is sitting on the parent's lap
- Play games – incorporate examinations into games
- Rehearse examinations on yourself, a parent or a cuddly toy
- Flexibility – examine available systems first
- Leave unpleasant examinations until last, e.g. throat examination
- Lots of eye contact, smiling and praise will work wonders.

Adolescents

It is important to respect the need for privacy and dignity of adolescents and older children. Appropriate explanations help. Some teenagers will prefer to be seen on their own, particularly for the examination. A chaperone will be needed if the patient is to be examined without family members present.

A PRACTICAL APPROACH

The detail of how to examine each system is important. Conventionally, we examine patients using a systems-based approach. However, the reality of examining children demands a more practical approach. Improvisation is needed, e.g. it is sensible to listen to a sleeping baby's heart at the start of an examination, rather than when the baby wakes up.

A practical approach to the examination of a child is shown in Box 1.2.

Box 1.2 Use your senses

1. LOOK	Observations: Sick or not? Bright and alert? Distressed? Appearance: colour, rashes, eyes Chest movement, respiratory effort Gait, coordination
2. FEEL	Fever, hands, pulse, perfusion Vocal fremitus, cardiac apex, abdomen
3. LISTEN	Cry, cough, stridor Heart sounds, breath sounds, bowel sounds
4. MOVE	Joints, coordination, neck stiffness
5. CHECK	Ears, nose then throat
6. LAST OF ALL	Plot the child's height and weight (and, for young children, head circumference) on the growth chart

Now write down all this information clearly and concisely.

Documentation

The history and examination should be clearly documented in the child's notes. Documentation is very important in all aspects of medical practice, especially in paediatrics. It is important not to lose sight of the day-to-day purpose for which records are made:

- To inform
- To communicate
- For continuity of care
- As a basis for planning care and treatment
- For evaluation of progress.

Principles of defensible documentation

- Identify the patient – write the child's name on each sheet of paper
- Date and time are important
- Identify yourself; if your signature is illegible, print your name clearly beneath your signature or use a stamp
- Write legibly
- Use only accepted abbreviations
- Never use the notes to make subjective or abusive remarks about the patient, parents or colleagues
- Be accurate; patients and parents are rightly angry when information about them is incorrectly or inadequately documented
- Take note of what is already documented, e.g. it is indefensible to prescribe penicillin to an allergic patient if that information is in the notes.

SUMMARY

The traditional history and systems-based examination have their role in the competent assessment of a child's illness. However, this highly structured approach may allow important detail to go unrecognized. It cannot be over-emphasized how important it is to let children and their families tell their story. Equally, time spent watching and observing a child is so much more important than quickly focusing on what may be an irrelevant detail of a systems examination.

Finally, consider what you have found from your history and examination. Are there any inconsistencies or concerning features? If so, consider whether the child could be at risk of harm. Take advice from an experienced colleague, and always act in the best interests of the child (see Box 1.2).

In the great majority of children, safeguarding concerns do not arise. The history and examination will usually be sufficient to determine a differential diagnosis, or at least to exclude a serious underlying problem.

You should summarize your clinical impression, any appropriate investigations and write down a clear plan. In the acute setting, this should include a 'safety net' - i.e. actions to be taken in the event of a change or deterioration in symptoms.

Children's place in society 2

(Lisa Jackson, Nandu Thalange)

CHAPTER CONTENTS

INTRODUCTION

An inquisitive visitor from a remote, isolated society might wonder why the Society for Protection of Animals has a royal charter whereas the Society for Protection of Children does not; why restaurants and pubs feel it is necessary to say that children will be welcomed (if they are well behaved); and why teenagers with as much interest and appreciation of the political world around them as most adults are not allowed to vote for the people that govern them. Despite lip-service being paid to the importance of children, society in western developed countries is adult-centred, and children's place in it is defined in terms of their relations with adults.

Society's responsibilities towards children are complex and sometimes contradictory. Children are our future and so need to be nurtured and at the same time they are vulnerable and so deserve protection. Society can discharge these responsibilities by supporting families. If families put their children's interests first and provide a stable, loving and stimulating environment, they will ensure the child's future health, development and social well-being. But children are also individuals and ought to be able to participate in society in their own right. Balancing these principles may be difficult.

THE UNITED NATIONS CONVENTION ON THE RIGHTS OF THE CHILD

A good starting point is to think in terms of children's rights. The 1990 UN Convention on the Rights of the Child (UNCRC) is the document on which the basis of children's rights, and their place in society, are founded (see www.unhchr.ch). It has been ratified by every country in the world with the exceptions of Somalia and the United States of America.

The UNCRC is a 'must know' for all doctors caring for children. It explains the responsibilities we have as health professionals caring for children, and provides a means to disentangle some of the complex ethical problems encountered in the healthcare of children.

The UNCRC begins by describing underpinning principles:

● The interests of children are paramount
● Children have the right to be supported in their own families and communities, but are not their families' 'property'.

It then lays out articles that cover rights of protection, participation and of provision. Below are listed some of those of relevance to child health.

Rights of protection

The right:

● To life (article 6)
● Not to be separated from their parents against their will except where to remain with them would harm the child (article 9)
● To special protection such as fostering or adoption when children are deprived of their family environment (article 20).

These rights reiterate the importance of families for the welfare of children. The right to be protected from:

● All forms of abuse (article 19)
● All forms of sexual exploitation (article 34)
● Economic exploitation (article 32)
● Exposure to illicit drugs (article 33).

These rights reflect the vulnerability of children and the responsibility of society to protect them. The most relevant for paediatric care are the articles protecting children from abuse, which includes physical, mental and emotional abuse, neglect, and sexual abuse and exploitation. Although paediatricians have a particular role in diagnosis and management, all doctors and healthcare workers have responsibilities for identification and prevention.

Rights of participation

● The right to an identity, i.e. a name, a family and a nationality (articles 7 and 8).

These may not seem relevant to healthcare but consider how many children change their surname, how often the surname a child answers to is different from the one stated on health records, and how often we call a child by a different name to the one they are familiar with.

● The right to express their views freely (articles 12 and 13)
● To have access to information (articles 13 and 17).

These are important general principles that are also directly relevant to children's health. Children should know about their health and contribute to decisions about their healthcare. In order to do this we need to be able to speak to children, provide them with written information, and listen to what they are saying, all in ways that are developmentally appropriate.

● The right of disabled children to enjoy life and participate actively in society (article 23).

This article describes the rights of disabled children to special provisions, but its inclusion as a right of participation reflects the view that disabled children should have the same status as any other child, or indeed as any other person. Participation is seen here as a positive property, in contrast to the negative notion of handicap (which describes how children's participation in society is limited by disability).

Rights of provision

- The right to the highest standard of health and the highest quality of healthcare attainable (article 24).

This article is the guiding principle for all those who care for the health of children. It describes the importance not only of treatment of illness, but of preventive and anticipatory measures, public health, nutrition, health promotion and information, all with an emphasis on primary healthcare.

- The right of every child to a standard of living adequate for the child's physical, mental, spiritual, moral and social development (article 27).

While article 24 underpins healthcare for children, this article is arguably the most important for children's health. It reflects the fact that poverty and deprivation have a pervasive detrimental influence on almost all aspects of children's health, well-being and development. The UK has very high rates of child poverty. Indeed, in 2008, the United Nations rebuked the UK for having unacceptably high levels of poverty for a wealthy country. Using the government's own definition of poverty, in 2010, 21.3% of children were living in poverty. In response, the UK government passed the Child Poverty Act (2010) which seeks to abolish child poverty by 2020.

PARENTS' AND DOCTORS' RESPONSIBILITIES AND THE CHILD'S BEST INTERESTS

While the UNCRC provides the basis for understanding society's care of children, the cornerstones of family and public law in England and Wales are the Children Acts of 1989 and 2004. It is within this act that the key principles of the child's best interests, the child's autonomy and the parent's responsibilities are described. These laws provide principles and guidance, but case-law will always play an important role in deciding on the best course of action in complex family problems.

Parents' rights and responsibilities

Children's best informed and most committed advocates are likely to be their parents. Of course, parents' decisions about children are influenced by their own personal attitudes and feelings. In most cases this is to be welcomed; it is the result of, and perpetuates, a diverse, multicultural, and pluralist society. Hence the importance of parental responsibility being enshrined in a wide range of laws and declarations (including the Children Act and the UNCRC). But at the other extreme, parents' own needs and desires might harm the child; this is child abuse, and society has an obligation to override the parents in order to protect the child.

The extremes are easy to understand, but there is a large grey area in the middle where the behaviour and decisions of parents conflict with the interests of the child in some way. Examples include physical punishment of children, parents condoning or encouraging truancy, cases where parents do not adhere to medical advice they have previously agreed was necessary for their child's health, or where parents present a child for medical diagnosis and treatment excessively and unnecessarily. The balance between a parent's rights and a child's interests can be very hard to determine. It is not a decision that an individual doctor, however experienced, can make alone because all of us are motivated by our personal or professional prejudices.

Physical punishment of children

Corporal (physical) punishment of children is still legal in the UK, although *public* chastisement of children less than 3 years of age is illegal in Scotland. The arguments for and against abolishing corporal punishment are well-rehearsed.

For:
- It is technically a form of assault which is illegal where adults are concerned
- It leads to a punitive form of child behaviour management, which is ineffective and potentially harmful
- There is no distinction between physical punishment and physical abuse of children
- It models aggressive responses to children that will influence detrimentally their responses to other people and their own children ('the cycle of abuse')
- It is a form of domestic violence
- Countries that have made this illegal have far lower rates of physical child abuse.

Against:
- There is very little direct evidence that it is harmful
- There is a large body of public opinion in its favour
- A law against corporal punishment would be impractical to enforce.

DUTIES OF MEDICAL CONFIDENTIALITY

Maintaining confidentiality is one of the fundamental duties of doctors. However, it is not absolute. There are circumstances where it is permissible, or even obligatory, to pass on medical information. Confidentiality may need to be broken if this would prevent harm to the patient or to others. This is why we have a duty to pass on information about child abuse. Even if our individual patient may be safe, there is a potential risk to others. The General Medical Council issued updated guidance on safeguarding and confidentiality in July 2012.

In contrast to other branches of medicine, where there is a direct two-way doctor–patient relationship, in paediatrics there are three parties involved: the doctor, the child and the parent(s). Occasionally a doctor can be in the uncomfortable position of being asked by the parent or child to keep some information confidential from the other, even though the doctor feels that to share that information would be in the best interests of all. Usually, discussing the benefits of sharing the information with the other party resolves the impasse. However, we must always be aware that our position as professionals and adults can seem very daunting to a child.

CONSENT

Similar principles apply to consent. Who should give consent to a medical intervention, whether this is a diagnostic test or some form of treatment? Going back to our first principles, children ought to have a say because they are individuals with their own rights, but, on the other hand, society endows a child's parents with authority to make decisions on their behalf because of their vulnerability and their unrealized long-term potential.

Legally, whatever the situation, parents can consent to treatment only if it is 'in the child's best interests'. Doctors must apply this test as well. In order to give consent there are three requirements:

● Adequate information
● Competence
● For there to be no coercion.

How can competence be assessed in a child or young person? Judges have described three tests which are equally valid for all vulnerable individuals including those with mental health problems and learning disabilities:

● The ability to understand and retain information
● To believe the information
● And to be able to weigh up the information and arrive at a choice.

These criteria are all highly subjective. Recent research has shown that we underestimate the competence of children of different ages to make informed decisions. Even at the same age, children's developmental abilities vary widely so we do need to make some judgement about their capacity to assimilate information and express a reasoned opinion.

After a famous court case – *Gillick v West Norfolk and Wisbech Area Health Authority 1986* - the law recognized that children aged under 16 years may have sufficient understanding and intelligence to consent to a medical intervention. They may do this against the wishes of their parents or without their parents' knowledge. For our part, it is vital that we record the evidence on which we base our assessment of the child's competence.

The law about refusing treatment is a little different. No-one under 18 years of age, whether they are competent or not in the *Gillick* sense, can refuse treatment that their parents' have agreed to. However, there are practical limits. No responsible doctor would force treatment on an investigation on a child who was violently struggling, and all doctors know young patients who refuse to take essential medications despite the best efforts of the parents and health workers to ensure that they do.

CHILDREN LIVING IN POVERTY AND MARGINALIZED GROUPS

An international view

In 1990, the United Nations set out its Millennium Development Goals. The fourth goal was to reduce mortality of children under 5 years by two-thirds, by 2015. Between 1990 and 2008, worldwide mortality in children under 5 years fell by 28%. Nevertheless, just under 8 million children under 5 years of age die each year, most from preventable causes. Of the 67 countries with high child mortality rates (accounting for over 95% of all deaths, worldwide), only 10 are on track to meet their Millennium Development Goal target. Many of these deaths are preventable by simple and relatively inexpensive measures, such as sanitation, immunization and oral rehydration.

This is an international scandal. In the longer term, the world economy operates in a way that keeps the poorest countries poor and does not reward expenditure on health and educational infrastructure. However, in the shorter term, it is not finance that is required, but organization and robust delivery systems – and leadership. Charismatic and outspoken leaders are making a difference with AIDS and HIV. Where are the leaders for children?

The other scourges of child health are the bedmates of poverty: war, conflict and violence. For children, these result in enormous social and health problems, including mental health problems, disrupted families and large numbers of orphaned and displaced children.

By comparison, the state of children in the UK might seem benign. However, the UK is not immune to child poverty. A survey by UNICEF in 2010 of child poverty in 21 European countries in the world placed the UK in the bottom four.

INEQUALITIES IN CHILD HEALTH

Social inequalities exist in almost all aspects of children's health. Babies from poorer backgrounds are born smaller, are more likely to die in infancy, and more likely to suffer from infectious diseases. In childhood, accidental injury is strongly associated with social class, as are mental health problems and suboptimal nutrition, with both obesity and poor growth being more prevalent. In young adulthood, teenage pregnancy, mental illness, drug abuse and death from injury and violence all show steep social gradients. Finally, many of the chronic degenerative diseases of old age, such as heart disease, stroke and chronic lung disease, are strongly influenced by adverse social circumstances in childhood (see Figure 2.1).

MARGINALIZED GROUPS OF CHILDREN

Ethnic minorities

Children from ethnic minorities are much more likely to be living in poverty, and have further disadvantages such as discrimination and racial abuse. English may not be their first language and they may have to struggle with conflicting cultural expectations.

There are other groups of children whose circumstances are detrimental to their health and well-being. These include refugees and asylum seekers, children whose parents are in prison, children from travelling families, and children being looked after by local authorities ('in care'). Preventive healthcare is less well covered, and mental and physical health problems are more common and less well managed in these children.

Children in lone-parent families

Many children live in families headed by a lone mother. In the UK these families have a very high risk of living in poverty (although in some other countries with a social benefit system that is more supportive of lone parents, this is not necessarily the case). The children have similar health disadvantages to other children living in poverty, and many studies have shown that the economic disadvantages suffered in these families determines the poor health experiences of the children rather than any deficit in parental care, or quality of family life.

Refugee and asylum-seeking children

Children from refugee and asylum-seeking families have greater health needs than indigenous children. There may be a number of reasons for this:

- **Separation from, or loss of parents** – causing emotional distress, attachment disorders in younger children, anxiety and worry, lack of protection and adult support
- **Under-nutrition** – with effects on growth, and function of various body systems, neurodevelopment and intellectual abilities

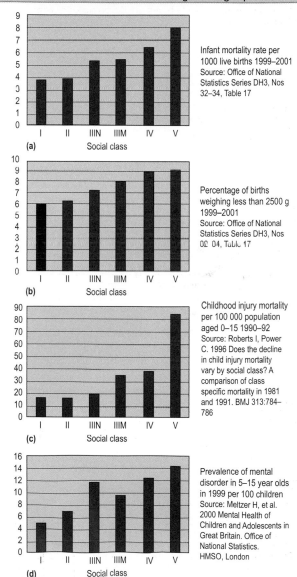

Infant mortality rate per 1000 live births 1999–2001
Source: Office of National Statistics Series DH3, Nos 32–34, Table 17

Percentage of births weighing less than 2500 g 1999–2001
Source: Office of National Statistics Series DH3, Nos 32–34, Table 17

Childhood injury mortality per 100 000 population aged 0–15 1990–92
Source: Roberts I, Power C. 1996 Does the decline in child injury mortality vary by social class? A comparison of class specific mortality in 1981 and 1991. BMJ 313:784–786

Prevalence of mental disorder in 5–15 year olds in 1999 per 100 children
Source: Meltzer H, et al. 2000 Mental Health of Children and Adolescents in Great Britain. Office of National Statistics. HMSO, London

Figure 2.1 Social class distribution of (a) infant mortality, (b) low birth weight, (c) injury mortality and (d) mental disorders.

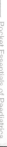

- Infections or parasitic infestations
- **Torture and physical abuse** – causing post-traumatic stress disorder, anxiety, depression, various physical consequences
- **Rape** – with risks of pregnancy, sexually transmitted infections, post-traumatic stress disorder, longer-term mental health consequences such as anxiety, depression, low self-esteem
- **Witness to murder, rape or violence towards others, including family members** – causing severe emotional distress, anxiety, post-traumatic stress disorder
- **Involvement in conflict** – children from conflict societies may be forced into participation in brutality, torture and fighting ('child soldiers'), with severe effects on mental well-being, notably post-traumatic stress disorder.

WHY IS THIS IMPORTANT?

There are several reasons why doctors looking after children need to be aware of these matters.

- Many children seen in clinics or hospital will come from poor, disadvantaged or marginalized families. It is important for doctors to be aware of the social conditions of their patients
- Knowing the effect of social circumstances on children's health will help us understand the reasons for some of their health problems, and may guide our treatments and advice
- Doctors have a duty to advocate for their patients. Knowledge of the effects of poverty and deprivation will inform the way that we advocate for individual children and their families
- Doctors have a wider duty of public health advocacy. This includes supporting measures to improve equity within society and to draw attention to the health consequences of poverty and discrimination. This is particularly relevant for paediatricians because children are a group who are not in control of their own social circumstances.

CONCLUSION

Children's place in society is a paradoxical one. On the one hand they are privileged with specific laws, provisions and services that reflect their vulnerability and their future potential, while on the other hand they are under-valued by their powerlessness in an adult-oriented society. This paradox is related to the ambivalence most adults feel about children themselves. Children's doctors have a duty to confront this ambivalence in themselves, in the general population, and in the laws and practices which govern our lives. By doing this we can make a difference to the lives of children and young people in our society and the wider world.

Further reading

United Nations Convention on the Rights of the Child. www.unicef.org/crc/.
Child poverty in the UK. Joseph Rowntree Foundation. www.jrf.org.uk.
Protecting children and young people: The responsibilities of all doctors. http://www.gmc-uk.org/guidance/ethical_guidance/13257.asp.
Millennium Development Goal 4 – Reducing child mortality. www.unicef.org/mdg.

The child with chronic disease 3

(Sarah Steel, Nandu Thalange)

CHAPTER CONTENTS

INTRODUCTION

Most children seen in primary or secondary care have an acute illness and most will make a complete recovery. When this does not happen, and ill health drags on, it impairs a child's natural, lively, sociable lifestyle. Care of these children and their families is as much about making life as normal as possible as about treating disease. This requires thoroughness, understanding and teamwork.

CHRONIC DISEASE

The prevalence of chronic disease in childhood is between 6% and 11%. Common chronic childhood diseases are listed in Table 3.1 and details of these conditions are found in the appropriate chapters. They produce a wide variety of clinical symptoms and require specialist assessment and management. Principles underlying the care of all children with chronic disease are highlighted in this chapter.

Some conditions are present at birth and result in lifelong disability. Others, e.g. Perthes' disease, asthma and epilepsy, may have an impact on health for a few years before resolving. Many conditions are life-threatening and a few lead to progressive disability.

Most children with chronic disease are managed as outpatients. It is better for children to be at home or at school as much as possible, and treatments are increasingly geared to this goal. Even highly complex interventions such as intravenous treatments and assisted ventilation can be managed at home by well-supported and trained carers and through the use of specialist home nursing teams.

THE CHILD'S PERSPECTIVE

Try to view the problem from the child's perspective. What professionals, parents or teachers might consider to be the major issues may well be at odds with the child's concerns and fears. Listening to the child is vital. Children will tell what it is that's bothering them if professionals take the time to ask and to listen. Children will often feel better simply for being listened to. If they will not talk to doctors they will often pour out their hearts

Table 3.1 Common chronic childhood diseases by system

System	Common chronic diseases
Respiratory	Asthma, cystic fibrosis
Cardiac	Congenital heart disease
Renal	Chronic kidney disease
Endocrine	Diabetes
Musculoskeletal	Developmental dysplasia of the hip, juvenile idiopathic arthritis, Perthes' disease, scoliosis
Gastrointestinal	Inflammatory bowel disease
Neurological	Epilepsy, cerebral palsy, muscular dystrophy
Developmental	Learning difficulties

to other team members such as nurses or therapists. Health professionals are in a powerful position to advocate for children and – sometimes – change their lives for the better.

AN APPROACH TO CHRONIC ILLNESS

An holistic approach views the child's needs in five domains: medical, educational, social, developmental and emotional.

Medical

The family's agenda

Consultation should start with the family's concerns. Initially these are likely to concern diagnosis and prognosis and, later, more practical problems. If family concerns are not dealt with, care will suffer. For example, professionals may be keen to emphasize the importance of regular physiotherapy or drug compliance, but the child may be more concerned that medication might be causing weight gain, or the parents that the child demands their attention for an hour each night at 3 a.m.

Diagnosis

This is usually established early in the illness but should be reviewed from time to time. Usually this means a quick review of notes to ensure that the diagnosis is secure. Medical knowledge moves on and these children may be under follow-up for many years. Re-investigation may be appropriate.

Systematic review

This is useful in the profoundly impaired child where any system and any aspect of care can be involved. Ask about basic functions: feeding, sleeping, bowels, bladder, mobility and self-care.

Medication

Medication regimes are often complex. Ask what medications the family are actually giving. Be open about compliance: 'Is he happy to take the medication?', 'Do you ever forget or get confused?'. Keep regimes as simple as possible. Use treatment charts or pill containers to help with this. Consider medication side-effects and drug interactions.

Monitoring progress

Shared health records and diary cards are often helpful, e.g. recording blood glucose results in children with diabetes, drug dosage changes or seizure frequency in epilepsy, or peak flows and treatment escalation rules in asthma. Physical examination at clinical review depends on the nature of the condition. Growth and development should always be monitored, and vision and hearing checked in children with neurological problems. In some cases regular investigations are necessary. An annual review of the whole case using a specific protocol is often good practice.

Prognosis

Consider the severity and outlook for this disease. Do professionals and family share a common understanding of these? If the prognosis is poor, is there an agreed plan for resuscitation or terminal care? Such issues demand high levels of trust between professionals, the family and the child. Integration and coordination of the healthcare professionals involved is crucial.

Information

Families and children should be advised where to find more information about the condition. Parent support groups often produce helpful literature and help lines. A suitable web site to inform their search for information is very useful.

Education

Going to school is important for every child's personal and social development, as well as for their education. This presents particular difficulties for children with chronic disease.

Medical needs in school

These may be as simple as access to an inhaler for asthma or as complex as gastrostomy feeds, buccal midazolam as emergency treatment for seizures, or upper airway suction to clear secretions. With proper planning, staffing and staff training these complex medical needs can be met in school. Whilst specialist provision may be necessary to deliver medical care, all school staff need to be aware of symptoms and to be able to offer first aid.

Therapy in school

Physical, occupational and speech therapy may be delivered in school. There is a need for close coordination of education and therapy needs.

Access to the curriculum

Children with disabilities will need a range of resources to access the curriculum (see Table 3.2).

Care needs

Children with chronic disease, especially neurological conditions, may need help with toileting, feeding and all other aspects of care.

Educational issues

School staff are often concerned at the prospect of having a child with acute medical needs in school. They fear for the safety of the child, the smooth running of the school and their own liability if problems arise. Some of these problems can be solved by careful communication between the health professional, family and teachers. Others require care plans, new facilities, extra staff or financial support. In the UK the education authority can assess needs and produce a formal *Statement of Special Educational Needs*. Currently, 2.7% of children have a formal Statement, although 21% are identified as

Table 3.2 Access needs in various disabilities

Nature of disability	Examples of access needs
Movement disorder	Level access, rails on stairs, desk height to suit wheelchair, some protection from boisterous playground activities
Difficulty with hand control	Laptop computer, special keyboard
Visual impairment	Large print material, bold bright materials, magnifiers
Hearing impairment	Amplification, give peers lip-reading education
Congenital heart disease	Modified physical education curriculum

having special educational needs. This is intended to clearly define resources needed by children with special needs. However, many feel that their children lack the right support. The current process is education led, and is time-consuming and bureaucratic, usually taking many months to complete.

To address these issues, in March 2011, the government published a green paper 'SEN and Disabilities' setting out plans to introduce a new single assessment process – the *Education and Health Care Plan* – that will be quicker and more straightforward to complete, by 2014.

Social

Children need the understanding, love and support of their families, and interaction with their peers, to achieve normal social development. Illness may compromise this. Thought must be given to how the child fits into their social context. This includes people – family, friends, relatives and the local community. It includes facilities – homes, schools and hospitals. Less obviously it may include the local Girl Guides and the benefit office.

Attitudes and expectations of the family towards the child may be complex – fear, ambivalence, and even dislike, particularly in siblings, may colour the family's attitudes. The financial implications of caring for a child with chronic ill health may be enormous. On average, it costs twice as much to bring up a child with a significant disability as it does a normal child. Meeting basic hygiene needs, costs of providing food, play equipment and transport, all play a part. Moreover, children with disabilities are more likely to live in poverty – Barnado's found that 30% of households lived in poverty, and 20% lived in substandard accommodation. Financial support is available in the UK through provisions such as the disability living allowance (DLA), and sometimes from charitable sources. The government plans to replace DLA with a new benefit, Personal Independence Payments, progressively from 2013–14. Local and national parent support groups can help integrate children into their communities.

Development

Child development is adversely affected by ill health, either through direct effects of the underlying condition such as cerebral palsy or autism, or as a consequence of the physical limitations imposed by the condition such as juvenile idiopathic arthritis or developmental dysplasia of the hip, limiting a child's motor abilities. Accurate assessment and appropriate and timely intervention are required to ensure the best long-term outcomes and to ensure carers do not have unrealistic expectations of the child.

Emotional

Children are essentially gregarious – they love to join in groups and find acceptance and security in being the same as everyone else. Chronic disease disrupts this. These children may look different, be more restricted in what they can do, behave differently, have a different relationship with their parents and have a different learning capacity to their peers. Small wonder then that some respond with anger, denial, frustration and refusal to cooperate with carers, whether family or professionals. The family will have their own difficulties in coming to terms with this. Some children are robust enough to join their normal peers. Some find peers in other disabled children. Some retreat to their family base. A psychologist who understands such issues can be an important part of the caring team.

For families struggling to cope, respite care can be an invaluable help, enabling the family and siblings to have some 'normal' time together. Since April 2011, local authorities in England have had a duty to provide a short break service for parents of disabled children. Many local hospices and organizations such as Barnado's also provide respite care.

INITIAL MANAGEMENT OF CHRONIC CHILDHOOD ILLNESS – BREAKING BAD NEWS

Telling a family that one of their children has a chronic disease or a chronic neurodevelopmental problem demands skill and empathy. Traditionally, we have referred to this process as 'breaking bad news', which has strong negative connotations, so the term 'sharing the news' is now preferred. The ground rules for these conversations are clear:

- Ensure that the right person breaks the news – usually a task for a senior doctor
- Make sure the case is known well and the facts are clear
- Arrange to see both parents together – this is very important and worth taking time and trouble to arrange
- Set aside uninterrupted time in a quiet room
- Having someone else present to support the parents may be helpful
- If the child is an infant, he or she should usually be present.

It is not appropriate for a senior house officer in a busy clinic to blurt out to a mother that her 4-month-old baby may have cerebral palsy. Once the conversation starts doctors should:

- Introduce themselves
- Check what the parents already know
- Warn the parents there is bad news to come: 'I am afraid we have some concerns about…'
- Be simple and direct about the news: 'I think your baby son has a condition called Down syndrome…'
- Allow time and silence for the news to sink in
- Check understanding: 'Do you know what I mean by Down syndrome?'
- Be prepared for an emotional response – and to offer comfort and sympathy
- Do not get too complex – this is not the time for a lecture on the prognosis of Down syndrome
- Be as positive as possible.

Although the family wants to understand the problem, their level of distress may make it hard to listen. Despite careful news sharing interviews, parents may walk away believing the very opposite of what has been said. Repeated advice and explanations are likely to be needed until the truth 'sinks in'.

When parents imagine their yet-to-be-born child, they expect to meet a healthy infant. If the child is born prematurely, or with a developmental or medical problem, they face an uncertain, perhaps frightening, and certainly daunting future. There is a psychological need to move on from the child they wanted, to the child they have. Parents often need much support during this transition.

Part of the way forward for all families is to grieve for the loss of the child who perhaps never was. This is hard. The parents may be thrown into the hectic life of caring for a child with special needs, and not have adequate time for themselves. If grieving does not take place, some parents embark on a quest for the miracle solution that will restore their 'lost' child, leading to excessive referrals and unnecessary, inappropriate and unproven treatments. Care and compassion may 'unlock' normal feelings of guilt, anger, sadness, failure, and lead to the 'discovery' of their special child.

The perceived vulnerability of the sick child may lead to the parental response of seeing their child as very special and precious. This sick role can persist throughout childhood, curbing normal social development and promoting dependence. Parents may need encouragement to allow the child to experience the hurly-burly of normal life.

The question of causation and blame will sometimes cause difficulties. The family may blame obstetric, paediatric or other health professionals, with or without just cause. If with justification, then explanation and apology are appropriate. Most parents want the truth, and an expectation that lessons are learned. Only if they meet a wall of silence do most families become entrenched. A sense of 'genetic' guilt can be destructive. Is it the mother's fault or the father's? Does it run in one side of the family?

Paradoxically, it may be as hard to cope with an apparently more minor problem. Sympathy and understanding from the broader social network may be lessened if it is not clear that the child has a difficulty, e.g. the hyperactive child may be thought of as naughty, and the blame laid at the parents' door.

Caring for siblings

Much of the above may apply to the siblings of the child. Parents and professionals may overlook the needs of unaffected siblings. Even young children may want to ask questions and to understand, and this helps them overcome natural feelings of apprehension, fear and even jealousy, and in turn makes them more understanding of their demanding and disruptive sibling. Support groups are available for siblings and can make a big difference.

WORKING TOGETHER FOR CHILDREN WITH CHRONIC DISEASE

For many families, accessing the care and support they need is a struggle. Teamwork is the key to planning and delivering services for these children and their families. Teams may be multidisciplinary health-based teams or multi-agency teams that include social services and education, according to specific needs. These teams must work with the primary health care team.

The asthma team in Case 3.1 constitutes the paediatrician, the asthma nurse and the school health adviser; the GP and practice nurse will also be involved. A cystic fibrosis team might include a paediatrician, dietician, physiotherapist, nurse specialist and psychologist. When children suffer complex neurodevelopmental problems lots of professionals may become involved. See Table 3.3 for a list of those involved in the care of chronically ill children.

Case 3.1 A girl with asthma

Jenny is an 11-year-old with asthma. She suffered post-viral wheeze as a toddler and had frequent hospital admissions during the winter months. She has not attended 30% of her schooling for the past 12 months and is becoming rebellious about taking her medication. Her care is reviewed using the following suggested plan.

Medical
The doctor in clinic reviews the diagnosis with a chest X-ray and respiratory function tests. The diagnosis of asthma is confirmed. The family express concerns about her persistent wheeze and resistance to using inhalers. She is worried because her inhaler makes her feel different in school and her mother is afraid the steroid inhaler will stop her growing.

The asthma nurse specialist talks to Jenny about her asthma. After advice and reassurance her treatment is modified to include a combination steroid/long-acting bronchodilator.

The family keeps a diary of peak flow measurements and inhaler usage which they bring to the clinic.

Education
Jenny attends her local primary school. Her mother has told the school that Jenny cannot join in physical recreation with her classmates. Jenny and the school are anxious about managing wheezing episodes and inhaler usage. The school health adviser negotiates an asthma care plan with the school. With this reassurance all parties agree Jenny can return to normal activities.

Social/emotional
Jenny's mother who has frightening asthma herself is very protective of Jenny. Jenny is not allowed to visit friends who have pets for fear of bringing on an attack. Jenny's sister is jealous of the attention Jenny attracts and is developing some behaviour problems. Jenny resents the impact of asthma on her life and is fearful of the long-term consequences. Usually these issues would be managed with discussion, reassurance and advice from the asthma team. On occasion a psychologist may become involved.

Development
Jenny is developing normally but there are concerns that she will fall behind if her poor school attendance persists.

Table 3.3 Professionals involved in the care of children with chronic disease

Professional	Aspect of care
Paediatrician	Diagnosis and general review
Orthopaedic surgeon	Scoliosis, hip dislocation
Orthotics	Footwear
Paediatric surgeon	Gastroesophageal reflux
ENT consultant	Recurrent otitis media
Audiologist	Hearing assessment
Ophthalmologist	Visual impairment
Orthoptist	Squint assessment
Child development unit	Therapy planning and implementation
Community paediatrician	Coordinating services
Physiotherapist	Physical therapy for movement disorder
Occupational therapist	Equipment, promoting use of hands
Speech and language therapist	Communication aids
Community specialist nurses	Support in school
Health visitor	Support and liaison
General practitioner (GP)	Primary care health problems
Clinical psychologist	Behaviour problems
Dietician	Nutritional needs
Social worker	Family support and respite
Educational psychologist	Planning appropriate education

The list in Table 3.3, although long, is by no means exhaustive or unrealistic. If families are to make any sense of this, the agencies must coordinate their activities and offer sensibly planned care. Usually care is supervised, at least in the early years, by a child development team – often staffed by a community paediatrician, a group of therapists and, on occasion, staff from education and social services. A *key worker* as the main link to the team is useful in helping families navigate the complex maze of health and social care. Combining professionals into mini-teams accessed from the same venue at the same time is also good practice. For example, an orthopaedic team might consist of an orthopaedic surgeon, a paediatrician, a physiotherapist and an orthotist. At school age, care may be planned by a school-based team, and in adolescence transfer to adult services needs further planning and teamwork.

Child development 4

(Richard Beach, Nandu Thalange)

CHAPTER CONTENTS

INTRODUCTION

Understanding the pattern and time frame of normal development is an essential part of paediatric medicine. Whilst it is such an important building block in understanding children's health, it may feel as though learning the sequence of early milestones is about as much fun as learning times tables at school. Like tables, however, a sound grasp of normal milestones is crucial when you are trying to make sense of child development.

Children follow a sequence of developmental skills. The age at which these skills are mastered can be compared within a large population of children, and normal ranges are described. This horizontal approach allows comparisons to be made with other children and is a good way of rapidly screening a population for those children who might be delayed.

For children who have delayed development it is important to compare the individual's performance with their own previous performance (vertical assessment). This provides individual specific information about the rate of progress that will help to encourage and inform parents and professionals working with the child. Slowing in the rate of a child's development is a worrying sign and may indicate a significant neurological disease.

In every developmental skill there may be differences in the quality of performance. Thus, most of us can kick a ball but, even with daily training, few of us could become a professional footballer. Certain skills are fundamental but as the tasks become more and more sophisticated, fewer individuals are able to acquire them.

Cross-sectional observation of many children at specific ages provides the basis of developmental tests such as the *Denver Developmental Screening test,* the *Abilities of Babies* and the *Abilities of Young Children* by Griffiths, the *Bayley Scales of Infant Development* and the *Schedule of Growing Skills.* Using these tests requires special training. All those working with children need to be able to perform an informal assessment of their development as outlined in this chapter.

Assessing an individual child's development depends on:

- How that child is developing over time
- How that child's development compares with other normally developing children of the same age.

Pitfalls

Many of the assessment tools we use today were devised several years ago. The authors may not have used populations that we would recognize as being representative today. For example, is the 'normal' population of a similar socioeconomic, gender and ethnic distribution to the local population? Skills and experience also vary with time. Few 4-year-olds today encounter shoe laces. Everyone prefers Velcro, so inability to tie laces may be due to lack of experience, rather than lack of skill.

The assessment

Doctors rarely have an opportunity to observe children in their normal surroundings. We rely on an accurate history and some form of structured observation.

Environment

A formal assessment of development may take between 30 minutes and 1 hour. It is important that the room in which the family is seen is 'child friendly'. There should be a small selection of age-appropriate toys. Medical equipment and other potential hazards should ideally not be visible and there should be at least one small chair and a table. It is important that the furniture and toys are set up so that it is possible to talk with the parent or carer and observe the child at the same time.

Taking a history

The history can give a picture of a child that cannot always be obtained from observation so it is important to allocate sufficient time. It is a good idea to have a format so that you can make sure that important details are not missed. This is covered in Chapter 1. Particular areas of importance when considering a developmental disorder are detailed below.

1. What are the parents' concerns?
2. The birth history; where, how, gestational age and birth weight are important details. Did the baby require neonatal intensive care? Has anyone expressed concern about the baby?
3. Social history and family tree; include a history of the parents' educational attainment and developmental concerns about other family members.
4. Find out if the child attends a playgroup or nursery; they may be with a child minder or family member for much of the day. Do they go to special groups and activities?

The developmental milestones are best asked about in a systematic way:

- **Gross motor skills.** Most parents can provide accurate information about the age of their child when they sat and walked. The Personal Child Health Record ('red book') is also a useful source of information
- **Fine motor skills.** Many parents find it difficult to remember dates when these milestones were achieved but are able to describe what their child can do now
- **Speech and hearing.** The results of hearing tests should be in the Personal Child Health Record. Most parents will remember when their child said their first word. They may recall that a professional expressed concern or told them that their child's language development was normal. Health visitors, nursery nurses and pre-school staff are very astute in detecting delay in communication skills
- **Play and social skills.** It is difficult to remember the fine detail of these rapidly evolving abilities and often an accurate picture of current skills is the most useful information. Ask about whether the children play with, or alongside, others. Are they very shy? Do they have difficulty in separating from a parent or carer? What do they like to play with? Is there imaginative play? Do they enjoy looking at books? Is there pointing, copying and anticipation?

The motor skills

Babies develop motor skills if:

- They have a normal central nervous system
- They have the motivation to practise new skills
- They have the opportunity to practise new skills.

Case 4.1 A boy who is not yet walking

Dillon was 32 months old and was visually impaired. He was not yet walking without holding onto furniture.

Case 4.2 A girl who does not crawl

Phoebe was 9 months old and had 3-year-old twin brothers. Her mum was extremely busy in the daytime and Phoebe spent most of her day in a buggy or the car. She was sitting independently but was reluctant to lie in a prone position and had no interest in crawling.

- Children who are visually impaired may lack confidence to walk independently (as in Case 4.1). They cannot see a really interesting toy so they may be less motivated to go in search of it.
- Case 4.2 shows an example of how a child has been given limited opportunity or motivation to lie in a prone position and to experiment with crawling.
- For some conditions, such as Down's syndrome, condition-specific developmental milestones are available.

THE MOTOR MILESTONES

Newborn to 3 months

Gross motor

Healthy term newborn babies have well-flexed arms, legs and spine and enjoy curling up, even on their tummies. If pulled into a sitting position by their arms they have head lag. They have persistence of the primitive reflexes. The primitive reflexes are:

A. **Grasp reflex.** Babies will grasp hold of an object stroked across the palm of their hands.

B. **The Moro or startle reflex.** A sudden noise causes babies to symmetrically extend their arms and legs.

C. **Rooting reflex.** If babies' cheeks are gently stroked they will turn their heads to locate the touch.

D. **Walking and placing reflex.** If babies are held upright and the sole of the foot is placed on a firm surface they will extend the leg; if the dorsal surfaces of the feet are stroked they will pick up their feet as if to walk.

Fine motor

Young babies have limited fine motor abilities.

3 to 9 months

Gross motor

The primitive reflexes begin to disappear. When held to stand, babies sag at the knees. Babies will support their heads when pulled to sit. They enjoy kicking their legs and waving their arms. By 6 months they can be pulled to sit with a straight back. In the prone position they will lift the head and shoulders off the floor so that they can look around. From 6 months they can kick their legs one at a time.

Fine motor

At first, babies find their hands and clasp them together. Finger play follows this. From 6 months, a palmar grasp is seen. They are able to transfer an object between hands. A hand is placed on the breast or bottle during feeding. Objects are briefly held.

9 to 15 months

Gross motor

By 9 months, babies are ready to set off to explore their world. They can sit unsupported and use their hands to manipulate objects. They attempt to crawl (or bottom shuffle). They enjoy standing and taking their weight through their feet, and by 12 months they can pull to stand, and may stand independently. By 15 months, most children will have started to walk. They are starting to crawl up stairs independently.

Fine motor

Pencils are held with a palmar grasp. To and fro scribbling starts. They may build a tower of 2 bricks. A pincer grip, enabling fine manipulation, emerges. They are able to drink from a cup with a lid.

18 to 30 months

Gross motor

By 18 months, most children can walk whilst carrying a toy; they are starting to climb onto the furniture and they can squat down to play. By 24 months, children's gait is more like that of adults. They no longer stand

and walk with their legs apart (wide-based gait) and can run (but may not be very good at stopping). By 30 months they can walk up stairs, run and enjoy simple playground equipment.

Fine motor

Hand dominance will start to emerge. Babies are able to feed themselves with a spoon then fork. Increasingly tall towers of blocks are built: 3 blocks high by 18 months and up to 7 blocks by 30 months. Manipulation of pencils becomes more refined with an established 'tripod' grip by 30 months.

36 to 48 months

Gross motor

By 3 years, children can jump with feet together. They can kick a big ball and they can walk backwards. They may be able to use a peddle car or tricycle. By 4 years, most children can stand on one foot and hop. They can throw and catch a large ball and stand on tip toes.

Fine motor

At 36 months, children are able to draw a person with a head and two to three other features. By 48 months they draw a person with limbs, toes and fingers. At 36 months, a circle and some letters are copied. By 48 months they are able to draw a house and copy more letters. By 48 months they are able to dress and undress other than deal with fastenings.

PLAY SKILLS

Play skills develop rapidly in young children. Children who are uninterested in play should cause concern. The most common cause of loss of playfulness is that the child is unwell. However, a child who is said to be uninterested may be unable to play because of a physical difficulty or a learning difficulty. Another possibility is that the child has had limited play experiences and has been emotionally deprived.

Television is not an adequate substitute for playing with, and talking to, a baby.

Experimental play

This is normal from 0 to 6 months. Babies reach out for an interesting-looking face or object and something happens.

Exploratory play

By about 6 months of age, babies become increasingly inquisitive about the world around them. They put objects to their mouths to suck and taste, and they learn to pursue interesting objects. At about 6 to 9 months, babies develop the concept of object permanence, i.e. an object will continue to exist even when it disappears from view. Before 6 months, babies lose interest if a toy is covered up, because for them that object has ceased to exist. Through exploration, they are learning about the world around them.

Imaginative play

This is over-and-above the functional play already described. By about 18 to 24 months, young children develop the concept that one thing can represent another, e.g. a doll can be a real baby that needs to be fed. This skill is linked to a growing understanding that we all have our own thoughts and that language is a necessary means for transferring those thoughts from one person to another. By 3 to 4 years, children are joining in complex collaborative imaginary games.

COMMUNICATION SKILLS

0 to 6 months

Babies show interest in sound from birth. They will stop what they are doing and learn to turn toward sounds. They cry to communicate pain, hunger and discomfort.

6 to 12 months

Babies begin to babble musically. They start to repeat syllables, e.g. 'da da', and they start to point to objects they want.

12 to 24 months

During this period most children will start to use occasional words with meaning. Initially these words will only be understood by a caregiver. Most children will have at least a few words by 18 months. Understanding of language always precedes spoken words, and by 18 months a child will be able to follow a simple command, e.g. 'give Daddy the biscuit'. At this stage, children are better at focusing attention on what they see rather than what they hear. It is normal for children to repeat words and phrases that they hear.

2 to 3 years

By 3 years, a child should be able to put three words together to express need, e.g. 'I want drink'. At this age it is common for children to have unclear speech. Words may be mis-pronounced, e.g. 'nepolant' meaning elephant. These mis-pronunciations are not of any significance. Similarly, grammar and tenses are immature. Children need lots of opportunity to practise these new skills, with listening and responsive adults as well as with their peers.

THE KEY MILESTONES

There are three milestones, which, if not met, should ring 'alarm bells'. These include:
- Not walking by 18 months
- Not talking by 24 months
- Global patterns of delay at any age.

Not walking by 18 months

Ninety-seven percent of children walk by the age of 18 months. Of the three percent who are not walking by this age the majority have low muscle tone often associated with ligamentous laxity. This is usually benign and may be familial. These children usually find it difficult to crawl and may get around by 'bottom shuffling'. It is important to detect those few children with serious conditions linked to delayed walking. These include cerebral palsy, muscular dystrophy and severe learning difficulties. Tip toe walking is usually a variant of normal development, but rarely, may be a sign of cerebral palsy (notably spastic diplegia). Upper motor neurone signs will usually be present, and it may be difficult to passively flex the ankle.

Not talking by 24 months

By 24 months children should be able to say a number of clear single words and are starting to link words. If this is not achieved the first thought should be – 'can the child hear?'. If hearing is normal then learning difficulties or autistic spectrum disorders are alternative explanations. Investigate other aspects of the child's development and enquire about restricted play and social interaction.

Global patterns of delay at any age

> **Case 4.3** A globally delayed 3-year-old
>
> Anna was 38 months old. Her mother had learning difficulties and long-standing mental health problems. Anna had older siblings. Her father had some learning difficulties and was the main carer within the family. Anna had been referred for assessment by the health visitor because there were concerns about the parenting capacity of her parents. Taking a history was difficult. Both parents had great difficulty in recalling important milestones and confused them with those of her siblings. Moreover, they did not have any particular concerns about Anna's development. However, whilst taking the history it was apparent that Anna had difficulty with maintaining interest in the age-appropriate play materials. She flitted from toy to toy and although she explored the toys in a rudimentary way she showed no evidence of pretend play. On formal assessment she appeared to be delayed by eighteen months to two years in all areas.
>
> By the age of 4 years, it became apparent that, although her parents undoubtedly found it difficult to meet her needs, Anna had quite significant developmental problems. Even with support, Anna did not show 'catch up' development and at school entry she required a high level of support in the classroom. Anna was diagnosed as having severe learning difficulties.

LEARNING DIFFICULTY (MENTAL RETARDATION)

Learning difficulties are defined by IQ. A *severe learning difficulty*, as in the above case, is defined as an IQ of less than 35, *moderate* as an IQ of between 35 and 50, and *mild* as an IQ of between 50 and 70. The lower the IQ the more likely an organic explanation exists for the child's difficulties. Increasingly, genetic causes of learning difficulties are being discovered. Inquire into alcohol use in pregnancy as fetal alcohol syndrome is a significant cause of mental retardation (see Chapter 18, page 266). A detailed family tree and questioning about the academic ability of relatives is useful; referral to a clinical geneticist may be of value, particularly if there are dysmorphic signs. Careful physical examination should seek any evidence of associated health problems and a careful search for dysmorphic features which might suggest a genetic problem. Investigation should be tailored to the individual case. See Table 4.1 for a list of tests, which should be considered.

Table 4.1 Investigations to be considered in a child with learning difficulties

Blood and urine tests
Full blood count and film
Haemoglobin electrophoresis
Thyroid function
ToRCH Screen
Creatine kinase
Uric acid
Calcium
Cholesterol
Low resolution micro-array (or Karyotype)
Specific genetic tests: Fragile X, MECP2 gene analysis, telomere analysis as indicated
Plasma and urine amino acids
Urine organic acids
Urine mucopolysaccharides
White cell enzymes
Acylcarnitines
Radiological investigations
Skull X-ray
MRI or CT scan
EEG
Retinal examination

OTHER COMMON DEVELOPMENTAL DISORDERS

Dyspraxia

> **Case 4.4** A boy with poor coordination
>
> Tom was referred for assessment by his school special educational needs coordinator because he was very clumsy. As a baby Tom had delayed motor milestones, and did not walk until 21 months. His speech was slow to develop, and he required speech therapy.
> At school, he had evident difficulties in concentration, and his writing and drawing was very immature.

Case 4.4 is an example of dyspraxia, which describes impaired execution and planning of motor tasks due to immaturity or impairment of the motor cortex, manifesting as clumsiness and impaired spatial awareness (motor dyspraxia), and impaired vocalization and tongue movement (verbal and oral dyspraxia). Affected children, more often boys (M:F = 4:1), are usually of normal intelligence.

Dyspraxia is usually associated with a history of infantile hypotonia, delayed motor milestones, difficulty in performing tasks such as getting dressed, doing puzzles or playing ball games. Pencil grip is often poor with very immature artwork and writing. Verbal and oral dyspraxia results in speech delay with impaired articulation of sounds. Treatment entails a coordinated approach using occupational, speech and physical therapy, and in the school-age child, appropriate educational support.

Delay in bladder and bowel control

These problems are common and distressing. The key milestones to be concerned about are not being dry by the age of 7 years and soiling after the age of 4 years.

Nocturnal enuresis

Enuresis is defined as involuntary voiding of urine after the age of 5 years – most commonly at night – nocturnal enuresis (as in Case 4.5). By the age of 5 years, 93% of boys and 97% of girls are dry by day and night. By the age of 10 years, half of those with enuresis at the age of 5 years will be completely dry. If the child has previously been dry, the condition is described as secondary enuresis, and may be triggered by urinary tract infection, emotional upset or rarely, neurological problems.

Case 4.5 A boy who wets the bed

Jamie, aged 7 years, was referred with bed-wetting. Until recently, he had been wetting the bed every night, but had since had a few dry nights. He had been dry by day since the age of 4 years. His mother had had enuresis when she was a girl. His GP had sent off several urine cultures which were negative. Examination of his lumbar spine and leg reflexes showed nothing untoward. He had no difficulty passing stool. The diagnosis of primary nocturnal enuresis was made, and dry bed training with a star chart and rewards for multiple dry nights were instituted. After 6 months, Jamie was having only infrequent episodes of enuresis.

In nocturnal enuresis, a careful history and examination are needed, but investigation other than urine dipstick testing is rarely necessary. The child with diurnal (daytime) enuresis, on the other hand, might need an ultrasound examination, including post-voiding to look for evidence of congenital anomalies and voiding dysfunction ('irritable bladder') (see Chapter 11, p. 125).

Children with enuresis are sometimes criticized and punished and have low self-esteem. It is important to emphasize that enuresis is involuntary, but that it normally resolves, and with some appropriate help, this might happen more quickly. In those children who develop secondary enuresis, consider the possibility of an organic cause, such as urinary tract infection, diabetes or a neurological disorder. Psychological distress (e.g. bereavement) may also manifest as secondary enuresis; however, in most children, enuresis (primary or secondary) is a benign variant of normal bladder control and is not associated with unhappiness or anxiety.

- **Treatment**: The child is the key partner, along with the parents and the doctor. Behavioural strategies that reinforce success are used in the first instance. Excessive fluid intake and use of stimulant drinks such as cola or tea is reduced. The child needs to void at bedtime, even if there is no urge to pass urine. Lifting the child again at the parents' bedtime may help. A dry night is applauded and celebrated, and if appropriate, a reward might be given. Use of star charts is helpful. The child should not be punished for wetting the bed. This approach, known as dry bed training, is effective in 80–90% of children within 6–12 months. Where simple measures are ineffective, referral to an enuresis service for consideration of behavioural and/or drug therapy may be appropriate.

Second-line treatment includes:

- Use of alarms that awaken the child on wetting. Alarms are effective, but often unpopular with the rest of the family!
- Desmopressin (DDAVP) to reduce urine output. This is effective in reducing enuresis, but there is a high relapse rate. It is best reserved for special occasions, e.g. sleep-overs or holidays.

Soiling after the age of 4 years

Soiling and encopresis are much commoner in boys. Most children who soil are constipated. The management of their soiling should focus on managing their constipation (see Chapter 13, p. 170).

Children who soil are frequently isolated by their peers and have a miserable time. This has a negative impact on the child's self-esteem. The psychological overlay in this situation should be addressed, otherwise the medical approach to managing their constipation is likely to fail. Clinical psychology support is invaluable.

Encopresis describes children who soil as part of a primary behavioural disorder. It may represent a toilet phobia or stress-induced loss of control. It may be done to provoke a reaction. These children are more likely to defecate in odd places, hide or smear their stools. Psychiatric and/or psychological support will be required.

Further reading

Enuresis & constipation – Education & resources for improving childhood continence (ERIC). www.eric.org.uk.

Safeguarding children 5

(Ros Proops, Jane Black, Richard Beach)

CHAPTER CONTENTS

Every week in the UK one or two children die as a result of child abuse. Many more suffer significant harm at the hands of their parents, carers or someone close to them. Only very rarely is the perpetrator a complete stranger.

High profile cases, including the tragic deaths of Victoria Climbié and 'Baby P' (Peter Connolly), have highlighted some important weaknesses in the procedures for safeguarding children in the UK. This has resulted in improved awareness and training for all who are concerned with the care of children and more stringent policies and procedures across institutions. The message is clear – safeguarding children is everyone's responsibility – and that includes you.

WHAT IS MEANT BY 'CHILD ABUSE'?

The Children Act 1989 introduced the concept of significant harm as the threshold that justifies compulsory intervention in family life in the best interests of children. Significant harm is defined as:

- **Physical harm** – including shaking, hitting, poisoning, non-accidental fractures, scalds and burns
- **Neglect** – described as the persistent failure to meet a child's basic physical and/or psychological needs likely to result in the serious impairment of a child's health or development
- **Emotional harm** – described as the persistent emotional ill-treatment of a child resulting in severe adverse effects on a child's emotional development. This includes the corruption and exploitation of children.
- **Sexual harm** – such as forcing a child to take part in sexual activities, whether or not the child understands or is aware of what is happening.

In order to protect children from significant harm, we must all be prepared to *think the unthinkable* and be prepared to question the information given to us about every child we see.

PHYSICAL HARM

> **Case 5.1A** A boy with a lump on his head
>
> Jack, a 4-month-old baby boy, was taken to his GP by his mother for a routine immunization. The GP noticed a large swelling on the side of his head. The boy's mother said she had not previously noticed it and had no idea how the lump arose. The GP sent Jack to the local hospital where a skull X-ray revealed a linear parietal fracture. The paediatrician was concerned that this might have been a non-accidental injury and admitted him for observation and further investigation.

What might make you suspect a child has suffered a non-accidental injury?

1. Factors in the history

- No explanation is given as to how a significant injury might have occurred.
- There are inconsistent or differing stories given about the cause of injury
- The explanation given is inappropriate for the child's expected developmental level. ('*Those who don't cruise, don't bruise*' – immobile children are not likely to accidentally sustain multiple bruises on their legs; by contrast, the shins of most 4-year-olds are covered in bruises.)
- The explanation given is incompatible with the injury sustained, e.g. an 18-month-old child has bilateral fractured femurs, where his mother says the injury happened when he did a 'roly-poly' on the kitchen floor.
- There is delay in presentation. The normal reaction when a child is injured is to seek medical advice at once. If a child is presented many hours or days later non-accidental injury is more likely.

There are also a number of risk factors which may make a child more vulnerable to abuse, including having very young parents; those living in poverty; a history of drug and/or alcohol misuse in the parents or carers; and a history of domestic violence in the household. Children with disabilities are also at increased risk. However, it is vital to be aware that child abuse is no respecter of social class and can occur in any household no matter how well off or educated the family concerned.

Sexual abuse may present in a variety of ways, including inappropriate sexual behaviour, psychological disturbance and anogenital soreness or discharge. Detailed physical examination looking for signs of sexual abuse should only be undertaken after specialist training.

2. Factors on examination

If child abuse is suspected the child should be carefully examined from top to toe. Is the child content in the carers company? Do they seem well cared for and appropriately dressed? Are they clean? Height, weight and head circumference should be measured and plotted on a centile chart. Whatever the presenting concern the whole child should be examined for bruises, scars or other injuries.

Bruising is common in active children – but is usually on the shins and perhaps the forehead. Bruising to less accessible sites such as the trunk (especially the back) and the cheeks and ears is suspicious of child abuse.

Although it is impossible to age bruises accurately, a pattern of bruising on different sites and of different colours should cause concern.

Always compare the injury with the history and attempt to reconstruct what might have happened. This can be particularly helpful in assessing burns and scalds.

Linear marks from straps or sticks and circular burns from cigarettes should be identified. On occasion forensic testing can link an injury to the weapon used in an assault.

Be careful about signs said to be diagnostic of abuse. Torn frenulum is a worrying injury often found in children who have died after abusive head injury. Nevertheless it can occur accidentally. Assess each case on its merits.

3. Investigation of suspected child abuse

Investigation like examination should check the whole child looking for unexpected injuries. In younger children a skeletal survey which takes radiographs of all the bones is helpful. Children with possible head injuries should have brain imaging and ophthalmic examination. Investigation should also be used to seek an explanation for symptom. For example, those with bruising require platelet estimation and clotting studies.

As with examination, some injuries detected by investigation are highly suggestive of abusive injury. Metaphyseal fractures and rib fractures on skeletal survey are good examples.

Don't forget that an injured child needs careful medical attention. Remember the possibility of unsuspected brain or abdominal injury.

Case 5.1B A boy with a lump on his head (cont'd)

Jack's paediatrician was concerned about his injury and made further enquiries.

Jack's mother was initially unable to give any explanation as to how the skull fracture occurred. Once on the ward, she mentioned to one of the nurses that her boyfriend sometimes got angry with Jack when he cried.

Further history revealed that the mother was herself only 18 and her boyfriend was not Jack's birth father. She admitted that he was sometimes violent towards her.

Comment

A skull fracture is a very serious injury in a young baby and may be associated with underlying subdural haemorrhage or other cerebral damage. With no adequate explanation it is highly probable that the cause is non-accidental. A history of domestic violence commonly accompanies non-accidental injury.

What should you do if you have child protection concerns?

1. Accurate documentation is essential

Whenever you take a history, it is vital that you always document what is said to you accurately. This is as essential in child protection cases as in any other area of medicine.

Ideally you should always document:

- *When* the history was taken – give date and time accurately
- *Who* gave you the information and who else was present (other relatives, nursing staff, etc.)

● *What* precisely you are told. Use quotations directly – it can prove very helpful when someone else reviews the history, and will be more accurate than your interpretation of what you have been told. For example, it is better to say 'Mum told me that "David fell down the stairs and hit his head"' than just 'David fell down stairs and hit his head'. After all, did you see it happen yourself?

Document your examination findings clearly and use drawings or body maps to indicate the site and extent of injury. Describe precisely what you have found, not what you are told/think is the cause. For example, a cigarette burn is a round, reddened raised lesion, approximately half a centimetre in diameter – but so might be a spot due to streptococcal infection.

2. Inform your senior colleagues

Always express your concerns with your consultant or other relevant senior colleagues. The key to protecting children is not only to think the unthinkable, but also to share your concerns with those in a position to take further action. They can arrange appropriate investigations and will know who else to inform. *Never assume someone else has done this for you.* Rarely, if you feel that a child, staff or others may be at immediate risk you should contact the police immediately.

3. Follow your local safeguarding children procedures

Nowadays all NHS organizations are required to have a written safeguarding children policy. Familiarize yourself with its contents and make sure you know where to go for advice if faced with possible safeguarding children concerns. All NHS bodies responsible for children must have a safeguarding team with a *named doctor* and *named nurse* available to give advice and support to employees.

All local authorities in Great Britain have a Safeguarding Children Board (a single board covers Northern Ireland), with a *designated doctor* and *nurse*, responsible for leading child protection in the locality. This role includes advising local safeguarding boards, working with public health to ensure awareness of safeguarding and related issues, such as domestic violence, providing advice to health providers, and feeding into health commissioning/provision.

Case 5.1C A boy with a lump on his head (cont'd)

Jack was observed on the ward overnight for any clinical effects of head injury. The following day he had a *skeletal survey* carried out. (This is a type of X-ray that looks at all areas of the body for evidence of any other bony injury. It may well require sedation and the expertise of a specialist radiologist for interpretation.) On this occasion it revealed several healing rib fractures and a healed fracture of the left upper humerus. A *CT scan* of Jack's head was reported as normal with no signs of cerebral haemorrhage.

What should happen once someone has raised the possibility of abuse?

Social services must be informed of your concerns, giving clear reasons as to why you feel the child has been, or is at, risk of being significantly harmed. This is usually the responsibility of the consultant in charge, or the GP dealing with the child, if the child presents in general practice and does not attend hospital. The procedures in your hospital will make this clear. However, many other people, including health visitors, teachers and members of the public, can and should notify social services if they are worried that a child might be being harmed.

Once social services are informed of significant concerns about a child, the following usually happens:

- A social worker will carry out *an initial assessment* of the family situation and the risks to the child/children
- A *strategy meeting* will be held to decide what further action should be taken. This generally involves key professionals involved in the case
- An *initial case conference* will be convened at which a decision is made as to whether or not a safeguarding plan should be instituted. This will ensure professional carers and the local authority work together in a planned way to ensure the child's continuing safety
- The progress of the safeguarding plan is reviewed at a *review case conference* about 3 months later. Once conference agrees that the child's safety is assured the plan can be discontinued.

Case 5.1D A boy with a lump on his head (cont'd)

Jack remained well while on the ward, and following a strategy meeting it was agreed that he might be at risk of further harm if discharged home to his mother and her boyfriend. He was therefore discharged from hospital to foster carers

A case conference took place 10 days later and a safeguarding plan was agreed because of the risk of continuing physical harm. Several months later Jack's mother left her boyfriend and moved back to live with her parents. Jack was eventually returned to his mother's care.

OTHER TYPES OF ABUSE

Neglect

Case 5.2 A girl left on her own

Kelly, a 3-year-old girl, was referred to social services by a neighbour who was concerned that she appeared to be left alone for prolonged periods in the house. She was noted to be extremely dirty and wearing clothes that were badly torn and did not fit.

When medically examined she was found to weigh well below the 0.4th centile for her age, and had marked speech delay. She had no idea what to do with crayons and paper or simple toys, and her behaviour suggested that she had never seen such objects before. She was placed in temporary foster care, where she rapidly gained weight and quickly learned to speak and play, although she had persistent difficulties interacting with other children and adults.

Emotional harm

Case 5.3 A boy who is a nuisance

Andrew, a 4-year-old boy, was constantly told by his parents that he was a nuisance and that they wished they had never had him. He had a favourite teddy bear which was given to him by his grandmother and that was his only real comfort. One day his father became very angry with him and burned the teddy bear in front of him as a punishment.

Sexual harm

Case 5.4 A girl with vulval soreness

Ebony, a 7-year-old girl, was taken to her GP by her mother because of recurrent vulval soreness. The mother was concerned that these episodes coincided with the girl's access visits to see her father. The GP referred the girl to a consultant community paediatrician and examination showed genital herpes. She later told a social worker that her father regularly asked her to sleep in his bed with him and had been doing so for 3 years since her parents had separated.

Fabricated or induced illness

Fabricated or induced illness (FII) – previously called Munchausen syndrome by proxy – is defined as illness which is fabricated or induced by a parent or carer. The carer, with a story of grave illness, brings the child to medical attention, often persistently. When the child is assessed they are found to be well with no evidence of ill health. The symptoms and signs cease when the child is separated from the perpetrator. The child may be subjected to numerous medical investigations before anyone raises the possibility of abuse. Presentations include seizures, suffocation, non-accidental poisoning and sudden infant death.

FII is *never* an easy diagnosis to make, and whenever the possibility arises doctors *must* work closely with other professionals, including the police and social services, to ensure that a detailed assessment is carried out and the case is appropriately managed.

You should consider FII when:
- There is persistent or recurrent illness
- The child looks well in spite of severe symptoms
- Investigations and treatment do not solve the problem
- The parent/carer is excessively attentive and cheerful, and reluctant to leave the child's bedside.

Clearly *all* of the above can, and do, arise in children with serious and real pathology. Always consider this diagnosis when a case seems unusual or the facts don't seem to fit the history given by the parent/carer.

THE CASE CONFERENCE

Case conferences are arranged by social services and are the place at which decisions are made as to whether or not a safeguarding plan is required and, if so, for what reason – physical harm, neglect, emotional harm or sexual harm.

Key professionals involved in the child's care are invited, such as the GP, health visitor (or school nurse, depending on the age of the child), paediatrician, teacher, and of course social worker. All are requested to submit a written report stating their involvement with the child to enable those present to make informed decisions about the level of risk to the child.

The parents are also invited and have access to all the reports provided for the case conference – hence the need to be factual and accurate when taking a history and documenting findings in the first place.

INFORMATION SHARING AND CONFIDENTIALITY

Many doctors worry that by providing information for social services they will be breaking their duty of confidence to their patients. However, it is clear that information must be shared between professionals in order to safeguard children. Indeed, sometimes it is only when information from a variety of sources is put together that people then recognize that a child is at risk of significant harm.

In order to understand some of the key issues around information sharing it is helpful to have an understanding of the law in relation to confidentiality. In July 2012, the General Medical Council issued guidance on safeguarding children for all doctors. You need to be aware of:

- The common law duty of confidence
- The Human Rights Act 1998
- The Data Protection Act 1998.

The common law duty of confidence

The doctor–patient relationship is viewed as confidential. However, disclosure of information is allowed under a number of circumstances. These include when the person to whom the duty is owed consents to the information being shared; and when there is an overriding public interest in disclosure, such as the need to protect a child from harm.

The Human Rights Act

This Act recognizes that everyone has the right to privacy and to respect for their private and family lives. However, this right is not absolute, and disclosure of information is justified when it will protect the health and welfare of the child or prevent a criminal offence.

The Data Protection Act

Essentially, this Act lays down requirements about the way personal information, held in computer or paper records, is handled and processed, including disclosure of that information. As with the Human Rights Act, disclosure of information is permitted if there are particular welfare concerns about a child and if it is felt that failure to disclose might result in harm to that child.

So whether you work in general practice, orthopaedics, radiology, obstetrics or paediatrics – or indeed any branch of medicine – *safeguarding children really is everybody's business.*

Further reading

Working together to safeguard children. 2010. Ministry of Education, UK.

Child protection companion. 2006. Royal College of Paediatrics and Child Health.

Welsh Child Protection Systematic Review Group. www.core-info.cardiff.ac.uk/.

Protecting children and young people: responsibilities of all doctors. http://www.gmc-uk.org/guidance/ethical_guidance/13257.asp.

Locomotion 6

(Kate Armon, Lisa Jackson)

CHAPTER CONTENTS

INTRODUCTION

Parents want normal, healthy children, and will worry if their child seems different to others. We are all made differently and the clinician must know what matters and what does not.

Children are active and lively and enjoy the freedom of running, jumping, climbing, and generally pushing their bodies to the limit. They often tolerate a great deal of pain before complaining. When they do complain of pain it is usually mingled with fear, e.g. that they will never enjoy football/dancing/riding again, so it is very important that you respond to and understand these fears.

History

See Table 6.1.

Examination

The examination of children with musculoskeletal problems is often opportunistic, as they may be in pain. Close observation that starts when

Table 6.1 Important features of a 'locomotor' or 'musculoskeletal' history

	Presenting symptom
Joints	Pain – where, when is it worst, does it wake the child at night, what brings it on, is there anything that improves it? Swelling Morning stiffness (this is different from pain) – 'It takes her an hour to get going and then she loosens up' Function – unable to weight bear, cannot do up buttons Joint distribution
Extra-articular	Fever Rash, hair loss, mouth ulcers Poor appetite Weight gain and growth Vision
Past history	Any precipitating or preceding illness Development
Family history	Complete family tree Ask especially about arthritis, psoriasis, systemic lupus erythematosus, maternal miscarriages, inflammatory bowel disease
Social	Functional ability – dress, feed, walk, etc. 'Is there anything that you want to do but can't?' School – ability and progress 'What are you into?' – can the child still do everything they wish to do, and as well as their peers?

the child and family walk into your consulting room is often the most useful examination technique.

Table 6.2 lists important features of the musculoskeletal examination. Remember the mnemonic GALS (*g*ait, *a*rms, *l*egs, and *s*pine).

The essence of the examination is engaging with the child and not losing their trust by hurting them. Perform a general examination, particularly noting any skin rashes. Watch the child walk (if the child is of walking age). Observe the bones and joints, look at and compare sides. Ask the child to move the joint (active movement), and then palpate and move joints for the child (passive). If it looks, feels and moves normally then it probably is normal.

Investigations

Try to subject children to investigations only where absolutely necessary. X-rays are important when looking for a bone or joint abnormality. A full blood count, blood culture and inflammatory markers (erythrocyte sedimentation rate (ESR) and C-reactive protein (CRP)) will help you to

Table 6.2 The musculoskeletal examination

Gait	The child must be in underwear/minimal clothing to observe lower limbs and spine fully Preserve dignity Look at position of knees, ankles and feet, freedom of movement
Joint (any)	Inspect – skin colour, muscle bulk, resting position Palpate – skin warmth, joint swelling (soft tissue, bone, intra-articular effusion), site of maximal tenderness, tendons Move – range of active and passive movement
Hands	Pattern of joint involvement, rashes, nails (pitting in psoriasis, nail fold infarcts in vasculitis) Can she make a fist with the distal phalanges tucked perpendicular to the palm? What is the grip like? Does the thumb oppose to the base of the fifth finger?
Arms (sitting up)	'Put your arms out straight, now turn your hands over' (elbow extension, supination/pronation), 'put your hands behind your head' (glenohumeral and sternoclavicular movement), 'stretch your hands to the ceiling' (proximal muscle strength) Move joints passively through their full range
Feet (lying down)	'Point your toes down, then bend them up' (ankle joint) Squeeze the metatarsophalangeal joints (gently) – for synovitis pain Test eversion and inversion of the heel and forefoot (subtalar and mid-tarsal joints)
Legs (lying down)	Normal muscle bulk? Any swelling, deformity? Equal leg length? – measure real and apparent shortening 'Hug your right knee into your chest' (knees and hips) then the left Check for knee effusion: compressing the bursa above the patella, gently press the patella with the other hand – does it bounce off the distal femur? If you stroke up the medial side of the knee, down the lateral side, can you see fluid bulging from side to side? (effusion)
Legs (standing)	Any valgus or varus deformity? (valgus – the distal part of the limb is angled away from the midline; varus – the limb is angled towards the the midline) Flat feet (loss of the medial longitudinal arch)? If so, get the child to stand on tip-toe – can you see the arch now?
Spine (standing)	Stand behind the child and look at how straight the spine is and whether the normal curves are present 'Bend forward to touch your toes' – this should result in a smooth curve with no lateral deviation (scoliosis) Observe the neck movements (forward and lateral flexion, extension, rotation)

distinguish a simple mechanical problem from an infective or inflammatory condition. Where juvenile arthritis or connective tissue disease is suspected, appropriate autoantibody tests are important. If an infective arthritis is suspected, the joint should be aspirated to culture the organism. This is usually done under general anaesthetic (unless you are caring for a very sensible and stoical adolescent, who may cope with local anaesthetic and Entonox). Technetium bone scans may show areas of acute inflammation or infection (a 'hot spot'). MRI scanning is extremely valuable in diagnosing most musculoskeletal disorders.

Principles of management

Children want to get back to 'normal' activity as quickly as possible and it is important that you discuss this with them.

- Will they get better? Almost always yes.
- How long will it take? Be realistic.

You should work towards recovery with appropriate therapy, including medication, physiotherapy, occupational therapy, orthotics and psychological support. The child and family need education and support about the condition, the impact on school and family life, and, very often, financial support (disability living allowance). Social services and voluntary organizations may be able to help (see also Chapter 3).

PACKAGING DEFECTS

'My baby's feet aren't right'

A baby in utero is in a very confined space towards the end of pregnancy, resting in a flexed 'fetal' position. This can result in several 'packaging defects', with the feet being affected most often. These foot postures are always mobile, can be passively corrected to a normal position, and will resolve spontaneously. They include talipes calcaneovalgus (foot turned upwards, dorsum lies next to shin, heels pointing outwards), and *postural* talipes equinovarus. In these conditions, the foot may be passively stretched into the appropriate position, without difficulty.

Talipes equinovarus (club foot) (Figure 6.1)

In true congenital talipes equinovarus the foot posture is rigid, and it is not possible to correct the position. It occurs in about 1:1000 live births, is twice as common in boys, and in about 50% is bilateral. It is increasingly treated successfully, without surgery, with weekly manipulations, serial full-leg plaster casting, and division of the achilles tendon. The correct position obtained at about 3 months is maintained with orthoses at night only; this is the Ponseti technique. Look out for associated spina bifida, neuromuscular abnormalites, chromosomal disorders and developmental dysplasia of the hip. The inheritance is multifactorial, with a recurrence risk of 1 in 50 if the infant is male and 1 in 20 if female.

'Funny toes'

It is common for one or two toes to be out of line with each other. Most commonly the third toe curls inwards and lies underneath the second toe. Sometimes the 2nd to 5th toes have a flexed posture (hammer toe). These deformities usually resolve by 18 months of age and parents may be reassured. If it is still present after that time, and *causing problems,*

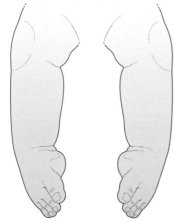

Bilateral talipes equinovarus
– Plantar flexion (equinus)
– Soles and heels point towards
  each other
– Forefoot adduction
– Shortened foot

Figure 6.1 Talipes equinovarus.

an orthopaedic surgeon should see the child. Toe syndactyly, particularly of the second and third toes, is common and requires no treatment.

Gait abnormalities

'My child doesn't walk properly'

There are several variations of normal posture. Most are part of normal development and resolve spontaneously. Those that are severe, persistent, painful or asymmetrical should be referred for a specialist opinion.

Bow legs (genu varum)

Normal infants are bow-legged when they start to walk. This results from bowing of the tibia, often associated with tibial torsion (twisting of the tibia inwards) such that when the upper tibia is forwards, the ankle joint is directed inwards. It usually resolves by 3 years. Rickets may be the cause (and is particularly common in dark-skinned races in the UK because of vitamin D deficiency) – look at the other bones, especially the ribs (thickening at the costochondral junction – 'rickety rosary') and take a wrist X-ray (widened, frayed metaphyses, osteopenia). Vitamin D deficiency is increasingly being recognized in the population at large. Frank signs of rickets, such as bow legs, are still unusual.

Knock knees (genu valgum)

A large proportion of children aged 2–7 years have knock knees (with knees together and ankles wide apart). The condition resolves with time, and parents require simple reassurance. Measuring the distance between the ankles is helpful. If the distance remains the same on an annual basis, the condition is improving because the bones are lengthening.

Pigeon toed (in-toeing)

There are three main causes of an in-toeing gait, which relate to the anatomical site of the abnormality (Figure 6.2):

1. The forefeet may point inwards (metatarsus adductus or varus); this commonly presents from birth to 5 years and slowly rights itself. Children are only noted to in-toe with their shoes off.
2. Medial tibial torsion will result in the top part of the tibia pointing forwards, whilst the bottom points inwards. This is common with bow-legs and usually corrects by about 5 years.
3. Children with persistent anteversion of the femoral neck commonly sit with knees bent and feet at either side of their hips. This is comfortable because internal rotation of the hip is easy, and external rotation is usually mildly reduced (difficulty sitting cross-legged). It normally corrects itself by 8 years.

Out-toeing

The infant or toddler may hold one or both legs in external rotation at the hip, such that the foot turns out. This normally resolves by 18 months. Examination reveals excessive external rotation of the hip on the affected side.

Toe-walking

This is common and normal if it starts early and involves both feet with normal balance and manoeuvrability. The child can walk with feet flat if asked to do so. A careful examination to exclude cerebral palsy is important (see Chapter 14, p. 197).

Flat feet (pes planus)

Foot posture varies with age. When children start to walk they do so on feet that appear flat, firstly because there is true flatness of the medial longitudinal arch, and secondly because a fat pad fills the arch. Eighty-five per cent of children develop a medial longitudinal arch by 8 years of age. At any stage the arch can be demonstrated by asking the child to stand on tip-toe. If the medial longitudinal arch does not form, this is abnormal, and may indicate a stiff forefoot with arthritis, or excess ligamentous laxity.

Flat feet are usually painless. Some do have discomfort, which is improved by wearing shoes with a good arch support (such as trainers), or putting arch supports in standard shoes. It is often associated with knock knees (genu valgum).

THE LIMPING CHILD

Transient synovitis of the hip

Case 6.1 describes the classical presentation of transient synovitis, which is the most common cause of acute hip pain in children. It occurs most often in boys (70%) in the 3–10-year age group and usually accompanies or follows a viral infection. Presentation is with acute-onset pain or limp. Pain may be referred to the thigh or knee. The child is not normally unwell, and is usually comfortable at rest. There may be a mild temperature and a decreased range of movement of the hip, particularly internal rotation.

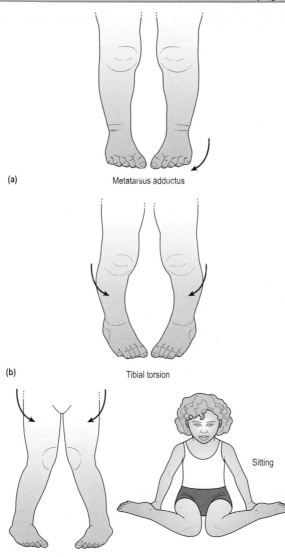

(a)   Metatarsus adductus

(b)   Tibial torsion

(c)   Femoral neck anteversion

Sitting

Figure 6.2 Causes of in-toeing: (a) metatarsus adductus; (b) tibial torsion; (c) femoral neck anteversion.

Tom is a 5-year-old boy who was brought to A&E because he would not walk. He had been completely healthy, but was noted to have had a cold the week before, and had started limping the day before. That morning he refused to get out of bed. He said that his right knee was hurting. He was still eating and drinking normally and did not have a fever. On examination, he looked well in himself, but was holding his right knee and hip slightly flexed. The knee had a normal range of movement and no swelling, but movement of the hip was limited and painful.

X-rays of the hip were normal, as were the full blood count and inflammatory markers (blood culture results were awaited). Transient synovitis of the hip was diagnosed, and Tom was asked to stay in bed until it felt better, which usually takes a few days. The doctor made sure that Tom's parents knew this was not going to cause any damage to the joint and that Tom would get completely back to normal. Paracetamol or ibuprofen was considered to help his pain. The parents were asked to return if Tom's temperature went up or if he got worse.

The main differential diagnosis is septic arthritis of the hip. This causes rest pain, a decreased range of all movements, and the child is febrile and unwell. If in doubt do a full blood count, inflammatory markers, a blood culture and an X-ray. A septic joint will be more likely if there is a neutrophilia and markedly raised inflammatory markers. Ultrasound scan may demonstrate an effusion in either condition, and a joint aspiration under ultrasound guidance with appropriate analgesia should be performed if in any doubt. Transient synovitis is managed with rest and non-steroidal anti-inflammatory drugs (NSAIDs) and will improve, usually within a week, with no long-term problems.

Legg–Calvé–Perthes disease (Figure 6.3)

This condition was simultaneously described by all three clinicians, Legg, Calve and Perthes, in 1910, and is an idiopathic avascular necrosis of the capital femoral epiphysis. Typically it presents in boys aged 5–12 years with a limp or pain of gradual onset. It is bilateral in 10–15%. There may not be much to find initially, but later there is a loss of internal rotation, muscle wasting and limb shortening.

X-rays may initially be normal and then show increased density in the femoral epiphysis, which becomes fragmented and irregular, and then gradually re-ossifies over a period of 18–36 months. There is little evidence that any interventions alter the natural history of the disease. The younger the child at disease onset, the better the outcome. The extent of the epiphyseal involvement and the sphericity of the femoral head and its congruency with the acetabulum at disease resolution predicts the development of early osteoarthritis. Long-term deformity, metaphyseal damage and degenerative osteoarthritis are complications. A large randomized control trial of bisphosphonate therapy in Perthes is currently underway, in an effort to improve the prognosis.

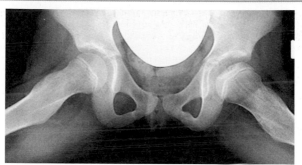

Figure 6.3 X-ray appearance of Legg–Calvé–Perthes disease.

Slipped upper femoral epiphysis (Figure 6.4)

A 10- to 15-year-old boy who is overweight is most likely to present with pain and limp from a SUFE. Restricted abduction and internal rotation is found, and it is bilateral in 30%. The onset is usually insidious, although it may be acute following minor trauma. The diagnosis is made on an X-ray (ensure that lateral views are obtained), which shows a posterior and inferior slip of the epiphysis on the metaphysis through the growth plate. Management is surgical, and usually consists of a pin to prevent further slippage.

Developmental dysplasia of the hip

Although a cause of limp, this condition should normally be detected after birth on routine neonatal examination (see Chapter 17, p. 248); however, late presentations with a limp do occur. DDH represents a spectrum of

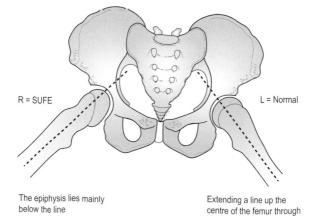

R = SUFE   L = Normal

The epiphysis lies mainly
below the line

Extending a line up the
centre of the femur through
the joint should bisect the
epiphysis

Figure 6.4 Slipped upper femoral epiphysis (SUFE).

disorders ranging from hip dysplasia, through subluxation to frank dislocation. The prevalence of the condition is about 1.5:1000 and is commoner in girls. Screening examination, with Barlow's and Ortolani's tests (see Figure 6.5), should enable early diagnosis and treatment with normal subsequent joint development. If the screening examination is abnormal the baby should have an ultrasound scan, which will give a detailed assessment of both the hip and the acetabulum. If hip dysplasia is confirmed, treatment should be supervised by a paediatric orthopaedic surgeon and physiotherapist. The infant will be put in a splint (usually a Pavlik harness, fitted expertly by paediatric physiotherapists), which maintains about 60° abduction and 90° flexion of the hip, but allows kicking of the lower leg. This maintains the femoral head within the acetabulum and allows each to grow normally. It may be required for 8–12 weeks and must be carefully monitored for fit as the child grows.

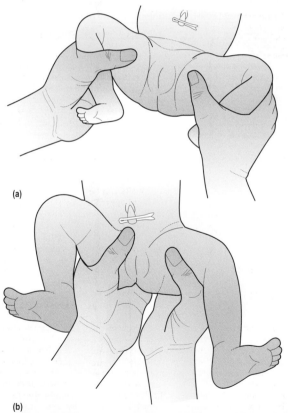

(a)

(b)

Figure 6.5 Tests for developmental dysplasia of the hip (DDH): (a) Ortolani; (b) Barlow.

Routine ultrasound scanning is offered at birth and at 6 weeks to those babies with a family history of hip dysplasia who have a higher risk of DDH. Asymmetry of the skin folds of the groin and thigh, limitation of abduction on the affected side, and shortening of the affected leg are all later signs of hip dislocation, as is a limp or abnormal gait when the infant starts to walk. If it is detected at this late stage, or if early intervention has failed, hip abduction using traction and a plaster hip spica may be tried, but complex surgery is usually needed.

Barlow test: Place the thumb on the inner surface of the thigh and the middle finger on the greater trochanter. Exert an outward and posterior force to dislocate posteriorly, and a 'clunk' is felt. Once pressure is removed the hip should relocate (Figure 6.5).

- **Ortolani manoeuvre:** The hands are placed in the same position as for the Barlow test. One hip at a time should be fully abducted in flexion. Abduction to 90° should be possible. Anterior pressure on the greater trochanter is applied and a 'clunk' will be felt as the hip relocates from a dislocated position.

THE PAINFUL LEG

Acutely painful limb – trauma

Children are frequently brought to the A&E department with a painful limb with a history of trauma. By and large, 'sprains' do not happen in young children, and if the child cannot weight bear or is unable to use the arm, the likelihood is that there is a fracture, and an X-ray is mandatory. Always consider carefully how the injury was said to have occurred and whether this is consistent with the findings (see Chapter 5) as non-accidental injury is an important differential diagnosis.

Acutely painful limb – infection

Osteomyelitis

Infections of the bone most commonly occur at the metaphysis of the distal femur or proximal tibia, but any site can be affected. The infection arises from haematogenous spread, and approximately 80% of infections are caused by *Staphylococcus aureus*. Other common pathogens include *Streptococcus pyogenes* and *Haemophilus influenzae*. In sickle-cell anaemia, *Salmonella* and *Staphylococcus* species occur more frequently.

Children with osteomyelitis usually have a high swinging fever with an acutely painful limb, which they are unwilling to move. There is often exquisite tenderness with associated swelling and erythema over the infection site, and moving the limb causes severe pain. In infants and young children the presentation may be more insidious (failure to feed, irritability, a limp or refusal to weight bear) and the diagnosis is difficult.

- **Investigations.** Blood cultures are frequently negative. There is a raised white cell count with a neutrophilia, a high ESR and CRP. X-rays are commonly normal initially, although there may be a visible soft-tissue swelling. After 7–10 days they may show an area of rarefaction followed by subperiosteal new bone formation. A technetium bone scan will show a 'hot spot' of increased uptake at the site of infection. Ultrasound may show early subperiosteal collections. The neighbouring joint may be aspirated, and fluid examined microscopically and cultured to exclude associated septic arthritis, particularly in the infant.

- **Treatment.** Effective, early antibiotic treatment improves the outcome, helping to prevent chronic infections with discharging sinuses or limb deformity. A broad spectrum cephalosporin given intravenously is used and refined when culture results and sensitivities aid rational antibiotic choice. Antibiotics are given intravenously until the clinical signs have resolved and the acute phase reactants returned to normal, followed by oral antibiotics, usually for a period of 4-6 weeks, guided by clinical response, and the severity of the initial infection.

Septic arthritis

Infection of the joint is most common in children under 2 years of age. It usually results from blood-borne bacteria, but may be caused by local penetrating injury, or in infants from metaphyseal spread from associated osteomyelitis. It is essential to treat the infection early and aggressively as destruction of the articular cartilage, growth plate and bone can occur. The causative organism is most commonly *Staphylococcus aureus*, but *Streptococcus pyogenes* and *Haemophilus influenzae*, amongst others, may occur.

- **Presentation.** Children present with an acutely painful, hot, erythematous, swollen joint, which they are reluctant to move. They are febrile and unwell. There is a detectable joint effusion, which can be aspirated under general anaesthetic and ultrasound guidance to identify or culture an organism.

  It is imperative in the neonate to consider other possible sites of blood-borne infection, such as the meninges (perform a lumbar puncture) and the urinary tract (collect and test urine).

- **Investigations and treatment.** Treatment is as for osteomyelitis. In the neonate an aminoglycoside such as gentamicin is added as Gramnegative organisms are more common. Orthopaedic intervention with a joint aspiration and washout is required.

'GROWING PAINS'

Preschool and early school-age children commonly have episodes of pain in the limbs, characteristically above and below the knee, and below the shoulder, usually manifesting as a dull and unpleasant ache, which wake them at night. Gentle massage or simple analgesia is usually sufficient. They are often worse after strenuous daytime activity. Musculoskeletal examination is normal. These pains are commonly referred to as 'growing pains' (or nocturnal idiopathic pain syndrome) and resolve with time.

ARTHRITIS

'My child has swollen, painful joints'

Children often present with joint pains, and the first consideration that arises, after acute infection has been excluded, is whether this is mechanical or inflammatory. Mechanical joint pains tend to occur towards the end of the day, or are made worse by activity; there is often a history of trauma.

In contrast, inflammatory polyarthritis is worse after a period of inactivity, and so is particularly bad in the morning. It may take some time for the joints to 'loosen up' in the morning (morning stiffness). On examination, finding erythema, heat, tenderness, a restricted range of movement, softtissue swelling or a joint effusion confirms inflammation. The causes of polyarthritis are shown in Table 6.3.

Table 6.3 Causes of polyarthritis

Category	Diagnoses
Infection	Bacterial – septicaemia/septic arthritis, TB Viral – adenovirus, coxsackie B, parvovirus, etc. Reactive arthritis Rheumatic fever Lyme disease
Juvenile idiopathic arthritis	See under 'Juvenile idiopathic arthritis'
Connective tissue disorder	Systemic lupus erythematosus Dermatomyositis
Inflammatory bowel disease	Crohn's disease Ulcerative colitis
Vasculitis	Henoch–Schönlein purpura Kawasaki's disease
Haematological disorders	Haemophilia Sickle-cell disease
Malignant disorders	Leukaemia
Other	Cystic fibrosis

Reactive arthritis

The commonest arthritis in children in the UK is 'reactive arthritis', secondary to an infection: post-streptococcal, post-viral and post-enteric. Although considered separately, Henoch-Schönlein purpura and transient synovitis are also post-viral in nature. Post-enteric arthritis is typically associated with salmonella, shigella and yersinia infections. Enthesitis (inflammation of tendons and ligaments close to their bony insertions) is a common feature. These children usually (95%) have the HLA B27 haplotype.

Juvenile idiopathic arthritis

Arthritis present for more than 6 weeks in a child under 16 years is classified as juvenile idiopathic arthritis (JIA), having excluded other causes.

The prevalence is 1 in 1000 in the UK (similar to diabetes), with an incidence of 10:100 000 per year. JIA is an autoimmune disease in which genetic and environmental factors combine in the pathogenesis. If a biopsy is taken, hyperplasia and inflammation of the synovium is found, which gives rise to the clinical signs.

History
JIA presents in various clinical patterns (Table 6.4). Children and their parents are concerned about the prognosis rather than the label, but the prognosis depends on the type of JIA. Ask about psoriasis.

Examination
This must include all the systems, since the disease can involve any system and extra-articular features provide helpful clues to aetiology. Each joint should be assessed in turn, including the often forgotten temporomandibular joints, and spine. See Figure 6.6 for the signs of JIA in the hands.

Table 6.4 Types of juvenile idiopathic arthritis

Type of JIA	Features	Prognosis
Oligoarthritis (60%)	Girls:boys 5:1, age 6 months to 6 years with 1–4 joints involved	Remission in 4–5 years usual One-third extend to polyarthritis
Polyarthritis (24%)	Girls aged 10–14 years with more than 4 joints involved	If rheumatoid factor positive, destructive and aggressive
Enthesitis related (7%)	Boys aged 10–14 years large joint arthritis and enthesitis common	Up to 60% develop ankylosing spondylitis
Systemic ('Still's disease') (9%)	Boys or girls aged 2 years Fever, malaise, salmon-pink flitting rash, hepatosplenomegaly, lymphadenopathy	Most remit after 3–5 years

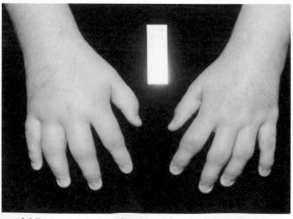

Figure 6.6 The hands in juvenile idiopathic arthritis (JIA). Note swelling of meta-carpalphalangeal and proximal interphalangeal joints.

Investigation

This includes full blood count, immunoglobulins, rheumatoid factor, anti-nuclear antibodies, CRP, ESR and radiography of affected joints for erosion and demineralization. Other investigations are undertaken according to the differential diagnosis. Septic or reactive arthritis must be excluded.

Treatment

Irrespective of the disease type, children with JIA require a multidisciplinary approach to management, involving doctors, physiotherapists, occupational therapists, social workers, orthotics, education, etc. It is a chronic condition that takes its toll on children and their families, and psychological input is often essential.

Treatment is aimed at controlling symptoms and gaining remission. This is one area of paediatrics where recent major advances have been made. Only 20 years ago the mainstay of treatment was corticosteroid therapy with all the attendant side-effects. The introduction of methotrexate has dramatically improved the outcome, and more recently the addition of biological therapy in the form of anti-TNF-α has revolutionized the lives of many children.

NSAID medication is the first line treatment, and in those with reactive arthritis may be all that is required. Those who do not improve will require intra-articular joint injections of corticosteroid. Where this does not completely resolve the arthritis, second-line therapy in the form of methotrexate is required (sulfasalazine may be tried for those with enthesitis-related arthritis).

Physiotherapy and judicious use of splinting is often beneficial once the acute arthritis is under control. Children with severe systemic features, serositis (pleura, pericardial, peritoneal) or multiple acutely inflamed joints need high-dose systemic steroids and early use of disease-modifying anti-rheumatic drugs. There is a large increase in biological therapies (monoclonal antibodies) used for the control of arthritis in adult patients, which are increasingly found to be effective in children, and which target different chemicals in the inflammation cascade. Therapy most commonly targets TNF α (e.g. Infliximab) interleukin 1 (e.g. Anakinra), or B lymphocytes (e.g. Rutuximab). The treatment goal is remission before evidence of joint distruction.

Complications

All children should be screened by regular slit-lamp examination for anterior uveitis, which is often asymptomatic. The autoantibody status should be checked because those who are antinuclear antigen positive are particularly likely to develop anterior uveitis (see Chapter 14, p. 212). In oligoarthritis, overgrowth of the bones surrounding the active joint may result in leg length discrepancy. Flexion contractures of joints may occur because the joint is held in the most comfortable position. Chronic disease can lead to joint destruction and the need for joint replacement. Osteopenia and growth failure may occur because of immobility, chronic disease and steroid use. Amyloidosis is, thankfully, rare.

HENOCH–SCHÖNLEIN PURPURA

This is a post-infective vasculitis (see also Chapter 11, pp. 127–128). There is often a preceding history of an upper respiratory tract infection. It peaks during the winter and is twice as common in boys, usually between 3 and 10 years old. The child presents with a rash, commonly on the extensor surfaces of the arms, legs and across the buttocks, which is initially erythematous, then maculopupular and non-blanching (purpuric). There is often a fever. Joint pain occurs in two-thirds, particularly of the knees and ankles. There is often periarticular oedema, rather than joint effusions. Colicky abdominal pain occurs in many children, and bleeding into the gastrointestinal tract may result in melaena. Intussusception is a rare complication. Renal involvement is common with 80% showing microscopic haematuria. Treatment is supportive. The blood pressure should be checked and urinalysis repeated until normalized. If the haematuria worsens, or proteinuria develops, a nephrologist should be consulted (see Chapter 11, p. 128).

SCOLIOSIS

'I'm concerned about my daughter's back'

Scoliosis is a lateral curvature of the spine that may be further subdivided into postural, which disappears on bending forward and is likely to resolve with time (the cause may be leg length discrepancy), and structural.

Structural scoliosis, where there is rotation of the vertebral bodies, can be identified when the child bends forwards – the curvature remains, and a rib hump develops. Most are idiopathic (85%) and are seen in adolescent girls (4:1 female to male), 30% of whom have a positive family history. Some are congenital (secondary to a defect in the spine such as a hemivertebra) and the remainder are secondary to other disorders such as cerebral palsy, muscular dystrophy, neurofibromatosis or Marfan's syndrome.

Idiopathic scoliosis has a tendency to progress, and is monitored by serial X-rays. Treatment includes bracing to support the spine and/or major corrective surgery.

BACK PAIN

Back pain is uncommon in pre-adolescent children. The younger the child the more likely that significant pathology will be found. A careful assessment must be made. In the older child the causes include muscle spasm (often sports-related injury), poor posture, Scheuermann's disease (osteochondritis of vertebrae), spondylolysis (stress fracture of pars interarticularis), vertebral osteomyelitis or discitis and tumours.

OTHER PATTERNS OF LIMB PAIN

Chronic limb pain

If there is anything atypical about the history or examination, routine bloods and X-rays should be done in order to rule out a bone tumour (osteosarcoma and Ewing's tumour), or leukaemia (see Chapter 7). Bone tumours are rare and usually present with pain and swelling or occasionally pathological fracture.

Children with hypermobility may complain of generalized pains. Signs might include thumbs that can hyperextend onto the forearm, elbows and knees that extend beyond −10°, and hands that can be placed flat on the floor with legs straight. This needs to be explained, and physiotherapists may help with joint protection exercises.

Chronic pain syndrome

This is characterized by non-specific aches and pains in otherwise healthy adolescents in the absence of signs of pathological cause. Symptoms overlap with chronic fatigue, and excessive tiredness is often a feature. These children frequently miss a great deal of school. Management is by acceptance of symptoms, reassurance of no serious underlying abnormality, addressing psychological needs and a graded exercise programme.

Table 6.5 The Jones criteria for diagnosis of rheumatic fever	
Major	**S**ydenham's chorea 10%
	Nodules (subcutaneous)
	Arthritis 80%
	Karditis 50% (carditis)
	Erythema marginatum 5%
Minor	Fever
	Arthralgia
	Prolonged P–R interval on ECG
	Raised CRP and ESR
	Past history of rheumatic fever

Osgood–Schlatter disease

This is an over use syndrome commonly occurring in active teenagers around puberty. There is tenderness and swelling of the tibial tuberosity secondary to detachment of cartilage fragments (traction apophysitis). It is bilateral in 25–50%. Management consists of reducing activity and analgesia. Support splints may help.

Rheumatic fever

This is a form of reactive arthritis, and, although rare in the UK, is a major cause of heart failure in the developing world because of resultant mitral valve disease (see also Chapter 9, p. 98). It is a post streptococcal disorder characterized by a migratory transient arthritis, a skin rash, carditis, subcutaneous nodules and occasionally chorea. Treatment of streptococcal throat infections with penicillin has dramatically reduced the incidence in the developed world. The major and minor criteria are shown in Table 6.5. To make a diagnosis, two major criteria, or one major and two minor criteria, are required with supporting evidence of preceding group A streptococcal infection.

Treatment consists mainly of rest, eradication of persistent streptococcal infection and anti-inflammatory medication – usually high-dose aspirin. Complications such as heart failure, pericardial effusion and persisting infection can occur. Valvular damage, particularly to the mitral valve, may necessitate surgery.

Other resources

Musculoskeletal examination in children – Arthritis Research UK. A free DVD is available to illustrate proper examination of the child. www.arthritisresearch.org.

Blood and cancer 7

(Jo Ponnampalam, Nandu Thalange)

CHAPTER CONTENTS

INTRODUCTION

Abnormalities of the blood are found in a wide range of paediatric diseases, so examination of the cellular components and chemistry will often give helpful diagnostic information. Primary diseases of the blood, with the exception of iron deficiency anaemia, are individually quite uncommon. Their significance lies in their high morbidity (e.g. haemophilia) or severity (e.g. acute leukaemia).

KEY CONCEPTS

Blood diseases generally present with evidence of failure either of the cellular components leading to anaemia, leucopenia or thrombocytopenia, or the clotting cascade with resultant easy bruising, and mucosal and soft-tissue bleeding, or bleeding into joints – haemarthrosis.

ANAEMIA

Iron deficiency anaemia

As shown in Case 7.1, tiredness, lethargy and listlessness are suggestive of anaemia. Pallor may be harder to detect in darker skin but may be apparent to parents, and will be clearly evident from inspection of mucous membranes. A pale blue tinge to the sclera is characteristic of iron deficiency. The findings of tachycardia with a flow murmur reflect the compensatory increase in cardiac output.

Iron deficiency is suggested by microcytic, hypochromic anaemia, but thalassaemia (see below) may also cause this picture. Iron deficiency is confirmed by the low ferritin level. Ferritin is an *acute phase reactant* and rises with infection or inflammation, so may be misleadingly normal in the unwell child.

Case 7.1 A boy with iron deficiency anaemia

Rajesh, a 3-year-old boy of Indian origin, presented to his GP with an acute viral infection. He was sleeping for 14 hours at night, had two naps in the daytime and had little energy for play. He ate poorly, much preferring to drink milk. His GP found that his conjunctivae were pale blue with pallor of the buccal mucosa. His heart rate was 110 beats per minute at rest, and he had a short ejection murmur at the upper left sternal edge. His GP requested a full blood count, which showed Hb 6.5 g/dL, WBC 10.5×10^6/L and platelets 680×10^6/L. The MCV (mean cell volume) and MCH (mean cell haemoglobin) were low and the blood film confirmed microcytosis and anisocytosis. The ferritin level was also very low, confirming iron deficiency anaemia.

Iron deficiency causes a range of effects:
- Symptoms of anaemia (see above)
- Impaired or abnormal appetite
- Mucosal abnormalities, e.g. angular cheilitis and atrophic glossitis, pruritis vulvae
- Impaired cognitive and motor development in toddlers; impaired short-term memory in older children
- Impaired neutrophil and lymphocyte function.

Iron deficiency is extremely common, affecting 15–20% of children in the UK. The commonest explanation for iron deficiency anaemia in young children is inadequate dietary intake but other causes should be considered, such as:
- Malabsorption, e.g. coeliac disease (see Chapter 12, p. 172)
- Chronic blood loss from gastroesophageal reflux (see Chapter 13, p. 164) or Meckel's diverticulum, when ectopic gastric mucosa secretes acid, leading to ulceration and bleeding in the small bowel.
- Menstrual losses in older girls.

Iron deficiency may be prevented with adequate dietary intake in otherwise healthy children. Standard infant formulas and many weaning foods are iron-fortified. Premature infants are at higher risk and require supplementation with iron in the first months. Treatment of established iron deficiency usually requires a few weeks of oral supplementation with elemental iron.

Haemolytic anaemia

Haemolytic disease of the newborn

Case 7.2 A boy with jaundice

Oliver was noted to have early-onset jaundice within 12 hours of birth. He was promptly treated with phototherapy. Oliver's mother was known to have blood group O, rhesus positive, excluding rhesus incompatibility, but a direct Coombs (antiglobulin) test was positive. Oliver was found to have blood group A, rhesus positive, confirming the diagnosis of ABO incompatibility.

Haemolytic disease of the newborn is a condition of rapid red cell destruction in the fetus or newborn infant caused by maternal antibodies raised against the infant's red cells (see also Chapter 17, p. 252). Where a pregnant mother is blood group rhesus negative and the fetus rhesus positive, the leak of even a few fetal cells into the maternal circulation may be sufficient to trigger the production of IgG antibodies. These cross the placenta in the same, or more commonly in a subsequent, pregnancy to cause immune-mediated destruction of antibody-coated red cells. The same process occurs with ABO incompatibility (as shown in Case 7.2), although this usually causes milder haemolysis.

Clinical effects range from mild jaundice in the newborn period, sometimes associated with a greater drop in the physiological nadir of haemoglobin at around 10–12 weeks of age, to a severe fetal anaemia, with hydrops fetalis and fetal death.

Detection of potential rhesus haemolytic disease in 'at-risk' fetuses requires monitoring of maternal antibody status and fetal well-being. Treatment options include in-utero transfusion, and, if necessary, early delivery. First-line therapy in the affected newborn infant is phototherapy. If this is ineffective, exchange blood transfusion is performed in which blood is drawn from the infant and replaced with an equal volume of packed cells. Infants with haemolytic disease of the newborn require folate supplementation, and occasionally require late transfusion for correction of anaemia, typically at 6–8 weeks of age. Administration of anti-D immunoglobulin to rhesus negative women after pregnancy (including miscarriage and termination of pregnancy) reduces the risk of recurrence in subsequent pregnancies.

Haemolytic disorders of childhood

Haemolytic anaemias are characterized by shortened red cell lifespan, with a compensatory increase in erythropoiesis, increased synthesis of bilirubin, and anaemia. Presentation may occur at birth with early-onset or severe neonatal jaundice, with inter-current infection provoking haemolysis or aplastic crisis, with symptoms of anaemia, with specific complications such as dactylitis in sickle-cell anaemia (see below), or by chance, following routine investigations (see Case 7.3).

Haemolytic anaemias may arise from:

- Structural membrane abnormalities of the red cell, e.g. hereditary spherocytosis
- Abnormalities of haemoglobin, e.g. thalassaemia, sickle-cell anaemia
- Metabolic abnormalities of the red cell, e.g. glucose-6-phosphate dehydrogenase (G6PD) deficiency or pyruvate kinase deficiency
- Hypersplenism and immune-mediated haemolysis.

General principles of treatment of haemolytic anaemias

- Folic acid requirements are increased due to high red cell turnover, and supplementation is usually required to optimize erythropoiesis
- Chronic anaemia is usually well-tolerated and transfusion is done as infrequently as symptoms allow
- Transfusion may be required for acute haemolytic crises. These occur secondary to inter-current infection, notably with parvovirus which causes a temporary depression of erythropoiesis – *aplastic crisis*. In G6PD deficiency (an X-linked condition, therefore very rare in girls) a variety of oxidant drugs will provoke acute haemolysis

- Blood transfusions ultimately may lead to iron overload, particularly in thalassaemia, requiring use of iron chelation therapy with desferrioxamine administered by overnight subcutaneous infusion 5–6 days per week. Newer oral agents, deferiprone (DFP) and deferasirox (DFX), approved for use in 2006, are available. DFP is less effective than DFO in treating liver disease, and so is usually used in combination with DFO. DFX is as effective as DFO, but long-term efficacy and safety is not yet established, and use is not recommended in patients with cardiac involvement. All chelation agents have significant side-effects, notably agranulocytosis with DFP.
- Symptomatic pigment gallstones require cholecystectomy
- Bone marrow transplantation may be appropriate for thalassaemia and severe sickle-cell disease

Hyposplenism secondary to progressive splenic infarction in sickle-cell disease, or following splenectomy, is treated with prophylactic phenoxymethylpenicillin ('penicillin V') and pneumococcal immunization due to the risk of overwhelming pneumococcal infection.

Case 7.3 A boy with severe haemolysis

Craig was admitted to hospital at the age of 4 years with severe gastroenteritis. He was noted to have pallor, splenomegaly and mild jaundice. A urine dipstick was positive for urobilinogen and haemoglobin, but negative for bilirubin, suggesting haemolysis. His blood count showed anaemia (Hb 4.7 g/dL), with spherocytes and red cell fragments on his blood film. A Coombs test was negative, excluding autoimmune haemolysis. Examination of parental blood specimens showed that his father also had mild anaemia with spherocytes, suggesting the diagnosis of hereditary spherocytosis.

Hereditary spherocytosis

Thalassaemia

Thalassaemia is the commonest single-gene disorder worldwide. A gene deletion results in reduced synthesis of either alpha- or beta-globin chains, producing alpha- or beta-thalassaemia, respectively.

Normal individuals have four alpha-globin and two beta-globin genes. Alpha- and beta-globin chains combine to form $\alpha_2\beta_2$ tetramers. Loss of a single alpha gene is asymptomatic, but loss of impairment of two or three alpha-globin genes results in alpha-thalassaemia trait and haemoglobin H disease respectively, characterized by hypochromic microcytic anaemia. Haemoglobin H is a β_4 tetramer which results from inadequate alpha-globin synthesis. If all four alpha chains are affected, no normal haemoglobin is made, resulting in fetal death from hydrops fetalis.

Similarly, partial or complete loss of a single beta-globin gene produces beta-thalassaemia trait, whereas if both genes are affected, beta-thalassaemia major results. Beta-thalassaemia major may be partly ameliorated by persistence of fetal haemoglobin.

There is considerable variation in ethnic distribution of the different abnormal genes, with the Mediterranean, Middle East, Indian subcontinent and South-East Asia most affected.

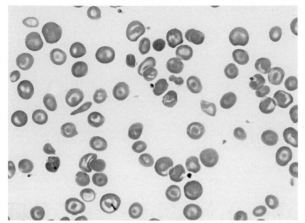

Figure 7.1 Blood film of patient with thalassaemia showing characteristic findings of hypochromic, microcytic anaemia with target cells and faint basophilic stippling.

Clinical features result from increased erythropoiesis occurring in the bone marrow and in extramedullary sites such as the liver. This process is driven by erythropoietin produced in response to relative tissue hypoxia.

The hallmark of thalassaemia major is hypochromic, microcytic anaemia, which may be severe, with associated hypersplenism due to increased red cell destruction (see Figure 7.1). Beta-thalassaemia also produces skeletal abnormalities, most notably frontal bossing, due to hyperplasic marrow, and growth failure.

Sickle-cell disease

Sickle-cell anaemia results from a glutamate to valine substitution in position 6 of the beta-globin gene. When present in the homozygous form

---

Case 7.4 A boy with sickle-cell crisis

John, aged 4 years, and his family were refugees from Sierra Leone. He was admitted to hospital with severe abdominal pain. On examination he was jaundiced with pallor and tachycardia, and he had severe upper abdominal tenderness, despite morphine analgesia, with what appeared to be a massively enlarged spleen. An urgent blood count and film showed sickle cells with severe anaemia (Hb 3.8 g/dL) and thrombocytopenia. A diagnosis of splenic sequestration crisis, secondary to sickle-cell anaemia, was made. He was treated with oxygen, analgesia, intravenous fluids, broad-spectrum antibiotics and repeated transfusions, and eventually made a full recovery. Homozygous sickle-cell anaemia was later confirmed. He was treated with regular folic acid and penicillin and periodic blood transfusion for symptomatic anaemia.

this renders the red cell prone to sickling. Common triggers are hypoxia, dehydration and fever, and the result is less compliant sickle-shaped red cells which occlude small vessels causing tissue ischaemia and end-organ damage. The sickle cells are rapidly removed from the circulation causing anaemia and hypersplenism (as shown in Case 7.4). Ultimately, hyposplenism results from recurrent splenic infarction. Hydroxycarbamide (see below) may help preserve splenic function, thereby reducing infection risk.

There are a number of clinical problems particular to sickle-cell disease:
- Vaso-occlusive crises leading to:
  - Severe bone pain, including foot and hand involvement in young children (dactylitis)
  - Avascular necrosis of bone
  - Renal injury leading to haematuria and progressive loss of renal concentrating ability
  - Stroke-like episodes
  - Priapism
  - Retinopathy
- Sequestration crises where large amounts of blood are sequestered to the spleen or liver, leading to anaemia, shock and severe abdominal pain
- Sickle chest in which widespread pulmonary infiltrates occur, leading to respiratory failure
- Infection with encapsulated organisms notably *Pneumococcus, Haemophilus* and *Salmonella,* due to progressive infarction of the spleen, leading to hyposplenism
- Impaired growth with delayed puberty (special growth charts are available in the UK for children with sickle-cell anaemia).

Hydroxycarbamide is now established as an effective treatment for sickle-cell disease. It is a ribonucleoside reductase inhibitor which inhibits cell division, and is widely used for the adult conditions chronic myeloid leukaemia and polycythaemia rubra vera. Randomized trials have shown that it is effective in reducing painful crises, dactylitis, episodes of sickle chest, and transfusion requirements, with an overall survival benefit. It has several actions:
- Increasing fetal haemoglobin
- Reducing rate of sickling
- Decreasing leucocytes, thereby reducing marginating neutrophils, which adhere to vascular endothelium and are implicated in painful crises and sickle chest.

Use of hydroxycarbamide in trials was associated with a 60% reduction in hospital admissions. Its use is indicated in patients with more than three admissions per year with painful crises, over the last 2 years, two or more episodes of sickle chest, or severe impairment in normal life due to pain. However, in May 2011 the outcome of a randomized control trial of hydroxycarbamide in children aged 9–18 months, treated for 2 years, showed very significantly improved outcomes compared with placebo, suggesting that it may have a wider role in the treatment of children.

Hydroxyurea is potentially leukaemogenic, and has significant toxicity. The most significant side-effect is myelosuppression. Skin rashes, nail discoloration, nausea/vomiting and diarrhoea may also occur. Frequent blood tests for monitoring purposes are required whilst on treatment.

BRUISING AND BLEEDING

Idiopathic thrombocytopenic purpura

> **Case 7.5** A girl with easy bruising
>
> Kara, a 4-year-old girl, developed an upper respiratory tract infection
> with fever from which she recovered within a few days. One
> week later she developed large bruises over her shins, knees and
> elbows, and smaller bruises over her thighs, buttocks and trunk.
> A single episode of epistaxis (bleeding nose) took 20 minutes to
> staunch. She appeared well apart from the bruising, and evidence
> of her recent nose bleed. She had no lymphadenopathy, fever or
> hepatosplenomegaly. Her blood tests showed Hb 13.5 g/dL, WBC 10
> $\times 10^6$/L with a normal differential white cell count and no blasts, but
> her platelet count was only 13 $\times 10^6$/L. Clotting studies were normal.

The acute-onset, easy bruising in Case 7.5 suggests thrombocytopenia,
which was confirmed. The most likely cause is *idiopathic thrombocytopenic
purpura* (ITP). If there is severe bleeding, platelets may be given. Most cases
of acute ITP resolve spontaneously over days or a few weeks. Treatment
with steroids or intravenous immunoglobulin will accelerate the rate of
recovery in most cases. Treatment is considered in children with a platelet
count below 30 $\times 10^{12}$/L with significant bleeding, depending on severity.
Steroids can disguise aleukaemic leukaemia, which may present with isolated thrombocytopenia, and bone marrow examination is recommended
before starting steroids. Treatment may incur significant side-effects and
will not reduce the risk of developing chronic ITP, which occurs in 10–30%
of cases and most cases can safely be managed conservatively.

Haemophilia

The two main forms are haemophilia A (80–85% of cases) and haemophilia B. Both are inherited conditions with X-linked recessive inheritance and consequently boys are affected, with deficient production
of clotting factors and an increased tendency to haemorrhage, either
spontaneously or after trauma. In haemophilia A, factor VIII is affected
(as in Case 7.6) and in haemophilia B, factor IX levels are reduced; both
are involved in the conversion of fibrinogen to fibrin in the clotting cascade.

> **Case 7.6** A boy with a large haematoma
>
> James, who was 3 years old and a known haemophiliac, presented
> with a large haematoma of his left thigh, after a fall. James had
> previously had an implantable venous access device (Portacath™)
> sited because of severe needle phobia, coupled with the need for
> frequent intravenous access. He received regular recombinant factor
> VIII to maintain levels at around 30% of normal. In view of the muscle
> haemorrhage, he received additional factor VIII to elevate his levels to
> 70% of normal and regular physiotherapy to maintain mobility.

Clinical manifestations may begin in early infancy or even in utero with intracranial haemorrhage or cephalohaematoma. Later, once the child begins to walk, haemarthroses or soft-tissue bleeds are more common and simple cuts and surgical wounds may bleed profusely. Head injuries carry an increased risk of intracranial haemorrhage. The severity is proportional to the factor concentration in the blood, with the most severely affected having levels <1% of normal values. The activated partial thromboplastin time (APTT) is prolonged.

Recombinant human factor VIII and IX is now available for intravenous injection either to treat an acute event or as regular replacement in severe cases. After intracranial haemorrhage – or, if surgery is necessary – factor VIII levels are restored to the normal range. In individuals with mild or moderate disease, factor levels can be temporarily boosted with intravenous DDAVP (desmopressin). Anti-fibrinolytics, such as tranexamic acid, are useful adjunctive therapy. Drugs with anti-platelet activity, such as aspirin and non-steroidal anti-inflammatory drugs (NSAIDs), must be avoided.

von Willebrand disease

The commonest inherited bleeding disorder, von Willebrand disease is caused by a relative lack of von Willebrand factor, which acts both as a carrier for factor VIII and to promote adherence of platelets to damaged endothelium. Milder forms are inherited as an autosomal dominant trait, the more severe as autosomal recessive. Clinical features include mucocutaneous bleeding and prolonged haemorrhage after surgery and trauma. There may be mild thrombocytopenia but more usually platelets are normal. APTT and bleeding times are usually prolonged, levels of von Willebrand factor and von Willebrand antigen are reduced and the ristocetin cofactor assay is abnormal.

Treatment with DDAVP boosts von Willebrand factor and factor VIII levels up to eight-fold. If ineffective, intermediate-purity factor VIII, and, in future, recombinant von Willebrand factor may be used.

BONE MARROW FAILURE

Bone marrow failure arises from disease affecting or replacing the bone marrow. All causes of bone marrow failure are rare. Marrow infiltration from acute leukaemia is the commonest cause. Aplastic anaemia presents in a similar way.

Aplastic anaemia

Aplastic anaemia results from reduced numbers of all haematopoietic cells – erythroblasts, myeloblasts and megakaryocytes – resulting in pancytopenia (as shown in Case 7.7). The majority of cases (50–75%) are idiopathic, but it may be congenital – Fanconi anaemia, or acquired following viral infection or toxin exposure.

The principal manifestations are symptomatic anaemia, infections secondary to leucopenia and bleeding secondary to thrombocytopenia. Treatment is with:

- Supportive therapy
    - CMV (cytomegalovirus) negative, leuco-depleted, irradiated blood transfusions
    - Prophylactic antifungal and antibiotic therapy
    - Aggressive treatment of intercurrent infection
    - Use of haematopoietic growth factors, e.g. G-CSF (granulocyte colony-stimulating factor), erythropoietin
- Immunosuppressive drugs, e.g. ciclosporin, anti-thymocyte globulin
- Bone marrow transplantation.

> ### Case 7.7 A girl with pallor and easy bruising
>
> Joanna presented at 14 years of age with very severe oral
> candidiasis, lethargy and malaise. On examination she was strikingly
> pale, and had a number of bruises, but no history of trauma. An
> urgent blood count showed pancytopenia (Hb 5.9 g/dL, WBC
> 1.1×10^6/L, platelets 6×10^{12}/L). Bone marrow aspirate showed
> hypocellularity. A diagnosis of severe aplastic anaemia was made.
> Joanna was initially treated with broad-spectrum antibiotics and
> amphotericin with initial clinical improvement but her cell counts
> did not recover with growth factor support and immunosuppressive
> therapy. Joanna was listed for urgent bone marrow transplant but
> died of overwhelming Gram-negative infection 3 weeks later.

Aplastic anaemia is severe, and without bone marrow transplantation
(BMT) the 12-month survival is under 10%. With BMT, survival is 70–90%.

MALIGNANT DISEASE

Childhood cancer is rare, affecting approximately 12–14 per 100 000 children each year. Nevertheless, it accounts for 20% of deaths in childhood between 1 and 14 years of age. Childhood cancer is 15–20% more common in boys. Major improvements in cytotoxic chemotherapy regimes and supportive care with antibiotics, blood products and nutrition have dramatically improved survival. More than 75% of children now survive at least 5 years after diagnosis. In 1971, fewer than 100 adult survivors of childhood cancer over 30 years of age were known in England and Wales. By 2000, this figure had risen to over 7000. However, these figures disguise major variation in outcome; for example, stage IV neuroblastoma carries a 5-year survival of only 25% whereas isolated retinoblastoma has almost a 100% cure rate.

Leukaemia accounts for around 30% of cancers, lymphoma a further 10% and central nervous system (CNS) tumours 25%. Embryonal tumours (neuroblastoma, Wilms' tumour, hepatoblastoma and retinoblastoma) account for 15%. The remaining 20% are made up of a wide variety of neoplasms with widely differing characteristics.

Risk factors

For the great majority of childhood cancers, there are no identifiable risk factors.

- **Radiation.** Radiation is a recognized cause of cancer, and children are more susceptible to the effects of radiation than are adults. Most evidence comes from high-dose, relatively short-term radiation such as following nuclear accidents or radiotherapy. The tumour most strongly associated with radiation exposure is papillary thyroid cancer. Risk can be reduced in the aftermath of exposure by taking potassium iodide. There is a lack of knowledge about the long-term risks of low-dose exposure, such as domestic radon, over prolonged periods.
- **Genetic factors.** Genetic factors may increase the likelihood of cancer through a range of mechanisms.
  - Abnormal chromosomal complement, e.g. Down syndrome (leukaemia), or Turner's syndrome (Wilms' tumour)

- Specific gene defects, e.g. mutations in Rb gene predispose to retinoblastoma
- Defects of tumour suppressor genes, e.g. *p53* mutations in Li-Fraumeni syndrome predispose to a wide range of cancers
- Syndromes with abnormal somatic growth such as neurofibromatosis or Beckwith's syndrome
- Defects of DNA repair, e.g. ataxia telangiectasia.

● **Infection.** Infection may be a major trigger factor for some forms of cancer, e.g. hepatitis B and hepatocellular carcinoma, AIDS and non-Hodgkin's lymphoma. Epstein–Barr virus has also been implicated in non-Hodgkin's lymphoma, particularly Burkitt's lymphoma.

● **Environmental factors.** Chemical and drug exposure may be implicated in the development of particular cancers, e.g. antenatal exposure to the barbiturate sodium pentothal (thiopental sodium) has been linked to brain and spinal cord tumours, and there is limited evidence suggesting a link between pesticide exposure and soft-tissue sarcomas.

Symptoms and signs

Symptoms and signs are non-specific and often relatively subtle in the early stages. Constitutional symptoms such as malaise, fever, pruritus and anorexia are common. Unfortunately many diseases are already advanced when first detected. Typical presentations include:

● **Visible or palpable mass.** The most obvious presentation of cancer is with a visible enlarging mass, such as a neck, soft-tissue or scrotal swelling, or incidentally recognized abdominal mass.

● **Headaches and neurological symptoms and signs.** Brain and spinal cord tumours produce elevated intracranial pressure and neurological symptoms or signs depending on their location and speed of growth. Epilepsy is an uncommon manifestation.

● **Local effects.** Osteosarcomas lead to pain and disability at the site of the tumour. Retinoblastoma causes visual loss. Wilms' tumour may produce haematuria.

● **Distant tumour effects.** 'Dancing-eyes syndrome' is a characteristic neurological syndrome arising from neuroblastoma. The mechanism is unknown. Tumours may also produce distant effects by impairing endocrine function or by secreting hormones. For example, hypothalamic tumours such as craniopharyngiomas will result in panhypopituitarism with failure of growth and puberty, hypothyroidism, diabetes insipidus and adrenal insufficiency (see Chapter 12). Pituitary tumours, phaechromocytomas and neuroblastomas may all secrete hormones causing distant effects. The most common functional pituitary tumour is a prolactinoma, which produces breast enlargement and galactorrhoea. Catecholamines from neuroblastomas or phaeochromocytomas may produce labile hypertension. These catecholamines may be detected in urine and are useful as tumour markers for diagnosis and monitoring.

● **Bone marrow failure** (see above). Bone marrow failure is seen most commonly with leukaemia, and results in anaemia with pallor, thrombocytopenia causing easy bruising and bleeding, or leucopenia resulting in severe infection. Bone marrow metastases, most commonly seen in neuroblastoma, may produce a similar picture. Bone pain is common.

Surveillance

Some children have an increased risk of developing cancer. For example children with Beckwith syndrome have a greater risk of developing Wilms' tumours of the kidney. Regular ultrasound scans to detect such tumours are necessary. Early detection facilitates treatment at an earlier stage. Children who have recovered from cancer are at risk of relapse and second malignancy and undergo regular surveillance.

Diagnosis and staging

Diagnosis, classification and grading of malignant disease require a range of investigations, including a tissue sample (bone marrow aspirate or tissue biopsy) for confirmation of the primary disease, and quantification of local and distant tumour spread by use of ultrasound, CT and MRI or nuclear medicine scans. Histology and molecular genetic studies shed further light on the disease, and frequently determine the approach to treatment.

Having established a diagnosis, and determined the extent of disease, treatment options may then be considered. Treatment has to take account of the effect on the child, e.g. cranial radiotherapy in infants and very young children (<6 years) has very severe effects on brain development and is not recommended.

Treatment

Treatment of childhood malignancy is a complex area, but the principal elements of management are:

- Chemotherapy
- Radiotherapy
- Surgery
- Supportive and palliative care
- Surveillance for recurrence or further malignancy
- Surveillance for 'late effects'.

Presentations of principal childhood malignancies

Leukaemia

Around 2–4/100 000 children per year develop acute leukaemia and over 80% of those have acute lymphoblastic leukaemia (ALL) (as in Case 7.8), most of the rest having acute myeloid leukaemia (AML). The peak incidence is between 2 and 5 years, and although there is an increased incidence in children with chromosomal disorders, e.g. Down syndrome, or with immunodeficiency, this condition mostly occurs in previously well children.

Common clinical features are lethargy, pallor, easy bruising, bone pain and swelling of lymph glands, liver and spleen. Some children may develop infection due to neutropenia. Although primarily a bone marrow disease, the CNS (cranial nerve palsies or meningism), the testes (swelling, usually painless) and mediastinum (lymphadenopathy causing breathlessness) may all be involved at presentation.

There is usually leucocytosis due to blast cells (although normal leucocyte numbers may be reduced), anaemia and thrombocytopenia. Renal and hepatic function are sometimes affected. A secondary coagulopathy, or even disseminated intravascular coagulation, may be present. A lumbar

> ### Case 7.8 A boy with bone marrow failure
>
> Edward presented to his GP with pallor and numerous
> bruises. A blood count showed severe anaemia (Hb 5.0 g/dL),
> thrombocytopenia and numerous blast cells (WBC 145 × 10⁶/L)
> indicating leukaemia. He was urgently referred to hospital by which
> time immunophenotyping had confirmed ALL. On examination, he
> was miserable, with marked hepatosplenomegaly and some mild
> neck stiffness. He was commenced on broad-spectrum antibiotics
> and referred urgently to a specialist paediatric oncology unit where
> he underwent bone marrow aspirate and lumbar puncture. These
> confirmed total involvement of bone marrow with blasts, which were
> also present in cerebrospinal fluid, indicating meningeal involvement.
> Edward subsequently underwent intensive chemotherapy for a period
> of 3 years.

puncture is required as the finding of blast cells in the cerebrospinal fluid
is of grave prognostic significance and requires intensive CNS-directed
treatment.

Nearly all children in the UK are managed as part of a clinical trial. The
latest clinical trial, UKALL 2011, commenced in April 2012. UKALL 2003,
its predecessor, introduced assessment of minimal residual disease, which
is now accepted as standard therapy. Management requires exemplary
supportive care with antibiotics, transfusion of red cells or platelets and
avoidance of tumour lysis syndrome (acute renal failure secondary to large
elevation of uric acid following initiation of therapy) with copious fluids
and allopurinol (an inhibitor of uric acid synthesis). Multi-agent cytotoxic
chemotherapy is required involving four main phases: an induction phase
to bring the disease into remission, a maintenance phase lasting up to
3 years, intensification blocks of more aggressive treatment, and a phase of
treatment directed specifically at protecting the CNS. Over 90% of children
with ALL are now cured but relapse in the bone marrow, CNS or testes
remains a risk for several years after treatment finishes. Relapse requires
further multi-agent chemotherapy, usually with craniospinal radiotherapy, and in some cases bone marrow transplantation.

Innocent cervical lymphadenopathy

> ### Case 7.9 A boy with cervical lymphadenopathy
>
> Adam, aged 4 years, was referred with several hard, pea-sized
> lymph glands that had persisted for several months, after an
> episode of tonsillitis. He was otherwise well, and was on the 75th
> centile for height and weight. On examination, the glands were
> very hard and mobile – typical of innocent 'lead shot' glands.
> Adam's parents were reassured as to the innocent nature of
> the lymphadenopathy, and were advised that the glands would
> gradually involute over several months.

Cervical lymphadenopathy is universal in children. Prevalence studies indicate that up to 45% of otherwise healthy children have cervical lymphadenopathy at any one time. Usually (as in Case 7.9) the lymphadenopathy is bilateral, generalized and transient, in association with an infection, typically of the upper respiratory tract, and predominantly involving glands in the anterior triangle (see Figure 7.2 for an anatomical description of cervical lymph nodes). Unilateral lymphadenopathy signifies staphylococcal or streptococcal infection in 40–80% of cases. Subacute and chronic lymphadenitis occurs with cat scratch disease, toxoplasmosis and occasionally atypical mycobacteria. Persistent enlargement of glands in the supraclavicular region is much more commonly associated with malignancy. Malignant disease or mycobacterial infection is more likely if there are associated constitutional symptoms such as fever, night sweats, malaise and weight loss.

No investigation is necessary in the great majority of children, but where necessary, a blood count, ESR (erythrocyte sedimentation rate), serology for Epstein–Barr virus, toxoplasmosis and cytomegalovirus (causes of glandular fever), and *Bartonella henselae* (the cause of cat scratch disease), will exclude serious disease and may establish the cause. Fine-needle biopsy under ultrasound guidance, or excision biopsy of an affected gland, is rarely necessary. All biopsy material should be sent for histology and mycobacterial and fungal cultures.

Cervical lymphadenopathy secondary to malignancy is characteristically progressive, firm and frequently associated with constitutional symptoms. In the young child, neuroblastoma and leukaemia are the commonest causes, but in the older child and adolescent, Hodgkin's disease and non-Hodgkin's lymphoma are more common (Case 7.10).

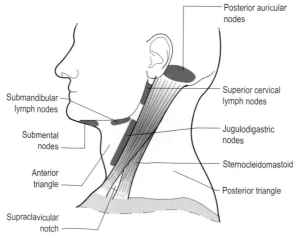

Posterior auricular nodes

Submandibular lymph nodes

Submental nodes

Anterior triangle

Supraclavicular notch

Superior cervical lymph nodes

Jugulodigastric nodes

Sternocleidomastoid

Posterior triangle

Figure 7.2 Anatomical landmarks of the neck.

> ### Case 7.10 A boy with cervical lymphadenopathy
>
> Peter, aged 14 years, presented with a progressively enlarging lymph gland in the supraclavicular region. He had drenching night sweats. The gland was painless, very firm, and the size of a chestnut when he was first seen by his doctor, but enlarged progressively over the next 3 weeks. A blood count and ESR showed a mild hypochromic, microcytic anaemia with an elevated ESR (106 mm/h). Lymphoma was strongly suspected, and a chest X-ray showed marked mediastinal lymphadenopathy. Peter underwent excision biopsy which confirmed non-Hodgkin's lymphoma.

Lymphoma

- **Hodgkin's lymphoma**. Hodgkin's lymphoma is distinguished clinically by the contiguous spread of disease from one lymph node group to the next, and pathologically by a unique histological feature, the Reed–Sternberg cell, an atypical histiocyte. About 50% of cases are triggered by Epstein-Barr virus infection, and probably represents an abnormal immune response in a genetically susceptible individual.

  Firm painless swelling of lymph nodes is the commonest presentation, particularly in the cervical region. Where the primary site is retroperitoneal or mediastinal other symptoms are more common, including cough, shortness of breath, fever, weight loss, sweating and pruritus.

  Chest X-ray and abdominal and pelvic CT scans are combined with a bone marrow aspirate and biopsy to stage disease extent. If available, positron emission tomography CT (PET-CT) scanning offers superior detection of affected tissues, and is valuable for monitoring treatment response. MRI scanning may be used for suspected brain or spinal cord involvement. Excision biopsy allows tissue diagnosis. Treatment requires a combination of chemo- and radiotherapy. Refractory or relapsed lymphoma is treated with aggressive chemotherapy and salvage bone marrow or stem cell transplantation.

- **Non-Hodgkin's lymphoma**. Non-Hodgkin's lymphoma (NHL) arises from B- or T-cell lines, including primitive precursors. T-cell lymphoma is uncommon. Although arising in lymphoid tissue, extra-nodal spread is common. Thirty-five subtypes of non-Hodgkin's lymphoma are recognized. Some cases are triggered by Epsten-Barr virus, notably Burkitt's lymphoma. Human T-cell leukaemia/lymphoma virus type 1 (HTLV-1) is predominantly seen in patients of Japanese or Afro-Caribbean origin. *Helicobacter pylori* infection of the stomach may cause mucosa-associated lymphoid tissue (MALT) lymphoma. Antibiotics are curative in 70-80%.

  Features vary with the primary site. Bone pain, skin lesions and testicular swelling mark more widespread disease. Bone marrow involvement may be substantial, particularly in T-cell disease, overlapping with T-cell leukaemia.

  A cervical lymphoma presents with painless neck swelling, as in Case 7.10. Mediastinal involvement leads to general malaise, shortness of breath and signs of pleural effusions or superior vena caval obstruction. Abdominal lymphoma causes nausea and vomiting, bowel disturbance including obstruction, pain, weight loss, melaena, ascites and fever.

  Treatment is with a multi-agent cytotoxic chemotherapy regime similar to that for acute leukaemia.

Case 7.11 A boy with elevated intracranial pressure and ataxia

Aaron, aged 6 years, started to awaken with headaches. He was very miserable and frequently vomited. His symptoms worsened, prompting referral to hospital. He was noted to be mildly ataxic. Fundus examination proved impossible, but in view of the history, he underwent an urgent CT scan. This showed a cerebellar tumour with hydrocephalus. Biopsy showed a juvenile pilocytic astrocytoma. He underwent surgical debulking and post-operative cranial irradiation.

Brain tumours

Children usually present with symptoms of rising intracranial pressure, particularly headache and vomiting. Features in the history that should elicit concern are a short history of headaches, with progressive symptoms, particularly if associated with functional impairment such as difficulty walking, unsteadiness, etc. (see also Chapter 14, p. 187).

As Case 7.11 shows, manifestations of cerebral tumours are primarily related to anatomical site and pressure effects – tumours may obstruct CSF (cerebrospinal fluid) flow leading to hydrocephalus (see Chapter 14, p. 187). This may lead to a rapid rise in intracranial pressure.

Other presentations of brain tumours include:

- Focal neurological signs such as hemiplegia or cranial nerve palsies
- Rapidly rising head circumference in an infant
- Ataxia due to cerebellar dysfunction
- Seizures (rarely)
- Neck stiffness (posterior fossa tumours)
- Temporal visual field loss (lesions affecting the optic nerves or chiasm, e.g. hypothalamic tumours)
- Papilloedema
- Percussion of the skull may reveal a 'cracked-pot' percussion note, typical of hydrocephalus.

Investigation of a suspected brain tumour is with a brain scan. An MRI scan is preferable, but often a CT scan can be done much more quickly. Tissue diagnosis of the tumour is usually indicated, although the risks of surgery may preclude a biopsy, particularly for brain stem tumours. Tumour markers such as alpha-fetoprotein and human chorionic gonadotrophin may be elevated with germ cell tumours.

The therapeutic approach is determined by the site and extent of the tumour and its histological character. A small well-circumscribed astrocytoma in a peripheral cortical location may be entirely resected surgically with low recurrence risk. A glioma in the brain stem however cannot be resected without devastating damage and therefore treatment depends on radiotherapy. Adjunctive chemotherapy may improve survival rates if the histology is favourable.

Prognosis is extremely variable. Learning difficulties, residual weakness, cerebral palsy and epilepsy are all common sequelae.

Glioma

Gliomas arise from astrocytes and account for 50% of all childhood brain tumours. They range from benign, low-grade tumours, typically in the cerebellum or optic nerves, sometimes associated with neurofibromatosis, to aggressive high-grade tumours in the brain stem or cerebrum. Surgery is contraindicated in brain stem gliomas. Chemotherapy and radiotherapy may be employed, but often have only limited success. Slow-growing peripheral gliomas with clear resection margins have a 5-year survival rate in excess of 90%, compared with less than 5% for an aggressive anaplastic brain stem glioma. Use of newer agents, such as the alkylating agent temozolomide, or drugs targeting specific receptors such as vascular endothelial growth factor (e.g. bevacizumab) or epidermal growth factor (e.g. erlotinib), has improved prognosis somewhat for supratentorial gliomas, but the overall picture remains bleak for brain stem gliomas.

Medulloblastoma

Thirty per cent of brain tumours are due to embryonal primitive neuroectodermal tumours (PNETs), which, in the cerebellum, are referred to as medulloblastomas. Medulloblastomas account for 90% of all PNETs. For a case history of medulloblastoma, see Chapter 14, Case 14.2, p. 187. PNETs are malignant with a propensity to metastasize within the brain and spinal cord. Treatment of medulloblastoma entails surgery, followed in children over 4 years by craniospinal radiotherapy.

Craniopharyngioma

> ### Case 7.12 A girl with growth failure
>
> Sunila, aged 7 years, was seen with a 2-year history of growth failure. Her mum had also noticed that she did not seem to see as well on the left side, and would occasionally bump into things. She was found to have bilateral optic atrophy with visual field loss, which was worse on the left side. She underwent an urgent CT scan which showed moderate hydrocephalus and a large midline tumour with calcification, indicating a craniopharyngioma. She underwent subtotal resection with radiotherapy. Subsequently, Sunila developed panhypopituitarism, epilepsy and significant learning difficulties, and was registered blind.

Craniopharyngioma, an embryonal tumour, arises in the suprasellar region, and is a benign tumour, but with a high rate of local recurrence. As in Case 7.12, progressive growth failure, often going back a number of years, is the earliest sign. The tumour contains solid and cystic elements, often with calcification, readily seen on CT scan. Treatment is with surgery and post-operative radiotherapy. Proximity to the pituitary gland and optic chiasm commonly leads to panhypopituitarism and/or blindness.

Neuroblastoma

Neuroblastoma (as in Case 7.13) is a tumour of neural crest cells and arises from the adrenal glands or sympathetic nerve root ganglia. The tumour secretes catecholamines, whose metabolites, vanillylmandelic acid and homovanillic acid, may be measured in urine.

Case 7.13 A boy with 'panda eyes'

Sachin, aged 14 months, was referred urgently by his GP, with unexplained black eyes and failure-to-thrive. On examination he had a squint with periorbital ecchymosis. He was wasted and miserable, and his parents reported recent weight loss. He was initially investigated with a skeletal survey to look for evidence of non-accidental injury, and this showed apparent metastatic deposits in his ribs, pelvis and right femur. A cranial MRI scan also showed periorbital metastatic deposits. Urinary catecholamine metabolites were elevated and abdominal ultrasound showed a large retroperitoneal mass arising from the sympathetic chain. Biopsy confirmed neuroblastoma. In view of his metastatic disease, he had stage IV disease and was treated with intensive chemotherapy and subsequently surgery, followed by further cycles of chemotherapy.

With an incidence of around 1:100 000, neuroblastoma accounts for approximately 8% of all childhood tumours. It may present with an abdominal mass, nausea, vomiting or diarrhoea with failure to thrive, and signs of metastatic disease such as bone pain or proptosis. Fever and weight loss are common. Around two-thirds of primary tumours are abdominal.

Imaging with ultrasound and CT or MRI and bone marrow aspiration and biopsy determine the extent of tumour spread. The majority of children will undergo an MIBG (meta-iodobenzylguanidine) scan to permit accurate staging of the tumour. A biopsy is required to establish the histology and cytogenetics of the disease, notably the degree of amplification of the oncogene MYC-N, with more copies signifying a worse prognosis, and indicating the need for more aggressive chemotherapy. Histologically, neuroblastoma is a small round cell tumour, similar to lymphomas and Ewing's sarcoma. Staging is conventional on a I to IV scale according to disease extent. Uniquely, neuroblastoma has a stage IV 'special', which involves a localized primary with dissemination specifically to skin, liver and bone marrow in an infant. This widespread form of the disease often undergoes remission either spontaneously or with minimal chemotherapy and therefore has an excellent prognosis.

After initial chemotherapy, the primary tumour is resected where possible, after which the more advanced stages will require further multi-agent cytotoxic chemotherapy, sometimes combined with stem-cell rescue therapy. Currently, clinical trials are underway testing the effectiveness of chimeric monoclonal antibodies against the ganglioside GD2, with promising early results, including patients who have relapsed post-bone marrow transplant.

Wilms' tumour

The differential diagnosis of an abdominal mass includes Wilms' tumour (Case 7.14), neuroblastoma, hepatoblastoma and non-Hodgkin's lymphoma.

Wilms' tumour is an embryonal renal tumour with an incidence of approximately 8 per million. It accounts for about 6% of childhood tumours. Patients with abnormalities of chromosome 11 have an increased

Pocket Essentials of Paediatrics

> ### Case 7.14 A boy with a mass
>
> Toby, aged 6 years, was referred by his GP subsequent to the
> discovery of an abdominal mass after presenting with pallor and
> anorexia. On examination the mass was very firm, and occupied
> the entire right flank up to the midline. Urinalysis showed blood 2+.
> An urgent ultrasound showed a large tumour arising from the right
> kidney. Urine was sent for catecholamine metabolites, but was
> negative. A biopsy confirmed Wilms' tumour (nephroblastoma).
> Staging of the tumour showed local invasion, but the tumour was
> apparently confined to the abdomen without distant metastases
> (stage III). Histology was unfavourable, so Toby underwent
> chemotherapy followed by surgery and radiotherapy.

risk of Wilms' tumour, as well as other abnormalities, including hemihy-
pertrophy, aniridia, genitourinary abnormalities and learning difficulties,
most notably Beckwith syndrome. Familial Wilms' tumour accounts for
around 2% of all cases.

The majority of patients with Wilms' tumour do well, with survival
rates over 60%.

Osteosarcoma and Ewing's sarcoma

> ### Case 7.15 A girl with a painful limp
>
> Kirsten, aged 12 years, was referred with a very painful limp
> affecting her right leg, making it increasingly difficult for her to
> weight bear, and disturbing her at night. The pain had initially been
> attributed to a sporting injury, but was failing to improve. X-ray
> showed evidence of new bone formation and lytic lesions with a
> classic 'sunburst appearance' in the lower femur, characteristic
> of osteosarcoma. Kirsten underwent staging scans, including a
> chest CT scan and a radionuclide bone scan, to look for evidence
> of metastatic disease. She underwent aggressive chemotherapy
> followed by limb-sparing surgery.

Bone tumours may be primary or secondary. Secondary bony metastases are commonly seen with neuroblastoma.

The majority of osteosarcomas occur in adolescents and young adults,
presenting with limb pain, swelling or limp (Case 7.15). The metaphyses
of long bones are most commonly affected and metastases may occur in
the lung. Disease is confirmed radiologically with X-ray, bone scan and
CT scan of the chest. After preliminary chemotherapy, surgical resection is
attempted, with limb preservation where possible. Further chemotherapy
is usually required.

Primary Ewing's sarcoma may affect bone or soft tissue, causing pain,
swelling and systemic upset such as fever and weight loss. Metastases
occur in lungs, bone, bone marrow and lymph nodes. Radiological staging

with PET-CT or MRI is required with bone marrow aspiration and biopsy. Tissue biopsy is required for histological confirmation. Treatment is with multi-agent chemotherapy and surgical excision of residual primary disease. In more advanced disease, high-dose marrow ablative chemotherapy is combined with autologous bone marrow rescue. With modern treatment, 5-year survival is now 50-75%, with better survival in younger patients (<15 years).

SUPPORTIVE AND PALLIATIVE CARE

Supportive care comprises a package of care to support the child with cancer and their family, medically, emotionally, socially and financially.
Medical care includes:

● Treatment to protect the child from foreseeable complications, e.g. rehydration, and allopurinol to prevent tumour lysis syndrome (see above), or prophylactic antibiotic and antifungal therapy to protect the neutropenic child after intensive chemotherapy
● Prompt treatment of possible and confirmed intercurrent infection
● Treatment of pain and nausea
● Replacement of blood products
● Nutritional support to maintain weight and growth
● Monitoring for side-effects and complications of treatment.

It is also vital to support the child and their family by giving clear, consistent and accurate advice and support, providing access to psychological support and helping the family access financial support such as the Disability Living Allowance (to be replaced with a new benefit, Personal Independence Payments from 2014).

Sadly, many children with malignant disease cannot be cured, and effective palliative therapy is essential. Common symptoms are fatigue, pain, dyspnoea, nausea and vomiting, anorexia and constipation, with accompanying anxiety and fear. The goal is not to prolong life, but to enhance it, by freeing the child from these distressing symptoms as far as possible. This may involve selective use of chemo- or radiotherapy, transfusions and nutritional support, as well as conventional symptomatic therapy. Involvement of the child is crucial in alleviating anxiety and fear, by allowing them to participate in decisions about their care. There are now children's hospices in many parts of the country, which offer high-quality palliative care in and out of the home.

LATE SEQUELAE OF CANCER AND THEIR TREATMENT

The most serious consequence of childhood cancer is relapse or occurrence of a second malignancy. The occurrence of a second malignancy may be due to an underlying cancer predisposition, or due to effects of treatment, e.g. thyroid cancer and radiotherapy to the neck or certain chemotherapeutic agents.

Patients treated for Hodgkin's disease appear to be at very high risk of second malignancies, particularly women, in whom the combination of alkylating agent chemotherapy and radiotherapy hugely increases the risk of breast cancer. A third of women who received treatment for Hodgkin's lymphoma before the age of 7 years will develop breast cancer within 25 years, compared with the background risk of 2% by age 50 years.

Intellectual function may by impaired by neurosurgery, chemotherapy or radiotherapy involving the brain and spinal cord. Such damage is irreversible.

Specific problems may occur following chemo- or radiotherapy; for example:

- Cardiomyopathy (anthracyclines), pulmonary fibrosis (bleomycin), renal impairment (ifosfamide), deafness (platinum), etc.
- Cranial radiotherapy also commonly leads to hypopituitarism with growth failure, hypothyroidism and hypogonadism, although precocious puberty may also occur, particularly in girls
- Infertility is very common secondarily to chemo- or radiotherapy and pituitary dysfunction. It is important to address fertility issues, as they are a significant cause of psychological morbidity
- Spinal radiotherapy will impair spinal growth, resulting in relative skeletal disproportion, with short stature.

Skin 8

(George Millington, Nandu Thalange)

CHAPTER CONTENTS

INTRODUCTION

All children will have a condition affecting their skin at some time. Most conditions are acute and transient, such as the exanthem accompanying acute viral infections like parvovirus, rubella and measles (see Chapter 16). These skin manifestations serve as a useful diagnostic guide but may not require specific treatment. Some, such as atopic eczema, will be chronic and potentially debilitating without appropriate management. Still others will be permanent and require care of the skin lesion and also of potential complications such as the epilepsy seen with port wine haemangioma in Sturge–Weber syndrome (see also Chapter 14, p. 204).

INFLAMMATION

Chronic skin inflammation is usually due to eczema, although more rarely psoriasis is the cause. Self-limiting acute inflammatory disorders are commonly due to allergic or hypersensitivity reactions. The distribution of the rash is often highly characteristic and suggests the diagnosis (Figure 8.1).

Atopic eczema

Eczema is often described as the 'itch that rashes'. *Itch* and *dryness* are key components of atopic eczema. *Secondary infection,* usually with *Staphylococcus aureus* and streptococci, is common, and should be suspected whenever the skin is weeping and crusted (as in Case 8.1). Viral superinfection, such as with herpes simplex or varicella, may cause dramatic exacerbations with marked systemic upset – *eczema herpeticum.*

Eczema is the commonest skin complaint of childhood, affecting 10–15% of all children. Eczema is an inflammatory eruption, with erythema and papules or vesicles on a dry background. Secondary scaling and crusting occur commonly, progressing to lichenification in chronic cases. Although a chronic condition, 90% of cases remit by 15 years of age.

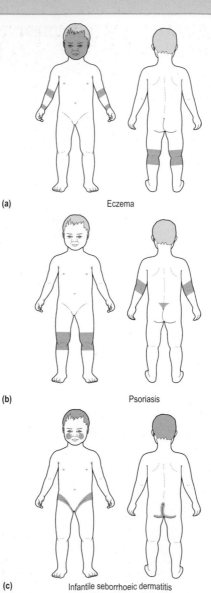

(a)　　　Eczema

(b)　　　Psoriasis

(c)　　　Infantile seborrhoeic dermatitis

Figure 8.1 Distribution of rash in various skin conditions.

Case 8.1 A girl with a dry itchy rash

Jade, a 14-month-old girl, was taken to the GP because she was distressed, miserable and would not sleep. She had a longstanding dry itchy rash over the wrists, in front of her elbows, behind her knees, and behind her ears. Recently the rash had become vesicular with weeping and crusting. She had previously had episodes of wheeze with viral infections and a single episode of a red blotchy rash after eating egg. Her mother had asthma and her father suffered from seasonal rhinitis.

The 'itch–scratch cycle' is a key factor. Dry skin itches and the child scratches. The trauma of scratching releases inflammatory mediators, causing more itch and may also break the epidermal barrier and lead to infection. The distribution of the rash varies with age, the face, head and trunk being more commonly affected in young infants, while the extensor and flexural surfaces of the limbs are more commonly affected in older children. There is a genetic predisposition in many cases with a history of eczema or other atopic diseases in close family members.

Trigger factors are not always obvious but include secondary staphylococcal infection, over-washing with soap, stress resulting in scratching, or, occasionally, dietary allergens such as egg or cow's milk protein.

Contact eczema or dermatitis is uncommon in childhood although an allergic causation should be considered. This may be obvious, as e.g. with nickel sensitivity when the rash is limited to the area in contact with nickel. Common culprits are watchstraps or earrings. In some cases, biological detergents, or lanolin, found in many emollient creams, may cause contact dermatitis.

Seborrhoeic dermatitis has overlapping features but it appears preferentially on the scalp with a yellowish greasy appearance, often with more scaling, and it usually appears early in infancy. Scabies can resemble eczema due to the combination of scratching and inflammation/superinfection.

● **Treatment:**

Management involves:

● Attempting to reduce the itch by reducing bathing and avoiding biological detergents
● Wearing loose clothing (preferably cotton)
● Managing dryness with emollients, used in place of soap, and applied copiously to affected areas. Wet wraps may help to seal in moisture
● Reducing inflammation by application of topical steroids; use of the more potent creams and lotions should be restricted to short courses to reduce the risk of side-effects
● Calcineurin inhibitors (tacrolimus, pimecrolimus) are recommended as second-line treatment by NICE (NICE clinical guideline 57, December 2007). These anti-inflammatory agents are effective, and do not thin the skin, unlike steroids. The commonest side effect is stinging after application, which quickly disappears. They may increase vulnerability to infection, and should not be applied to broken or obviously infected skin. There is a theoretical risk that they may increase skin cancer risk, so ideally should not be applied to sun-exposed areas over an extended period, and should not be used in conjunction with ultraviolet light treatment

- Anti-pruritics, usually antihistamines, which may help reduce itch, especially at night when the sedative effect is also potentially beneficial for sleep
- Avoidance of known allergens, which include measures to reduce exposure to house dust mite where appropriate
- Treatment of infection due to bacteria with short courses of oral antibiotics. Long-term use of topical antibiotics in combination with steroids is associated with antibiotic resistance.
- Phototherapy with ultraviolet (UVB) light is beneficial in some cases. Typically, 15–30 treatments are required.
- Severe cases may merit the use of oral steroids, azathioprine or ciclosporin.

Seborrhoeic dermatitis

Seborrhoeic dermatitis is usually a mild inflammatory disorder affecting sebum-rich areas of the scalp, face and trunk. Infection with the yeast *Malassezia furfur* is implicated in the pathogenesis. *Malasssezia* expresses lipases which act on sebum, releasing inflammatory fatty acids, in addition to activating the alternative complement pathway. The resultant inflammation ranges from mild dandruff to severe erythroderma. Clinical features depend on the site of infection:

- *Scalp:* involvement manifests as scaling and inflammation with the appearance of dandruff, but it may progress to a red, scaly, weeping rash. The rash may extend around the ears and onto the forehead. In infants, scalp involvement has the classical appearance of cradle cap with thick yellow scale.
- *Ears*: The skin around the ears may ooze and crust, and the ears may swell.
- *Face:* The nasolabial folds and inner eyebrows are most commonly involved. Eyelid involvement (blepharitis) may be troublesome.
- *Chest and back*: well-demarcated scaly red patches are seen on the central part of the chest and between the shoulder blades.
- *Flexures*: flexural involvement affects moist skin folds, particularly the groin, axillae, abdominal flexures and under the breast. Groin involvement is especially striking in infantile seborrhoeic dermatitis.

Seborrhoeic dermatitis may be especially severe in HIV infection, due to the unchecked proliferation of yeasts.

Treatment of the scalp is with medicated shampoos. Skin involvement responds to combined steroid/antifungal creams. In severe cases, a course of oral itraconazole may be necessary.

Infantile seborrhoeic dermatitis is a benign self-limiting variant affecting infants. It usually occurs in the first 3 months of life. Despite the florid appearance of the rash, the child is well and in no discomfort, in contrast to eczema. Treatment with a topical combined antifungal steroid cream is effective. Cradle cap may be treated by bathing with olive oil or other emollients or using an antifungal shampoo.

Psoriasis

Although more common in adults, 25% of individuals affected by psoriasis develop their first lesions in childhood. Around 1–3% of children are affected. Usually it develops as round red raised papules or plaques with a silvery-grey scale. The scalp, elbows, knees, lumbosacral area and the extensor surfaces of limbs are most frequently affected and distribution is often approximately symmetrical (see Figure 8.1). Less commonly seen is the guttate form with multiple small drop-like lesions, which more commonly occurs in adolescents. Associations include nail discoloration and pitting and a form of polyarticular arthritis (see Chapter 6, p. 52). Simple treatment of psoriasis entails adequate use of moisturizers, and sun exposure. Medical therapy is primarily aimed at symptom control. The mainstays of treatment are topical vitamin D analogues (e.g. calcipotriol) and topical coal tar preparations supplemented by short courses of topical corticosteroids. Ultraviolet B treatment (narrowband or broadband) is used in short courses for more severe cases (over the age of 14 years). Second-line treatment consists of disease modifying drugs – methotrexate is used in the first instance; ciclosporin is an alternative, if it is not tolerated. Acitretin, or other vitamin A analogues, may be used in boys, but the teratogenic potential makes use in girls undesirable. Use of second-line agents precludes the use of UV therapy due to the potential risk of skin cancer. Biologic therapy with monoclonal antibodies is reserved for third-line treatment. NICE has approved the following agents: Etanercept, adalimumab, infliximab and ustekinumab for psoriasis.

Pityriasis rosea

Pityriasis rosea is a self-limiting inflammatory skin disease, common in adolescence. A large red patch on the trunk – the *herald patch* – is followed 48–72 hours later by numerous small oval, rose-pink macules or papules, with scaling. The lesions on the trunk commonly follow the lines of the ribs, giving a characteristic '*Christmas tree*' distribution. A viral aetiology is likely, but unproven. The rash remits in 1–2 months. Troublesome itch may be alleviated with aqueous cream; otherwise no treatment is required.

Urticaria and angio-oedema

Urticaria (commonly known as 'hives') is a relatively common dermatosis, affecting over 20% of people at some point in their lives. It is three times more common in atopic individuals. Urticaria is characterized by short-lived erythematous, intensely itchy swellings, known as wheals. It is a consequence of histamine release by mast cells in the skin. Angio-oedema is a related condition, with larger non-erythematous swellings, usually of the lips, tongue or extremities. Histamine release may be triggered by allergy, exercise, physical pressure, and even sunlight (solar urticaria). Allergens can be environmental, in food, drugs, or secondary to infection. In the common idiopathic form of urticaria/angio-oedema, it is unusual to identify a trigger. This is by far the commonest situation in children. Blood tests or skin prick tests are usually fruitless. Treatment is with non-sedating antihistamines, such as ceterizine. Angio-oedema may affect the tongue or throat. This may be alarming to the patient, but is rarely life-threatening. This is in contrast to hereditary angio-oedema (usually due to C1 esterase inhibitor deficiency), in which attacks are usually severe.

For acute angio-oedema, a short course of prednisolone is usually advised. If severe, iv chlorpheniramine may be used, and in life-threatening angio-oedema, adrenaline is indicated.

Episodes of urticaria/angio-oedema usually last from a few days to a few weeks. By definition, urticaria lasting more than 6 weeks is deemed chronic, and allergy is rarely the cause.

Erythema multiforme

Erythema multiforme is an acute hypersensitivity reaction. An infectious trigger is common; particularly mycoplasma and herpes group viruses. Drugs may also cause erythema multiforme. In a half of the cases no cause is identified.

The rash is dramatic, with sudden onset of macules, vesicles and urticarial elements, but *target lesions* are the hallmark. Target lesions are red 1–2 cm macules with a discolored purpuric or bullous centre. Involvement of the palms and soles of the feet is common. Accompanying fever, arthralgia and malaise usually occur. Symptomatic relief with paracetamol is normally the only treatment required, although in severe cases steroids may be used. Resolution takes 2–6 weeks.

Occasionally, the rash may be severe and involves the eyes, oral and nasal mucosa and anogenital region – *Stevens–Johnson syndrome*. Stevens–Johnson syndrome is a severe condition, which, rarely, may be life threatening. *Mycoplasma pneumoniae* is not infrequent as a causative organism. Treatment comprises supportive care to maintain hydration, nutrition and comfort. Intercurrent mycoplasma infection should be sought and treated. Intravenous methylprednisolone or immunoglobulin may speed remission.

Erythema nodosum

Large, tender, red patches over the shins may accompany infection or inflammation. Erythema nodosum may also occur secondarily to drug sensitivity. The lesions appear in crops lasting a few days and they are usually associated with systemic symptoms such as fever, arthralgia and malaise. The commonest infectious precipitants are *Streptococcus* and *Mycoplasma*. Tuberculosis, sarcoidosis and inflammatory bowel disease are important causes.

SKIN INFECTIONS

Bacterial infections

Impetigo

Case 8.2 A boy with lesions around his mouth

Andrew, a 3-year-old boy, developed a single red spot by his upper lip. Within 2 days, similar lesions around his mouth and over his cheeks had become vesicular, then pustular, and finally crusted. Yellow serous discharge had given the lesions a golden hue and separation of some of the crusts had left a raw weeping area.

The golden crusts seen in Case 8.2 are typical of impetigo, caused by *Staphylococcus aureus* or sometimes *Streptococcus*. The rapid spread is facilitated by auto-innoculation of the infection by rubbing and scratching. Skin swabs should be taken, and 'best-guess' systemic antibiotics commenced (e.g. co-amoxiclav) until culture and sensitivity results are available. Recurrence is common, often due to persistent nasal carriage.

Erysipelas and cellulitis

Erysipelas is a superficial well-demarcated streptococcal infection, typically on the face, with associated oedema due to involvement of lymphatic vessels. Cellulitis is a deeper infection of the skin, caused by staphylococci or Group A streptococci.

Both cause a warm, red, painful swelling of the skin with fever and malaise. They occur as a primary infection or secondarily to minor trauma. Treatment is with systemic antibiotics, if necessary, by the intravenous route.

Staphylococcal scalded-skin syndrome

Infection of the skin with specific phage types of Group II staphylococci may result in scalded-skin syndrome. The child is often very unwell with fever and severe malaise. Cleaving of the epidermal layer by endotoxin causes large sheets of skin to blister and then separate, leaving raw weeping denuded areas resembling scalds. Treatment is with emollients, (e.g. a 50:50 mix of liquid and white soft parafin), analgesia, fluid replacement and intravenous antibiotics. On occasion, skin loss may approach 100%.

Acne

Almost all children suffer some degree of acne in adolescence. Acne results from obstruction of pilosebaceous follicles by sebum. Acne is worst where there is a higher density of sebaceous follicles – the face, upper chest and back. Secondary infection of the obstructed follicles, notably *Propionobacterium acnes*, produces a marked inflammatory response with pustules. The child or teenager with acne has a mixture of closed and open comedones (whiteheads and blackheads), pustules and erythema. Acne is associated with other signs of excessive sebaceous secretions with generally greasy skin and hair.

● Treatment:

Treatment is directed at treating infection with topical antibiotics (e.g. erythromycin) or antiseptics (benzoyl peroxide). Topical retinoids, such as tretinoin, may be useful as these are antiinflammatory and comedolytic, and reduce follicular proliferation. Oral antibiotics, such as minocycline, and retinoids are frequently needed for severe cases.

Viral infections

Herpes simplex

Infection with herpes simplex virus type 1 is ubiquitous in children. In a minority, it causes a severe acute febrile illness with gingivostomatitis. Painful ulceration of the buccal mucosa results in erosion and haemorrhage. Dehydration may occur as swallowing is painful, and thick secretions may build up in the mouth. Treatment is with analgesia, fluids, oral hygiene and oral aciclovir.

Secondary or recurrent herpes labialis results in tightly grouped painful vesicles ('cold sores'), with crusting over the lips and perioral region, and may be treated with oral aciclovir.

Molluscum contagiosum

Case 8.3 A girl with lesions on her fingers

Gemma, a 5-year-old girl, was taken to her GP. She had had several small raised lesions on her fingers for many months. They were approximately 2–5mm in diameter, raised, with a central dimple ('umbilication') and pinkish-grey in colour. There was no itch but one or two lesions had become red and tender before disappearing over a few days.

Molluscum contagiosum is caused by a poxvirus and spreads by auto-inoculation. Uncommonly, secondary infection may occur, causing spreading erythema and tenderness, but more usually the lesions are relatively asymptomatic, as in Case 8.3. Healing, sometimes preceded by an episode of inflammatory change, occurs spontaneously, often after 18 months to 2 years.

Viral warts

Warts are intra-epidermal lesions due to the human papilloma virus. They occur most commonly on the hands, where they form raised hyperkeratotic lesions 2-4 mm in diameter, and on the soles of the feet, where they become embedded by trauma, causing painful plantar verrucas. Two-thirds resolve within 2 years. Salicylic acid paste or cryotherapy with liquid nitrogen may accelerate resolution.

Fungal infections

There are two principal causes of cutaneous fungal infections of the skin in children – *Candida* and dermatophytes.

Candidiasis

In candidiasis, the skin is inflamed and erythematous with neighbouring *satellite lesions* – small red spots adjacent to the affected skin. Candidal infections usually affect moist areas such as the perineum or around the mouth, particularly in infants. Treatment is with a combination steroid/antifungal cream such as clotrimazole-hydrocortisone.

Dermatophytes

Dermatophytes cause a number of superficial fungal infections:

- **Scalp ringworm** (tinea capitis): well-circumscribed, itchy bald patches, with scaling causing scarring alopecia. Green fluorescence is commonly seen under ultraviolet light, depending on the infecting organism
- **Ringworm** (tinea corporis): itchy erythematous patches, typically originating in the groin or axillae, extend across the trunk
- **Athlete's foot** (tinea pedis): the toe webs are usually affected with moist, white, 'blotting-paper' skin. The infection may extend over the sole of the foot, and occasionally, the nails are affected.

Diagnosis is made on skin scrapings or nail clippings. Treatment is with topical or oral imidazoles. Treatment of scalp ringworm is with a 4-week course of terbinafine (though unlicensed in children). Shorter regimes using terbinafine or itraconazole may be effective. Topical imidazoles are usually effective for tinea corporis and tinea pedis.

SCABIES

Sarcoptes scabiei is a highly infectious 8-legged mite, less than 0.5 mm in diameter, which burrows through the stratum corneum to cause recurrent crops of intensely itchy erythematous papules and vesicles. Scratching leads to excoriation with weeping, crusting and secondary infection. Linear burrows are characteristic but are readily seen in only 10–20% of cases. Usual sites in infants are the head, neck, hands, feet and face and, in older children, finger and toe webs, axillae, flexures, wrists and genitals. Microscopy of skin scrapings reveals the mite if there is diagnostic doubt.

Treatment is with:

- Topical application of malathion or permethrin to the entire body (index case and all household members)
- Washing of all clothing and bedding.

HAEMANGIOMAS

'Strawberry' naevus

Case 8.4 An infant with a red swelling of the eyelid

Kerry, a 3-week-old infant, presented with a red swelling of the eyelid, first noticed by the parents 2 weeks beforehand. It had spread from pin-point size to involve most of the upper eyelid. The child was well, with a 1 cm raised red-purple swelling comprising a leash of small capillaries, which partially blanched on pressure.

The finding of a rapidly swelling telangiectatic lesion early in infancy (as in Case 8.4) suggests a *'strawberry' naevus.* Strawberry naevi are present in up to 3% of babies and are especially common in preterm infants. The lesion appears at, or shortly after, birth. Lesions grow quickly, reaching a maximum size by 6–12 months of age, after which spontaneous involution begins. Complete resolution usually occurs by age 9–10 years, and there is usually no residual trace – except sometimes a patch of pale or slightly atrophic skin. Complications, including erosion with secondary haemorrhage, and infection, occur in about 5%. Very large cavernous lesions may cause platelet trapping in the abnormal vessels, leading to thrombocytopenia and bleeding – the Kasabach–Merritt syndrome. Many haemangiomas respond favourably to propranolol. Steroids may be tried in resistant cases, but side effects are problematic. Pulse-dye laser may be used after infancy, if lesions are in difficult locations, such as the eyes, mouth and ears. Laser therapy is less effective after age 6 years.

Port wine stains

Port wine stains are flat, small-vessel, capillary haemangiomas present at birth. They are often a deep purple shade, and usually flat, but bulky lesions are occasionally seen. They may be quite disfiguring, particularly on the face. When found over the upper cheek and forehead they may be associated with an intracranial vascular malformation – Sturge–Weber syndrome – with epilepsy and learning difficulties (see Chapter 14, p. 204). Early laser therapy is recommended for port-wine stains to achieve the best cosmetic effect.

ALOPECIA

Alopecia – loss of hair – may be diffuse or patchy.

Diffuse hair loss

Growing or *anagen* hairs normally constitute 80–90% of scalp hair, with the remainder – *telogen* hairs – being shed. A number of factors may affect the normal hair cycle of hair growth and loss; however, because of the long duration of hair growth, the effects are apparent only 6–12 weeks after the initial trigger, when there is widespread hair loss and thinning, but not bald patches – *telogen effluvium* – when the majority of hairs are in telogen. Precipitants include stress and illness. Normal hair growth resumes within a few months.

Diffuse hair loss also occurs secondarily to hypothyroidism, with zinc deficiency, and after chemotherapy.

Patchy hair loss

Circumscribed areas of hair loss leading to bald patches are divided into scarring and non-scarring alopecia.

Alopecia areata

The alopecia areata described in Case 8.5 is the commonest cause of non-scarring alopecia in children. The marginal exclamation-mark hairs, where the base of the hair tapers towards the scalp, and which may easily be pulled out, are characteristic. Nail pitting may be seen. There is an association with autoimmune conditions such as vitiligo and hypothyroidism. The majority of children recover completely, and the value of treatment is uncertain, but where desired, intradermal steroid injection has been used.

> ### Case 8.5 A girl with hair loss
>
> Kirsty, aged 12 years, presented with hair loss, leading to circumscribed bald patches over her scalp. There was no scarring or inflammation. On inspecting the scalp with a hand lens, 'exclamation-mark' hairs were seen at the edge of some of the lesions.

It is important to differentiate alopecia areata from traumatic hair loss due to tight hair bands, and from other causes of alopecia such as ringworm, or tinea capitis (see above), which are characterized by scarring.

HEAD LICE

The ectoparasitic louse, *Pediculus humanus capitis*, infests the scalp. The louse feeds on the scalp, and its saliva produces itching and inflammation. These lice are transmitted by personal contact or via fomites, such as combs and cuddly toys. Humans are the only host, and the lice live for only a short time off the scalp.

Each louse may live for several weeks, and a single louse may lay up to 120 ova. The ova, known as *nits* are attached to the hair follicles close to the scalp.

- **Treatment:**
- Malathion and dimeticone shampoos may be purchased 'over the counter'. Malathion is ovaricidal and may reduce re-infection
- Isopropyl myristate and cyclomethicone solution
- Coconut, anise, and ylang ylang spray
- Regular wet combing with a fine-toothed comb, preferably after application of a hair conditioner, facilitates removal of nits
- Washing of combs, brushes, bedding, towels and soft toys is usually advised, but of doubtful value.

Further reading

The British Association of Dermatologists has an outstanding website with excellent online resources. www.bad.org.uk.

Circulation 9

(Rahul Roy, Richard Beach, Graham Derrick)

CHAPTER CONTENTS

INTRODUCTION

Heart disease causes dread in parents and carers. This is usually because their experience of heart disease is in adults whose ischaemic heart disease causes chest pain, peripheral oedema or sudden death. In developed countries cardiac problems in children are usually congenital and present with heart murmur, breathlessness or cyanosis. Recent advances have made congenital heart disease an eminently treatable condition, and many children with murmurs have normal hearts and need no treatment at all. Do not forget when talking to families how frightening talk of heart problems will be.

HISTORY

Serious heart disease in children presents with poor growth, breathlessness, pallor or cyanosis. In babies this causes feeding problems – breaking off in mid-feed, with panting or 'grunting' respiration and sometimes sweating. Murmurs (e.g. ventricular septal defect, VSD) may not be evident at birth, but may be apparent by the time of the 8-week check. Older children with heart disease may lack energy and tire easily.

Ask about any episodes of cyanosis, pallor or distress. Check for a family history of cardiac problems in children. Reassure the family that the grandfather's recent heart attack is unlikely to be relevant. Ask about any previous treatments or heart operations.

EXAMINATION

Make a non-threatening start by feeling the radial and then the brachial pulse. Remember that the pulse is faster in infants than in older children and adults. Some irregularity of the pulse (sinus arrhythmia) is normal in healthy children. The character of the pulse may be abnormal in aortic stenosis (low volume) or patent ductus arteriosus (PDA; collapsing or 'bounding' pulse).

Palpating the femoral pulses feels intrusive to the child – leave it until the end, but do not forget to do it. Radiofemoral delay is not of use in paediatrics as most children are too small for the delay to be perceptible.

Ideally the examination can now proceed through inspection of the praecordium, palpation, auscultation and percussion, but in an active toddler you may need to grab opportunities to examine as they present. Remember that children who have had cardiac catheterization may have impalpable pulses and small scars in the groin or antecubital fossa over the femoral or brachial artery. Listen to the heart sounds at each of the four sites shown in Figure 9.1. At each site listen carefully for first and second heart sounds. In the pulmonary area it should be possible to hear the pulmonary and aortic components separately. An extra sound at the apex following the second sound is the third sound. This is usually physiological in children. In children with a cardiac failure there may be a gallop rhythm produced by third and fourth sounds. Finally, listen for heart murmurs. Try to decide where the murmur is best heard, how loud it is and whether it is a pansystolic (i.e. beginning with, and not separate from, the first heart sound) or an ejection systolic murmur. Diastolic murmurs are rare in childhood, but listen carefully all the same.

Blood pressure measurement is important in children, but is best left until last as it may be distressing. In infants, blood pressure can be measured using an automated blood pressure machine – palpation techniques are unreliable. In older children the blood pressure can be measured using a stethoscope in the normal way, but the correct size cuff must be used. The cuff should cover two-thirds of the length of the upper arm, and the bladder should encircle at least 80% of the arm. Centile charts for blood pressure are available in the UK. Blood pressure should be measured in the right arm in almost all circumstances, and both arms if there are thoracotomy scars.

The following scheme is recommended.

Inspection

- Central cyanosis – look at the tongue; measure oxygen saturation if in doubt
- Jugular venous pressure – the short neck and skin folds in infants only allow this examination in older children

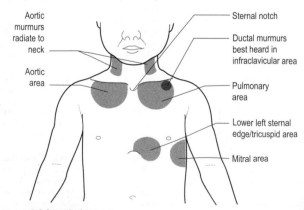

Figure 9.1 Auscultation points.

- Look at the chest wall for operative scars – a left or right thoracotomy scar may be easily overlooked because the incision is posterior and can be hidden by the arms – lift the arms and look round to the scapula
- Before examination, plot growth on the chart as children with heart disease may fail to thrive, and measure the respiratory rate.

Palpation

- Examine the hands and look for:
  - Finger clubbing – finger clubbing suggests chronic disease
  - Splinter haemorrhages if there have been concerns about endocarditis – though in children these are as likely to be traumatic.
- The pulse – establish the rate, rhythm and nature of the pulse; in young children the brachial pulse is easier to identify than the radial pulse
- Feel for the apex beat
- Feel for thrills over the chest wall and over the right carotid. Thrills palpable in the sternal notch can be present in both aortic or pulmonary stenosis.

Auscultation

For auscultation points see Figure 9.1.

- Heart sounds – establish the volume and nature of the sounds. Variable splitting of the second sound and a third heart sound may be normal variants in children
- Murmurs – intensity
- Timing (systolic/diastolic)
- Area of maximum intensity
- Radiation
- Listen to the lung bases
- Listen to the back of the chest as some murmurs are best heard in the back, e.g. coarctation of the aorta

To complete the examination:

- Palpate the abdomen for hepatomegaly – a sign of heart failure
- Feel the femoral pulses and check the blood pressure in the right arm.

INVESTIGATIONS

A chest X-ray will allow assessment of cardiac size and pulmonary vasculature. An ECG may give information on the relative size of the cardiac chambers and on cardiac strain. Characteristic abnormalities are seen with some congenital heart defects, e.g. superior QRS axis and ostium primum atrial septal defect (ASD) or tricuspid atresia. Transcutaneous oxygen saturation, ideally in the right arm, will more reliably detect cyanosis. If saturation is less than 95%, in the absence of a sufficient alternative explanation, echocardiography is indicated. An echocardiogram allows accurate diagnosis of cardiac anatomy and a useful assessment of cardiac function. Cardiac catheterization accesses the heart through a catheter usually inserted into the femoral artery. This technique enables therapy, e.g. balloon atrial septostomy, to create an artificial ASD in transposition of the great vessels, as well as aiding diagnosis.

It is likely that motion-tolerant pulse oximetry of newborn infants will be introduced during the currency of this textbook, following the publication of a major trial in over 20 000 newborn infants, in November 2011, which demonstrated effectiveness in early detection of severe congenital heart disease. The UK National Screening Committee is currently considering its nationwide introduction.

HEART DISEASE IN INFANTS

The neonate with a heart murmur

The circulation alters dramatically at the time of birth as the umbilical cord is cut and the lungs, rather than the placenta, become the source of oxygenated blood. Turbulent flow during these changes leads to transient murmurs in the neonate. A neonatal murmur may also be the first sign of significant congenital heart disease leading on to cyanosis or cardiac failure if undiagnosed. Check carefully for possible cardiac symptoms – see below. If the baby remains asymptomatic, and careful assessment discovers no abnormality, then a transient pulmonary flow murmur is likely. This will normally resolve within 48–72 hours of birth. An echocardiogram is essential if there is clinical uncertainty.

Changes in the circulation at birth (Figure 9.2)

1. The umbilical cord is clamped and cut, cutting off flow to and from the placenta.
2. The lungs become aerated and pressure in the pulmonary circulation drops.
3. Extra blood pours into the lungs as a result of this drop in pressure and returns via the pulmonary veins to the left atrium.
4. This changes the relative pressures in the left and right atria, and encloses the foramen ovale by a flap valve effect.
5. Normal lung function produces a marked rise in the oxygenation of the neonatal blood.
6. Muscles in the wall of the ductus arteriosus contract and lead to a physical, and later anatomical, closure of the duct.
7. The pulmonary pressure continues to drop over the first 1–2 months of life.

> **Case 9.1** A baby with collapse (left ventricular outflow tract obstruction)
>
> Edward, a 4-day-old baby, was discharged from the maternity unit after a normal routine examination, only to collapse within a few hours. He was rushed to the A&E department. He was pale and shocked with weak, thready brachial pulses, but no palpable femoral pulses. He was grunting with tachypnoea and marked respiratory distress.

The baby in Case 9.1 was urgently intubated and ventilated, and resuscitated with fluids - including saline and bicarbonate because of a severe metabolic acidosis. The differential diagnosis was thought to be overwhelming sepsis, congenital heart disease with cardiac failure or a metabolic disorder. In view of the impalpable femoral pulses, a prostaglandin E_2 infusion was commenced. Coarctation of the aorta was confirmed by echocardiography and Edward was transferred urgently to a children's cardiac unit.

Left ventricular outflow tract obstruction may arise from hypoplastic left heart syndrome, critical aortic stenosis or, as in Case 9.1, coarctation of the aorta. The left ventricle fails to eject blood into the obstructed aorta, and the circulation is maintained by blood flow through the ductus arteriosus, bypassing the obstruction. When the ductus arteriosus closes, catastrophic collapse occurs, with pulmonary oedema, pallor, shock and acidosis. In hypoplastic left heart syndrome, children are born without an effective left ventricle and rely on the right ventricle to perfuse both

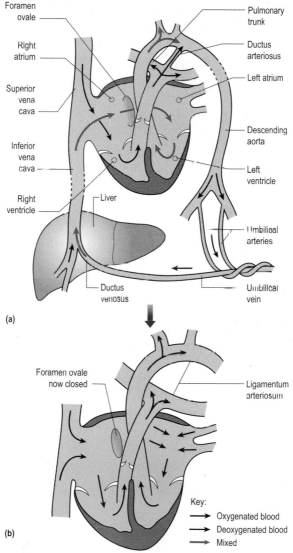

Figure 9.2 Changes in the circulation at birth. (a) The fetal circulation; (b) the new-born circulation.

lungs and systemic systems. Using prostaglandin E$_2$ to keep the ductus arteriosus open may sustain life until palliative surgery may be performed. There is practical and ethical debate as to the advisability of surgery for these children, as the prognosis remains guarded.

Case 9.2 A blue baby (congenital cyanotic heart disease)

Emma, a healthy term neonate, was noted to be cyanosed by her midwife at 6 hours of age. There was no breathlessness and the baby had taken a feed. On examination, there was a soft systolic murmur. Pulse oximetry showed an oxygen saturation of 66%. Oxygen administration did not improve this significantly.
A diagnosis of probable cyanotic congenital heart disease was made, and a precautionary prostaglandin E$_2$ infusion commenced, pending echocardiography.

Children with neonatal cyanosis need an urgent diagnostic work-up (as in Case 9.2). If lung perfusion depends on a PDA, these children may deteriorate rapidly when the duct closes.

Transposition of the great vessels and tetralogy of Fallot account for over 90% of cases of cyanotic congenital heart disease. Transposition of the great vessels is the commonest cause of cyanotic congenital heart disease at birth.

In transposition of the great vessels, the left ventricle is connected to the pulmonary artery, feeding oxygenated blood back through the pulmonary artery to the lungs. The right ventricle returns deoxygenated blood to the aorta; thus there are two independent circulations. Common mixing through the ductus arteriosus or an associated VSD allows ingress of oxygenated blood into the systemic circulation. An arterial switch operation in the neonatal period is the treatment of choice.

In Fallot's tetralogy the combination of a VSD and right ventricular outflow tract obstruction restricts blood flow to the lungs and leads to right ventricular hypertrophy, with a right to left shunt through the VSD producing cyanosis. The more severe the pulmonary stenosis, the earlier the presentation with cyanosis. Typically, cyanosis becomes evident at 3–6 months of age. Treatment requires surgery to close the VSD and relieve the right ventricular outflow tract obstruction by muscle resection, valvotomy and patch enlargement of the valve itself. This is normally undertaken in the first year of life.

Case 9.3 A breathless baby with failure to thrive (congenital acyanotic heart disease)

Adam, an 8-week-old infant, was failing to grow as expected. Feeding was becoming more difficult and he seemed pale, breathless and sweaty after feeds. Examination revealed tachycardia and tachypnoea even at rest. There was no cyanosis, but he had a loud pansystolic murmur, audible at the apex, with an overlying thrill. The liver was enlarged 3 cm below the costal margin, confirming cardiac failure. Echocardiography showed a large VSD.

Other more complex congenital heart lesions, such as tricuspid atresia, Ebstein's anomaly, or pulmonary atresia, cause cyanosis by a combination of limiting pulmonary blood flow and common mixing of oxygenated and de-oxygenated blood. Surgical treatment may include creating a shunt between the arterial and pulmonary circuits to maintain lung perfusion. These shunts, if successful, will produce an audible, continuous murmur best heard over the surgical scar – a useful tip in an examination.

VSDs (such as in Case 9.3) are the commonest congenital heart defect. The communication between the ventricles leads to blood flow from the high-pressure left ventricle to the low-pressure right ventricle. Infants do not usually present in the neonatal period when the left and right pressures are similar, but, as the pulmonary artery pressure drops, pulmonary blood flow increases with resultant pulmonary hypertension and pulmonary oedema.

Cardiac failure is treated initially with diuretics. Some VSDs can get smaller or even close spontaneously with time and even large lesions may be treated medically in the first instance. Surgery is indicated if medical treatment fails, or if it is predicted that the VSD will not close because of its morphology. PDA is the other principal cause of left-to-right shunt, and may present in the same way.

PDA is especially common in premature infants, as the mechanism for duct closure is immature. In these babies increased pulmonary blood flow as a result of left-to-right shunting through the duct may complicate pre-existing lung disease and lead to ventilator dependence. Symptomatic pre-term infants may be treated medically with indomethacin or ibuprofen, which inhibits prostaglandin synthesis leading to duct closure.

HEART DISEASE IN CHILDREN

The older child with a heart murmur

Murmurs are often heard at routine checks before children go to school or while they are being examined during intercurrent illnesses.

The innocent murmur

Innocent ejection systolic murmurs are caused by turbulent blood flow within any part of the circulation. See Box 9.1 for the characteristics of innocent murmurs.

It may also be possible to hear turbulent flow in the venous return from the head and neck. This produces a continuous murmur usually heard

---

Box 9.1 Characteristics of innocent murmurs

- Asymptomatic
- Localized to the left sternal edge
- Postural – volume varies with sitting/standing (not invariably true)
- Short duration
- Soft in quality
- No radiation
- Otherwise normal examination with normal cardiac impulse and no palpable thrill

under the clavicle, variable with respiration and position of the neck. These murmurs disappear when the child lies down.

With experience and a careful clinical examination it is possible to define an innocent murmur without the need for further investigation, but any murmur that does not obey these rules must be investigated.

Left-to-right shunts

Ventricular septal defects (VSDs) are due to defects in the septum separating the high-pressure left ventricle from the low-pressure right ventricle producing high flow if large or very turbulent flow if small. Large VSDs present in the neonatal period with heart failure as described above. Smaller lesions, which are not haemodynamically significant, may produce an impressive pansystolic murmur in an asymptomatic toddler or older child ('Maladie de Roger'). The murmur is harsh, high pitched and often associated with a thrill. These may close spontaneously through childhood and no treatment is usually necessary.

Patent ductus arteriosus (PDA) is usually asymptomatic if it presents with a heart murmur in mid-childhood. The physical signs of PDA are only collapsing or 'bounding' pulses if the left-to-right shunt through the duct is large, because the blood ejected into the aorta rapidly runs through the PDA into the low-pressure pulmonary circulation. There is usually a continuous 'machinery' murmur under the left clavicle. This does not sound like a venous hum, being much louder, and does not go away when the child lies down. Treatment can be usually accomplished safely and effectively via cardiac catheterization.

Atrial septal defects (ASDs) are also asymptomatic in childhood but troublesome to adults if they are allowed to persist until the third or fourth decade, when atrial enlargement can precipitate atrial arrhythmias. There is a left-to-right shunt at atrial level but with relatively low flow due to the low-pressure gradient. The physical findings are subtle – the key sign is a palpable right ventricular parasternal impulse and the wide and fixed splitting of the cardiac second heart sound heard over the pulmonary area. Otherwise the ejection systolic murmur could easily be confused with an innocent murmur – emphasizing the importance of listening to the heart sounds in children. An ostium primum ASD is a much more significant defect that requires surgery in early childhood, and may be associated with an apical pansystolic murmur in addition, from left atrioventricular valve incompetence.

Outflow tract obstruction

Coarctation of the aorta arises where the thoracic aorta is constricted at some point. It presents in the neonatal period if severe, or may present with a heart murmur alone, often heard over the back in the older child. Hypertension proximal to the coarctation may be observed. Poor femoral pulses, or a marked difference between the blood pressure in the upper and lower limbs, help to make the diagnosis. Coarctation may become more severe as time passes and may result in left ventricular failure. Treatment is surgical. Coarctation is very rare in girls, and may indicate Turner syndrome.

Aortic or pulmonary stenosis arises due to congenital narrowing of the atrioventricular valves, and produces ejection systolic murmurs. Aortic or pulmonary valve stenosis may also produce an ejection click – an additional sound after the first heart sound heard distant from the maximal intensity of the murmur, often at the apex of left lower sternal edge and before the onset of the murmur. Aortic stenosis murmurs are best heard in the aortic area, and may transmit to the neck. There is often a thrill over the murmur, and in the right carotid. Listen carefully for an early diastolic murmur indicating accompanying regurgitation. (It is best heard at the left sternal edge with the child sitting forward in full expiration.) The murmur of pulmonary stenosis is heard in the pulmonary area and radiates to the back. These conditions may present with symptoms in the neonatal period but more frequently turn up in mid-childhood. Monitoring is needed. Valves can be dilated with a balloon attached to a catheter. Open surgery and valve replacement are rarely needed in childhood.

Arrhythmias

> ### Case 9.4 An infant with a rapid heart beat
>
> Robin, an 8-month-old infant, presented with a sudden onset of pallor, altered consciousness and grunting respirations. On assessment, his pulse could not be easily palpated. Capillary refill was 6 seconds. On auscultation, the heart rate was extremely fast and on ECG was in excess of 250 beats per minute with narrow QRS complexes.

If the complexes on the ECG are narrow, as in Case 9.4, the arrhythmia is most likely to be a supraventricular tachycardia – the commonest pathological childhood arrhythmia. Broad complex tachycardia may be supraventricular or ventricular in origin. If the heart beats fast enough there is no time for refilling and the circulation fails, as in this case. It can occur at any age, including in utero, when treating the mother may control it. There is rarely a structural defect. Management is to restore sinus rhythm with vagal manoeuvres, medication or if necessary DC cardioversion (see Appendix I, p. 287).

Ninety per cent of children will have no further attacks after infancy, and preventative treatments may often be stopped after then. The main differential diagnosis is a symptomatic sinus tachycardia where the heart beats rapidly in response to shock, fever and severe systemic illness. Sinus tachycardia rarely exceeds 200 beats per minute, whereas supraventricular tachycardia usually exceeds 220 beats per minute.

CHEST PAIN IN CHILDREN

This is a common referral to paediatricians. Although children describe their chest pain as 'heart pain', the causes of chest pain in children very seldom include cardiac disease, yet referrals to cardiologists are common. Sources for chest pain in children include musculoskeletal, oesophageal, pleural and airway. Rarely cardiac chest pain can be caused by pericarditis, myocarditis, or extremely rarely aortic dissection or ischaemia. A careful history, ECG and chest X-ray should be enough to exclude a cardiac cause for chest pain without the need for specialist opinion. Echocardiography seldom assists this evaluation and should not routinely be offered.

RARE PROBLEMS

Hypertension in childhood

Severe hypertension is rare in children but can be devastating, presenting with visual loss, stroke or cardiac failure. Causes of severe hypertension include coarctation of the aorta, renal abnormalities, notably acute glomerulonephritis, steroid therapy, hyperlipidaemia and endocrine conditions such as phaeochromocytoma.

Elevated blood pressure may also complicate diabetes, obesity, hyperlipidaemia and chronic renal disease. Blood pressure monitoring is facilitated by reference to blood pressure centile charts.

The lesson is to measure blood pressure in children, particularly if there is some clue in the history such as abdominal pain, headache, breathlessness and visual problems, or steroid therapy.

Infective endocarditis

Infective endocarditis is an infection within the heart – usually affecting the heart valves. Abnormal blood flow through the heart caused by congenital anomalies increases the risk of bacterial colonization in the circulation infecting the heart. Clinical signs include fever, anaemia, arthralgia, splenomegaly, microscopic haematuria and changing heart murmurs.

The most common organism causing endocarditis is *Streptococcus viridans*. Bacteria are shed into the circulation during dental manipulations and surgical procedures, particularly those involving the bowel or the urinary tract. Tattoos and piercing may also result in a breakdown of the body's defences. However, antibiotic prophylaxis for dental, surgical and other procedures is no longer recommended by NICE because evidence that this practice prevents endocarditis is lacking.

Rheumatic fever

Rheumatic fever is the commonest cause of heart disease in children worldwide. It is a complex multisystem disease which may involve the heart, joints, nervous system and skin with various non-specific inflammatory changes (see Chapter 6, p. 57).

Sudden cardiac death in childhood

Sudden cardiac death in childhood is exceptionally rare. It may follow:
- Myocarditis
- Hypertrophic obstructive cardiomyopathy
- Aortic stenosis
- Inherited prolonged QT syndromes
- Late complication of Kawasaki's disease due to occlusion of coronary aneurysms (see Chapter 16, p. 238)
- Commotio cordis – ventricular fibrillation triggered by a sudden blow to the chest, usually during sport. It is much more common in males, with a mean age of death of 15 years. Defibrillation is life-saving.
- Idiopathic – 'sudden adult death syndrome'.

For patients with hypertrophic obstructive cardiomyopathy and inherited prolonged QT syndromes, screening of relatives with ECG and echocardiography is indicated.

Respiration 10

(Chris Upton, Nandu Thalange)

CHAPTER CONTENTS

INTRODUCTION

Respiratory illnesses, affecting the upper and lower respiratory tract, are the commonest cause of hospital admission in childhood. They are also an extremely common cause of primary care consultation. Coughing and snuffles are very common in children, especially during the winter months. Many children suffer wheeze and breathlessness as well. These symptoms are often caused by common viral infections, as the child acquires immunity in the early years. A complex interaction of inherited, environmental, allergic and social factors leads to significant morbidity in a few. The ability to distinguish mild from severe, and acute from recurrent, is the key to successful management.

HISTORY

Cough, snuffles, wheeze, breathlessness and stridor are the common respiratory symptoms in children. Wheeze is an expiratory whistling noise, but members of the public do not always understand the term. Even experienced doctors may on occasion get confused between expiratory wheeze and inspiratory stridor. Be careful, then, not to make assumptions. Ask about the nature of any cough as this is helpful in reaching a differential diagnosis. Upper airway coughs are often 'barking' in nature – like a seal rather than a dog. The cough associated with lower airway obstruction, such as bronchiolitis or asthma, is often described as 'hacking' or 'dry'. A 'fruity' cough may indicate suppurative lung disease such as bronchiectasis.

Noisy breathing and rattly chests are common in younger children and do not necessarily indicate troublesome underlying pathology. They may upset parents or grandparents more than they do the child. Consider whether the symptoms affect the child's day-to-day life and activities. Do they sleep normally, or are they woken by cough or wheeze? Do they manage regular attendance at school or nursery? Can they exercise normally, particularly PE and games? The infant equivalent of exercise is feeding, so ask if there is any difficulty with feeding, or slow weight gain.

Enquire particularly about the pattern and duration of any symptoms. Do they persist every day, or only occur episodically, e.g. with viral upper respiratory tract infections (URTIs)? A family or personal history of asthma or allergy such as eczema, hay fever or food allergy, may point towards asthma as the diagnosis. Ask about environmental precipitants such as passive smoking and exposure to dust or other inhaled allergens, including pollen and pet dander. Psychological and emotional factors need to be considered, as these are common triggers of airways obstruction.

Less common symptoms from respiratory disease include *chest pain, vomiting* and, in infants, *apnoea*. Young children with airways obstruction will sometimes refer to chest tightness as pain. Severe pain localized to the chest wall on deep breathing or coughing is called pleuritic pain, and is characteristic of acute lobar pneumonia with pleural involvement. Vomiting is frequent in young children with respiratory disease. Babies with gastro-oesophageal reflux may present with wheeze and cough; conversely, children with other respiratory conditions may vomit as a result of the large intrathoracic pressure swings affecting lower oesophageal ('cardiac') sphincter tone. Very young children, with conditions that usually cause cough, may present with apnoea instead. It is a common symptom in whooping cough and may be the presenting symptom in bronchiolitis, especially in ex preterm infants.

Remember that children with non-respiratory disease, such as diabetic ketoacidosis or panic attacks, may present with respiratory symptoms. On the other hand, some children with respiratory disease, especially pneumonia, may present with abdominal pain, or high fever alone, and little or nothing in the way of respiratory symptoms.

EXAMINATION

Use the scheme 'inspection, percussion, palpation and auscultation'. Start your examination by observing the child at rest. Is there tachypnoea (see Table 10.1), recession or other evidence of respiratory distress, e.g. head bobbing in a baby or nostril flaring in a toddler? Does the child look anxious? Is there an audible noise during respiration (see Table 10.2)? Do not

Table 10.1 Respiratory rates at different ages

Age	Breaths per minute
Neonate	40–60
Infant	30–40
5 years	20–25
10 years	15–20

Table 10.2 Audible respiratory sounds

	Quality	Loudest	Pathology
Wheeze	High pitched, tuneful	Expiration	Narrowing of mid-sized airways
Stridor	Crowing and harsh	Inspiration	Narrowing of larynx or trachea in the neck
Rattle	Moist/bubbling	No change with respiratory cycle	Collection of secretions usually in the upper respiratory tract

forget that tachypnoea may be due to fever or acidosis when there is no respiratory tract pathology.

Recession is a key physical sign in infants and young children. It describes the in-drawing of soft tissues around the chest by negative intrathoracic pressure generated by airway obstruction or reduced lung compliance. It may be seen in adults but is common in children because both soft tissues and the thoracic cage are more compliant. The resultant recession may be subcostal, intercostal or suprasternal. In addition, in neonates, the whole sternum may be sucked in – sternal recession, sometimes associated with grunting.

In older children you should complete a formal examination of the respiratory system including checking for clubbing (see Table 10.3) and cyanosis, percussion and auscultation. Look for chest deformity – Harrison's sulci or pectus carinatum ('pigeon chest'). These indicate chronically increased airway resistance – most commonly due to asthma.

In young children, particularly under 2 years, respiratory examination needs to be opportunistic and percussion is rarely of value. Audible crackles in the chest do not always mean lung consolidation or infection, particularly in the young child. They are often heard in wheezy children where they may be due to oedema and mucus in the small airways (see Table 10.4). Think about whether there are other signs of consolidation, such as reduced air entry or bronchial breathing. Examination of the ears and throat is a challenge in a fractious toddler – it is best left until last.

Table 10.3 Causes of clubbing

System	Cause
Cardiac	Cyanotic congenital heart disease
Bacterial endocarditis
Respiratory	Bronchiectasis
Cystic fibrosis/ciliary dyskinesia
Tuberculosis
Empyema/abscess, malignancy
Gastrointestinal	Inflammatory bowel disease, chronic active hepatitis
Primary sclerosing cholangitis
Other	Familial

Table 10.4 Severity of respiratory distress	
Grade	**Characteristics**
Mild	Tachypnoea Mild recession No effect on feeding or speech
Moderate	Tachypnoea Moderate or severe recession, struggles to feed, cannot speak in full sentences Oxygen may be needed to maintain saturation
Severe	Tachycardia, gasping, speechless, frightened May be pale and quiet or agitated and hypoxic despite oxygen Chest may be silent and respiratory effort flagging Impaired consciousness

Ears, nose and throat

A successful ENT examination requires younger children to be held gently but firmly by the parents (Figure 10.1).

Ears

Ask the parents to sit the child on their lap at 90° to their chest. With one arm, ask them to gently hold the child's head against their chest. Their other arm should hold onto the child's free arm. Gentle traction should be applied to the ear. The pinna should be pulled in an upward and outward direction. The auriscope should be gently held in a pincer grip. The ring finger of this hand should rest on the cheek of the child while the auriscope is within the ear. This allows the examiner's hand to quickly follow any sudden movements the child may make.

Throat

This is an unpleasant examination. It should be left until last. A tongue depressor is necessary for a complete examination. If throat disease is suspected, it is useful to have a swab to hand. A child may comply with throat examination once. They may resist a further request a few minutes later for a throat swab.

INVESTIGATIONS

Chest X-ray

This simple investigation is easily obtained in hospital but may be overused. Consider what you hope to learn before requesting a radiograph. It is not necessary, for instance, to X-ray every wheezy child, unless the episode is moderate or severe, or there are focal signs. Do not send an unstable child, particularly with upper airway obstruction, across the hospital to the X-ray department – stabilize the child first or request a portable X-ray. If there is any question of an inhaled foreign body, a single film is never sufficient. Except in those who require immediate bronchoscopy, X-ray screening in the young child, or inspiratory and expiratory films in the cooperative older child, are needed to confidently exclude or confirm a foreign body.

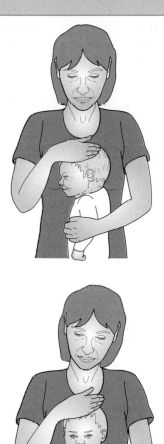

Figure 10.1 Positions for the ear and throat in the ENT examination.

Blood gas

Blood gas is a useful examination to assess the severity of a respiratory illness but is only needed in those with severe distress. Capillary samples are normally adequate, unless there are concerns about hypoxia, but arterial punctures are difficult and painful, and may aggravate hypoxia. Radial or brachial samples should be collected where needed.

Other blood tests

Blood tests are generally over-used. A blood count and C-reactive protein measurements in children with fever and cough are unhelpful at distinguishing common viral infections from more significant bacterial lower respiratory tract infections. A high lymphocyte count will help corroborate a diagnosis of whooping cough. Urea and electrolyte measurement is really only needed if there is coexistent severe vomiting or dehydration, or in children requiring intravenous fluids. Blood cultures are necessary if a child with pneumonia is very toxic and there are concerns about associated septicaemia. IgE and blood allergy tests may help confirm atopy in the child with probable asthma. Only occasionally does it directly influence management, e.g. the wheezy baby with eczema and milk allergy. Rarely, immune function testing may be required in children with true recurrent bacterial lower respiratory tract infections (see Chapter 16, p. 241).

Respiratory secretions

These are under-used. They are often forgotten as young children either cannot or will not produce sputum. Sputum culture, if available, is more helpful than blood culture. If persistent bacterial bronchitis is suspected a cough swab is a useful alternative to sputum culture and is invaluable in monitoring conditions such as cystic fibrosis and other forms of bronchiectasis. Immunofluorescence testing of nasopharyngeal aspirates is useful in infants with bronchiolitis to confirm or exclude respiratory syncytial virus (RSV) infection. A nasopharyngeal aspirate or pernasal swab is used to test for whooping cough.

Lung function testing

Peak flow measurements can be used in most children from about 5–7 years and are helpful in diagnosing and monitoring the severity of asthma. The child takes a deep breath, and then breathes out quickly through the mouthpiece of the peak flow meter, ensuring a good seal. The best of three measurements is taken.

Spirometers are now available in simple portable format, with computerized screens, which are fun for young children to use. They enable children as young as 5 years to perform previously complex lung function measurements. Analysis of a flow volume curve from such a spirometer can be very helpful in excluding or confirming airways obstruction.

UPPER RESPIRATORY TRACT INFECTIONS

Upper respiratory tract infections (URTIs) may be summarized as snuffles, fever and misery.

Viral URTIs are the commonest conditions encountered in primary care. Adults are immune to most of the upper respiratory tract viruses in their immediate environment – they only produce symptoms when they contract a new virus. Children have to acquire immunity to a host of viruses in their first few years, and have, on average, six to ten episodes of infection annually. Changes of environment – such as starting at the nursery or school – will produce an even higher infection rate. Although often trivial illnesses in medical terms, the symptoms of snuffles, fever and sore throat may make young children thoroughly miserable.

Nasal obstruction may cause feeding problems in babies as they are obligate nose breathers. Symptomatic treatment includes paracetamol for the relief of discomfort and fever. Decongestant nose drops and oral decongestants are ineffective and best avoided. Saline nose drops are probably as effective as more expensive proprietary remedies.

Influenza

Flu, caused by the influenza virus types A, B and C, is a seasonal infection striking in the autumn and winter months. Influenza A is classified according to two key proteins – haemaglutinin (types H1–H3), important for infectivity, and neuraminidase (two types, N1 and N2), which determines viral replication. Neuraminidase is the target for the drugs oseltamivir and zanamivir. Influenza B also expresses neuraminidase, and hence is susceptible to antivirals. Influenza type C is a very mild, non-epidemic infection

Type A is marked by *antigenic drift*, ensuring on-going susceptibility to seasonal flu, from year to year. Periodically, major *antigenic shift* occurs, probably due to recombination with avian and human flu types in pigs. Major antigenic changes herald worldwide pandemics, such as the recent H1N1 'swine flu' pandemic. This predominantly affected young people (peak age 12–17 years) and was, for the most part, a mild disease, with symptoms indistinguishable from seasonal flu. However, in those with pre-existing conditions, the disease could be severe or fatal.

Influenza has a short incubation period (1–3 days), followed by sudden onset of fever, cough, coryza and myalgia. Vomiting, and less commonly diarrhoea, may occur. Myalgia is more common with influenza B, and creatine kinase may be elevated. Influenza is highly infectious, with rapid spread by respiratory droplet transmission. Symptoms typically remit in 5–7 days.

In those with severe disease, symptoms of rapidly progressive respiratory failure develop, typically 3–5 days after symptom onset, principally due to viral pneumonitis, but, in a third bacterial super-infection occurs. Multi-organ failure may supervene, and extracorporeal membrane oxygenation is required in severe cases.

Mortality

Aside from viral pneumonitis, death follows secondary bacterial pneumonia, notably with pneumococcus (particularly serotype 1), *Haemophilus influenzae* B and *Staphylococcus*. Rarely, frank myocarditis occurs, and is rapidly fatal. A necrotizing encephalopathy, characterized by widespread changes in the brain stem, thalamus and cerebellum, with normal cerebrospinal fluid (CSF) and negative virological studies in CSF, also occurs rarely.

Prevention and treatment

Immunization of vulnerable children (e.g. those with asthma, congenital heart disease, diabetes or renal disease) is recommended. Pregnant women are at high risk of severe complications of influenza and should be offered immunization. Immunization of pregnant women also affords some protection to infants in the first few months after birth.

In epidemic situations, for children over 12 months, with increased vulnerability to infection, presenting within 48 hours of onset of flu symptoms, NICE recommends use of oseltamivir or zanamivir to ameliorate the illness. Post-exposure prophylaxis is recommended in unimmunized children 13 years and over, in at-risk groups.

Tonsillitis

Bacterial tonsillitis is hard to distinguish on clinical grounds from viral URTI as both conditions may produce a red throat with enlargement of local glands. It is often assumed that a white exudate over enlarged and inflamed tonsils is suggestive of bacterial infection but controlled studies have not shown this. Most tonsillitis in young children is viral and even if streptococcal infection is confirmed there is little evidence that antibiotics do anything other than reduce the risk of post-infective complications such as rheumatic fever or nephritis. Antibiotics are only necessary if the infection is slow to settle and there are concerns about secondary problems such as quinsy or nephritis. Avoid ampicillin or amoxicillin, as glandular fever may be the cause – look for generalized lymphadenopathy or hepatosplenomegaly (see Chapter 16, p. 237).

Otitis media

This presents with fever, misery and acute pain in the involved ear. Any viral URTI may produce a pink or red drum, but check for pain and look for evidence of loss of light reflex and bulging of the drum. The evidence suggests that paracetamol is as effective as antibiotics in treating otitis media and an initial period of observation with analgesia is recommended. Nevertheless it is hard *not* to treat children with acutely inflamed tympanic membranes with antibiotics. Amoxicillin is usually the first-line treatment. Sometimes the tympanic membrane perforates during an acute infection, releasing a little pus which discharges from the ear. Perforation produces dramatic relief of symptoms and the damaged tympanic membrane usually heals spontaneously. Provided the ear discharge is transient and other symptoms resolve promptly no additional measures are needed. *Glue ear* may be a chronic consequence of otitis media or occur without acute infection. Hearing loss is the commonest symptom, and evidence suggests that prophylactic antibiotics for a few months can reduce the need for grommets or other surgery.

UPPER AIRWAYS OBSTRUCTION

Stridor and croup are important paediatric problems. The upper airway of children, being smaller than in adults, is more likely to obstruct with oedema of local tissues. Infections or allergies, which might produce hoarseness or loss of voice in an adult, may therefore produce alarming respiratory obstruction in a child. Acute severe stridor is an acute medical emergency. Management is described in Appendix I, p. 296.

Differential diagnosis of stridor

Croup, as is the diagnosis in Case 10.1, is the commonest cause of acute stridor. It occurs mainly in preschool children.

There is usually a viral prodrome, commonly with a barking cough. Parainfluenza virus is the commonest causative organism, and steroids are the mainstay of management. Meta-analysis of many trials has confirmed their efficacy and any child with croup severe enough to need hospital admission should receive steroids. Nebulized budesonide works more quickly than oral or parenteral steroids. In severe stridor, nebulized 1:1000 adrenaline (epinephrine), repeated as necessary, is useful as an emergency measure (see also Appendix I, p. 296).

Spasmodic croup describes the condition of a group of children with recurrent but often short-lived stridor. The condition is thought to be allergic – being commoner in those with other evidence of atopy.

> ### *Case 10.1* A boy with a barking cough
>
> Ahmed, aged 3 years, presented to hospital at 2 a.m. with his family. He was snuffly and miserable the day before, and was given some paracetamol for a mild fever at bedtime. At 1 a.m. he awoke with an alarming 'crowing' noise on inspiration, and a very loud, unusual cough – like a seal 'barking'. He and his parents were panic-stricken as he gasped for breath. On examination he was pale and frightened with a loud inspiratory stridor. He looked pink and well perfused. He was alert and cried when approached. He and his family were reassured by the calm gentle approach of the staff. He was persuaded to tolerate a saturation monitor which showed an oxygen saturation of 94% in air. As examination showed moderate recession, he was treated with nebulized budesonide.

Epiglottitis has become very rare following the introduction of *Haemophilus influenzae* b immunization. However, effectiveness of the vaccine has waned recently, prompting a booster, and children born abroad may not be immunized. Epiglottitis is a septicaemic illness, and good supportive care – as for any child with septicaemia – is needed. A third-generation cephalosporin such as ceftriaxone is used.

See Table 10.5 for the differences between croup and epiglottitis.

Bacterial tracheitis is a rare cause of stridor. The child is usually extremely ill with co-existent septicaemia and pneumonia. Pus is seen in the trachea at intubation. *Staphylococcus aureus* is the most likely organism, but other organisms, such as *Haemophilus*, *Moraxella* or *Streptococcus* may be responsible.

Inhaled foreign bodies may present with stridor. Other presentations include the asymptomatic child following a choking episode, cough, wheeze or hoarseness. The history may not be definite but the diagnosis should always be considered in such children. Prompt recognition and removal is essential, as they may prove fatal. Delay in removal may also cause long-term morbidity, such as bronchiectasis. Ninety-five per cent of

Table 10.5 The important differences between croup and epiglottitis

	Croup	Epiglottitis
Organism	Parainfluenza virus	*Haemophilus influenzae* b
Age	6 months to 3 years	3–7 years
Prodrome URTI	Usual	Uncommon
Onset	Days	Hours
Cough	Present	Often absent
Dysphagia	Absent	Severe with dribbling
Systemic	Mildly unwell	Toxic and ill
Posture	No preference	Sitting/leaning forward

Pocket Essentials of Paediatrics

inhaled foreign bodies in children are organic, most commonly peanuts, and are not radio-opaque.

Anaphylaxis

Anaphylaxis can present with severe upper airways oedema leading to obstruction. Wheezing and collapse with hypotension may also occur. Severe cases may require intubation. Adrenaline (epinephrine), given either intramuscularly or intravenously, may be life-saving (see also Appendix I, p. 286). Steroids may be required for the wheeze but anti-histamines really only offer symptomatic relief for itching. Recent studies in young children have shown that milk and egg are the commonest causes, as opposed to nuts in older children and adults. Following an episode of anaphylaxis, thought should be given to allergy tests to help delineate the cause. Adrenaline (epinephrine) pens are also dispensed in increasing quantities for use in the community. Although seemingly a sensible precaution, they require thorough training, with a care plan in place for use in the school or nursery, and evidence suggests that they are rarely used.

CHRONIC UPPER AIRWAYS OBSTRUCTION

Congenital stridor is seen in infants, and is most commonly due to **laryngomalacia.** The cartilaginous parts of the larynx and trachea are less firm than usual, and partly obstruct the airway on inspiration. If severe it may cause failure to thrive due to feeding difficulties, and is often worse with viral URTIs.

Rarer causes include vascular rings compressing the trachea from outside, mediastinal masses such as neuroblastoma (see Chapter 7, p. 74) and intrinsic airway conditions such as haemangiomas and webs. Babies with anything other than very mild stridor should have a plain chest X-ray and a barium swallow. A barium swallow is more effective than echocardiography in picking up vascular rings. Moderate to severe stridor requires direct laryngoscopy to look for intrinsic lesions such as airway haemangiomas. The prognosis for laryngomalacia is excellent, with the noisy breathing diminishing with age as the cartilage strengthens.

Snoring and obstructive sleep apnoea

Snoring is relatively common in children, and is usually benign. Snoring is characteristically episodic, and associated with upper respiratory tract infection, rhinitis or nasal obstruction. The commonest cause of chronic snoring is adenotonsillar hypertrophy. Snoring that is persistent and loud may be indicative of airway obstruction, which, in turn, may predispose to obstructive sleep apnoea (OSA).

OSA is relatively uncommon in children (incidence 0.8–2.0%). The commonest cause is marked adenotonsillar hypertrophy, typically presenting between 3 and 6 years of age. Congenital disorders that narrow the airway, such as achondroplasia, and disorders with reduced muscle tone, such as Down syndrome, predispose to OSA. In older children, morbid obesity is the commonest cause.

OSA may produce a range of symptoms. In the younger child, failure to thrive and behavioural problems may result. In severe cases, particularly in association with obesity, pulmonary hypertension and cor pulmonale may result from chronic hypoxia.

In addition to snoring, parents may report gasping, or pauses in breathing during sleep. Behavioural problems such as headaches, ADHD and enuresis are more common in children with OSA. Day-time sleepiness is less common than in adults.

Clinical signs may include visible tonsillar enlargement, glue ear (secondary to adenoidal hypertrophy), nasal obstruction with mouth breathing, and nasal speech and obesity.

Any child with chronic snoring should be evaluated with overnight pulse oximetry. Recurrent desaturations below 92% are suggestive of OSA. In the first instance, adenotonsillectomy is recommended. If symptoms of OSA persist, a formal sleep study in a specialist centre is usually recommended to confirm the diagnosis. Overnight continuous positive airway pressure (CPAP) may be appropriate for refractory cases.

CHRONIC COUGH

Chronic cough is defined as being present for more than 3 weeks. It has many causes. It may be associated with infection or inflammation, or it may be habitual, in which case the cough has a characteristic 'honking' or 'brassy' quality.

The assessment should inquire about the nature of the cough, any sputum production, and any associated symptoms or relevant past medical history. A paroxysmal cough suggests pertussis; night-time, or exercise-induced cough might suggest asthma; sputum production and fever suggest bronchiectasis or tuberculosis. Relationship to posture or feeds may occur with gastro-oesophageal reflux. A history of choking may indicate an inhaled foreign body. Immune deficiency or cystic fibrosis will usually cause failure to thrive. Tracheo-oesophageal fistula (see Chapter 17, p. 259), is associated with a characteristic 'TOF cough'.

Pertussis

Pertussis, or whooping cough, is caused by *Bordatella pertussis*. It invades the pulmonary ciliary epithelium causing bronchial congestion and inflammation, with peribronchial lymphoid hyperplasia (catarrhal stage 1–2 weeks). Wide-spread epithelial necrosis then ensues, with the characteristic coughing bouts (paroxysmal stage 2–4 weeks), and predisposes to atelectasis and bronchopneumonia. Paroxysms of coughing with a terminal 'whoop' are characteristic (as in Case 10.2). Children are unable to catch their breath and may become cyanosed. Apnoea occurs in young infants. Vomiting is common. Pneumonia accounts for 80–90% of deaths from pertussis. Seizures (3%) and encephalopathy (1%) may occur. The convalescent phase lasts from 1–2 weeks to many months. Use of antibiotics in the catarrhal stage may shorten the illness but, if started in the convalescent stage, has no effect

Case 10.2 A boy with coughing paroxysms

John, aged 5 months, was taken to his GP with a 2-week history of persistent coughing bouts. The bouts were associated with him going blue, and sometimes with vomiting. He was feeding poorly. His older sister also had a severe cough, which had been present for several weeks. Of note, John had not received pertussis immunization owing to parental concerns about vaccine safety. Whilst in the consultation, John had a coughing paroxysm with a classical whoop. He was referred to hospital for assessment where, after obtaining a pernasal swab, he was treated with clarithromycin. A blood count showed a marked lymphocytosis.

Pocket Essentials of Paediatrics

on the duration of illness, although infectivity to others is alleviated. In adults and older children, who are the usual sources of infection, the cough is a dry, repetitive, 'staccato' cough.

Large-scale outbreaks of whooping cough in Britain and the USA in 2011-12, to levels not seen for over 50 years, have led to concerns that the current whooping cough immunization schedule (see Chapter 1, p. 3) does not provide long-lasting immunity. The introduction of a further booster immunization for secondary school children and pregnant women is under consideration. Booster immunizations for healthcare workers have now been recommended.

THE WHEEZY CHILD

Wheezing is an extremely common symptom, occurring in about half of all children at some time in childhood. Many of these children have isolated episodes of wheezing in association with viral infections. Twenty to thirty per cent of children have either persistent or recurrent wheezing and only half of these turn out to have true 'asthma'. Attempts to delineate diagnostic groups more clearly are hampered by the lack of a truly robust definition of asthma in childhood. There is a group of children who wheeze only with viruses and who respond to bronchodilators, but lack interval symptoms and fail to respond to inhaled steroids. Definitions of asthma relying purely on bronchial hyper-reactivity will include those children with viral wheezing and overestimate asthma prevalence. Questionnaire studies of asthma prevalence are hampered by the same difficulties.

In practice this means that any child with acute wheezing can be treated in a similar fashion, but chronic management will depend more on the likely cause of the wheezing.

Acute wheezing

Bronchodilators through a large volume spacer have largely replaced nebulized treatment as the preferred option for initial treatment of acute wheezing in childhood. Careful assessment is needed and measures including oxygen and systemic steroids are needed in moderate to severe wheezing. See Figures I.14 and I.15 in Appendix I for full assessment and management.

> #### Case 10.3 A baby with acute respiratory distress
>
> Marcus was born at 30 weeks' gestation and needed ventilation for 3 days with respiratory distress syndrome. He was discharged at 6 weeks of age, 2 weeks before term. He was admitted at 8 p.m. one cold November evening aged 10 weeks. He had been chesty and snuffly for 48 hours with increasing cough and breathlessness. His feeding was disrupted. On examination he was breathing rapidly at 60 breaths per minute. He had severe recession. Auscultation revealed scattered fine crackles and some expiratory wheeze. He needed 40% inhaled oxygen to maintain oxygen saturation above 92%.

Bronchiolitis

Bronchiolitis is a term used to describe an acute respiratory infection, in children under 1 year, where wheezing may be present (as in Case 10.3). The cardinal signs are crepitations and expiratory wheeze with recession and, if severe, cyanosis. The baby initially has snuffles, which progress to a characteristic dry, hacking cough. RSV is the commonest cause of bronchiolitis, but is not a prerequisite for diagnosis. Treatment is supportive therapy with oxygen, nasogastric feeding and occasionally CPAP or even ventilation in those most severely affected (1–2%). Bronchodilators may help those with prominent wheeze, but controlled trials have failed to show clinical benefit of these or other treatments such as steroids, antibiotics, adrenaline (epinephrine) or specific antiviral treatment. Prophylactic treatment with the monoclonal antibody palivizumab is advocated for some high-risk infants, particularly those on home oxygen, to prevent life-threatening bronchiolitis.

In some parts of the world, the term bronchiolitis is used to describe any wheezy young child, which makes interpretation of the literature difficult. However, 50% of infants with bronchiolitis wheeze with subsequent viruses, as in the *episodic wheezing* group below. A proportion of these have atopy and would develop asthma anyway, so diagnostic categories are further blurred!

Persistent wheezing

Symptoms of chronic wheezing follow two common patterns, but with some crossover: episodic wheeze and chronic wheeze.

Episodic wheeze

Some children wheeze only with intercurrent infections with normal exercise and sleep symptoms in between times. This pattern tends to settle as the child gets bigger and is associated with small airways disease, whatever the cause. Low birth weight, prematurity, parental smoking and viruses such as RSV are common antecedents. They respond variably to bronchodilators. Steroids have not been shown to help children with mild to moderate viral wheezing. They should be used in severe wheezing as it is almost impossible to distinguish from acute asthma, but there is no evidence of benefit from prophylactic inhaled steroids in this group. Ongoing studies are examining the role of montelukast in this group. Management should focus on the acute episodes with bronchodilators early in the course of any infections and management plans, including the use of short-course oral steroids, but only for the more severely affected.

Chronic wheeze

This is classical asthma with frequent, often daily, symptoms, affecting sleep and exercise (as in Case 10.4). Background atopy is common. Management

---

> #### Case 10.4 A girl with chronic wheeze
>
> Helen was referred to hospital outpatients because of a long history of wheezing. Her mother said she had tended to be wheezy from about 6 months of age. She was admitted with an acute bout of wheeze following an upper respiratory infection at 18 months and spent 48 hours in hospital. For the last year she had had persistent wheeze. Three or four times a week she woke coughing and wheezing in the early hours. She was always worse after colds and got wheezy when she was very active at preschool. Her mother had had eczema as a child and her 9-year-old brother wheezed with URTIs. The family had a cat. Helen seemed worse when she visited her grandmother who had a parrot.

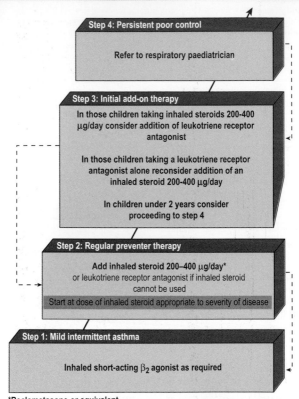

Step 4: Persistent poor control

Refer to respiratory paediatrician

Step 3: Initial add-on therapy

In those children taking inhaled steroids 200–400 µg/day consider addition of leukotriene receptor antagonist

In those children taking a leukotriene receptor antagonist alone reconsider addition of an inhaled steroid 200–400 µg/day

In children under 2 years consider proceeding to step 4

Step 2: Regular preventer therapy

Add inhaled steroid 200–400 µg/day* or leukotriene receptor antagonist if inhaled steroid cannot be used

Start at dose of inhaled steroid appropriate to severity of disease

Step 1: Mild intermittent asthma

Inhaled short-acting β_2 agonist as required

*Beclometasone or equivalent
Higher nominal doses may be required if drug delivery is difficult

Figure 10.2 Summary of stepwise management in children aged less than 5 years. (Reproduced from British Guideline for the Management of Asthma.)

is as outlined in current British guidelines for asthma management, with inhaled steroids being the mainstay. If there is doubt over a diagnosis of asthma, particularly in children too young to provide peak flows, a trial of inhaled steroids is a sensible way forward. Review the situation after 6 to 8 weeks – do not continue inhaled steroids if they are not helping.

See Figures 10.2 and 10.3 for a summary of stepwise management in children.

LOWER RESPIRATORY TRACT INFECTIONS

The hallmarks of lower respiratory tract infection (LRTI) are fever, breathlessness and cough. Acute LRTIs in childhood are mostly caused by viruses. Pneumonia tends to be a term used loosely when consolidation is present on a chest X-ray. Even in children with clear-cut consolidation present, a

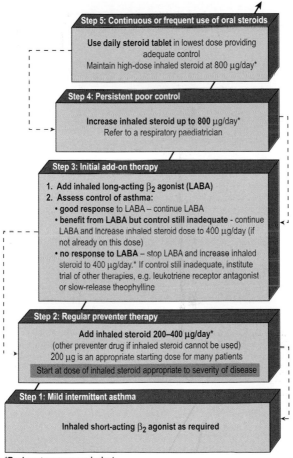

Figure 10.3 Summary of stepwise management in children aged 5–12 years. (Reproduced from British Guideline on the Management of Asthma.)

virus is still a common cause. However, as bacterial LRTI may have severe consequences, and it is difficult clinically and radiologically to tell the difference, antibiotics are routinely used for any LRTI.

LRTI in childhood tends to present in two ways. '*Atypical pneumonia*' has been a term used for a pattern of symptoms with fever, cough and variable with fever, cough and variable breathlessness, with or without evidence of airways obstruction in the form of recession. Crackles are audible but not usually bronchial breathing. The X-ray looks patchy, with reticular/nodular shadowing. Viruses are a common cause but bacterial LRTI with

> ### Case 10.5 A girl with pneumonia
>
> Savannah was a 7-year-old girl – usually very healthy – who
> presented with a 3-day history of upper respiratory tract signs. Six
> hours before admission she had suddenly become much worse.
> Her fever increased and she had a rigor. She was briefly delirious.
> On examination she looked unwell with a tachycardia (130 beats
> per minute) and rapid shallow respirations. Peripheral capillary
> return was 4 seconds. Initially there were no clues as to the
> aetiology of her deterioration but careful examination showed nasal
> flaring and an inverted respiratory cycle with a slight scoliosis to
> the right. A chest X-ray showed right upper lobe pneumonia.

mycoplasma or pneumococcus may present this way. In primary care,
amoxicillin is usually the recommended first-line antibiotic. In secondary
care, if the child is unwell, treatment to cover mycoplasma is appropriate;
azithromycin or clarithromycin are commonly used. This presentation is
more common than classical lobar pneumonia, so the term 'atypical' tends
to be avoided now.

Classical lobar pneumonia is due to extensive alveolar consolidation, and
airways obstruction is not seen. The child presents unwell with a fever and
there may be no symptoms to point to the respiratory tract (as in Case 10.5).

A chest X-ray should always be included in a septic screen of a child with
no clue as to the aetiology of the infection. Pleuritic chest pain is common,
and respiratory distress with nasal flaring, and sometimes cyanosis, is a late
symptom. The classical signs of a dull percussion note, reduced air entry,
bronchial breathing and crackles may be heard, especially if it is lower lobe
in origin. In upper-lobe pneumonias, in particular, no signs may be found
and diagnosis is based on the radiology. If the child is toxic with a high fever,
or has a pleural effusion, admission for intravenous therapy is needed. In the
UK, benzylpenicillin is the first-line treatment, but in some parts of the world
pneumococcal resistance is a problem and other agents are required.

Most children respond to treatment in 24–48 hours and can be allowed
home on oral antibiotics. Beware of children whose fever does not settle
in 48 hours, particularly if they have a pleural effusion. Empyema is still
a relatively common complication. Controversy exists as to the best management, with some advocating early surgical intervention and others the
insertion of a fine chest drain and the use of urokinase. Either way, the
long-term outlook is usually good.

UNCOMMON SERIOUS INFECTIONS

Tuberculosis

Tuberculosis (TB) has become more prevalent in the UK recently. Some of
the rise is associated with HIV infection and some with immigration from
high-risk countries. The primary infection causes relatively few symptoms,
although a primary complex (peripheral lung lesion with hilar lymphadenopathy) may be visible on chest X-ray. Reactivation causes chronic
cough with weight loss and general malaise. Diagnosis is by a combination of radiological findings, culture of sputum, or gastric washings, blood
tests (e.g. the T-spot test, which measures the gamma-interferon response

to TB), and skin testing using the Mantoux test. Local advice is needed regarding best drug combinations as multi drug-resistant TB is unfortunately becoming more common. Three or four drugs are usually used.

HIV infection

HIV infection is usually acquired perinatally in childhood. It should be seen less often following the introduction of universal HIV screening in pregnancy in the UK. It may remain asymptomatic for many years in childhood, but if untreated it may present in the first few months with severe respiratory disease. The protozoan *Pneumocystis carinii* is the commonest cause of severe pneumonia. High-dose intravenous co-trimoxazole is the treatment of choice, but mortality remains high. Avoidance of breast-feeding, delivery by caesarean section and prophylactic zidovudine have been shown to reduce perinatal acquisition of HIV dramatically. In those infected in childhood, combination anti-retroviral therapy has improved prognosis (see Chapter 16, p. 242).

CHILDREN WITH SPECIAL NEEDS

Special-needs children are very prone to LRTI. There is a combination of factors, including poor clearance of secretions, poor gag reflex, choking, gastro-oesophageal reflux and poor respiratory reserve due to scoliosis. Quality of life may be improved by consideration of these factors. Broad-spectrum antibiotic cover using co-amoxiclav, for example, is often used. Senior help is always required when considering the appropriate treatment of severe LRTI in children with limited life expectancy.

CYSTIC FIBROSIS

Cystic fibrosis (CF) is the commonest genetic condition seen in Caucasian populations. It is inherited in an autosomal recessive fashion with the CF mutation present on the long arm of chromosome 7. Over a thousand mutations are known, with AF508 being the commonest, accounting for 80% of mutations in the UK. Affected individuals may have compound heterozygosity for two different mutations. The cellular transport mechanism that is affected is primarily a chloride channel – cystic fibrosis transmembrane regulator (CFTR). CFTR maintains an ionic gradient over the surface of the cells lining the epithelium, which keeps the cell surface moist. When CFTR malfunctions, respiratory and other epithelial surfaces dry out, resulting in tenacious, viscid secretions (see Box 10.1).

Box 10.1 Clinical presentations of cystic fibrosis

- Meconium ileus
- Failure to thrive (due to pancreatic insufficiency)
- Loose smelly stools (due to pancreatic insufficiency)
- Chesty cough (sticky secretions in the respiratory tree)
- Family history
- Screening
- Late presentation (may be recognized only in adult life; finger clubbing is an important sign)

Newborn screening for CF was introduced across the UK from 2007 but should be remembered as a possibility in children born before that date. Neonatal screening is based on newborn blood spots, which are screened first for raised immunoreactive trypsin (high concentrations of trypsin develop in obstructed pancreatic ducts, leading to pancreatic inflammation, and elevation of serum trypsin; the elevation persists for several weeks after birth), and then specific common genetic mutations. Screening is not 100% effective though, and one should remain aware of the possible clinical presentations.

Respiratory management

- Twice daily chest physiotherapy to help clear secretions
- Prophylactic antibiotics such as flucloxacillin, against *Staphylococcus aureus*
- Abolition of symptomatic cough wherever possible
- Monitoring of oxygen saturation
- Microbiological surveillance using cough swabs
- Radiological follow-up
- Lung function when old enough.

Respiratory deterioration is strongly linked with growth of *Pseudomonas aeruginosa*, and stringent efforts are made, using oral, intravenous and nebulized antibiotics, to prevent chronic infection.

Nutritional management

Maintaining adequate nutrition and growth is the key principle of management. Pancreatic enzymes before meals are given to the vast majority of patients who have pancreatic insufficiency (>85%). High-fat, high-calorie diets are the preferred option, to maintain nutrition and dietary supplements, and enteral feeding via gastrostomy is used if growth is failing. Fat-soluble vitamin replacement is also necessary. Complications should be treated vigorously (see Box 10.2). CF-related diabetes (CFRD) develops in a significant proportion of adolescents with CF. Annual screening with a glucose tolerance test is recomended from age 12 years, as patients are often asymptomatic. Untreated CFRD is associated with poorer lung

---

Box 10.2 Long-term complications of cystic fibrosis

- Sinusitis/nasal polyps (90% – especially when older)
- Abdominal pain – common
- Residual malabsorption
- Gastro-oesophageal reflux
- Distal intestinal obstruction syndrome
- Fibrosing colonopathy
- Liver disease (40% fatty liver, 5% cirrhosis)
- Diabetes mellitus (15% of 18–21 year-olds, 50% of 30 year-olds)
- Hypertrophic pulmonary osteoarthropathy
- Male infertility (nearly 100%)
- Psychosocial morbidity (100%)

function, more frequent chest infections and impaired nutritional status. Treatment is with insulin via multiple daily injections or an insulin pump.

Prognosis

Modern treatment of CF has been highly effective in improving life expectancy; nevertheless, mean survival is only 35 years. Consideration may be given towards a heart–lung transplant but this is now rarely needed in childhood.

Further reading

NICE Clinical Guideline 117, March 2011.

Homeostasis and the kidney 11

(Nandu Thalange, Lisa Jackson)

CHAPTER CONTENTS

INTRODUCTION

The body maintains stability of its many functions by means of a complex network of control systems. Such controls are present in every system controlling, e.g. heart rate, respiration and body temperature. This chapter is concerned with the systems that regulate aspects of the body's metabolic and biochemical functioning where failure of regulation causes disease in childhood.

THE KIDNEY AND URINARY TRACT

The kidney is central to water, electrolyte, acid–base and calcium homeostasis, as well as having a crucial role in regulation of blood pressure, and via the action of erythropoietin, manufacture of red blood cells. Kidney function depends on an unimpeded blood supply, functioning renal parenchyma, and an unobstructed outflow of urine. Any of these may be affected by congenital malformation or inherited disease, inflammation or infection.

History

Urinary frequency, dysuria and wetting are probably the commonest urinary symptoms. Children usually acquire daytime continence between 18 months and 3 years of age and night-time continence a year or so later.

By the age of 5 years, 95% of children are dry by day and 85% of children are dry by night.

Small volumes of dark urine suggest glomerulonephritis or dehydration. Large volumes of dilute urine suggest diabetes or excessive drinking. Red urine suggests blood, but certain colourings – particularly beetroot – can be deceptive. If there is frank haematuria ask whether it is present throughout the stream or just at the end. Terminal haematuria suggests a penile cause – a meatal ulcer or urethral trauma. Children may present with oedema when puffiness of the eyes and face is the presenting feature.

Examination

Most common renal problems produce few examination findings. Check the blood pressure and look for peripheral oedema. Interpretation of blood pressure values is aided by reference to published normal ranges for blood pressure. It is important to measure blood pressure, usually in the right arm, after a period of quiet rest, with the correct size cuff, and ideally to take repeated measures, as children are prone to 'white-coat' hypertension.

Palpate the kidneys and feel for tenderness in the loins. Inspect the back looking for a naevus that could overlie a spinal cord anomaly. Check the lower-limb reflexes. The external genitalia should be examined, but tact is needed and you may decide the examination should be deferred unless the history specifically suggests a genital problem. The examination is not complete without testing the urine with a multiple reagent stick (see Table 11.1).

Investigations

Urine microscopy and culture

Isolation of a pure growth of an organism together with elevated leucocytes from a properly collected urine sample is essential for the diagnosis of urinary tract infection (UTI). Urine collection bags are unreliable and should not be used. A 'clean catch' urine sample, after cleaning of the perineum, is preferred. A catheter specimen should only be taken if antibiotics are to be commenced because of the risk of introducing infection. A suprapubic aspirate is rarely required, and should be performed under ultrasound guidance – a catheter specimen is preferable in the urgent situation. Failure to collect a urine sample will make it impossible to diagnose UTI and may commit the child to unnecessary and invasive investigations.

Urine microscopy is also useful in the confirmation of haematuria, and to look for the presence of granular casts, seen in glomerulonephritis.

Imaging the urinary tract

Ultrasound is the key first-line investigation in any disorder of the renal tract. It will demonstrate renal size, anatomical abnormalities, including scarring, reflux and hydronephrosis, and renal masses. Serial ultrasound measurements may be used to monitor renal growth and appearances of hydronephrosis.

A DMSA (dimercaptosuccinic acid) renogram is a static radionucleotide scan. It is the gold standard for detecting renal scars and enables comparison of renal function on the two sides.

Table 11.1 Significance of urine dipstick test results

Test	Significance
pH	Normal urine pH ranges from 5 to 7. Inappropriately alkaline urine is found in some infections, and in renal tubular acidosis
Protein	Proteinuria is seen in a range of renal diseases, and is the hallmark of nephrotic syndrome. The presence of proteinuria may be indicated by very frothy urine
Blood	See Box 11.1 for causes of haematuria
Nitrites and leucocytes	Nitrites are products of bacterial decomposition of urea and suggest urinary tract infection. Their presence may be suggested by the smell of ammonia. The findings of leucocytes in urine also suggests infection or inflammation
Glucose and ketones	Glycosuria indicates blood glucose levels above the renal threshold for glucose reabsorption. The presence of glycosuria and ketonuria together strongly suggests type 1 diabetes
Bilirubin and urobilinogen	Urobilinogen is responsible for the normal yellow colour of urine, but if detectable on a reagent strip implies enhanced red cell destruction, as in haemolytic anaemia, or impaired clearance in bile, most commonly due to hepatitis. The finding of bilirubin in urine suggests hepatocellular dysfunction or obstructive jaundice. Urobilinogen may be absent from urine in obstructive jaundice, although the urine is dark due to the presence of conjugated bilirubin

A MAG3 scan is a dynamic renogram – the isotope can be seen to move through the kidney to the bladder and through voiding. It will distinguish urinary stasis and obstruction and also give information on reflux. This investigation requires control of voiding and thus is unsuitable in children who are not toilet-trained.

A micturating cystogram (MCUG) involves catheterization and radiographs as the child voids urine. It may be indicated after UTI in infancy to detect urethral valves in boys, and reflux in infants of either sex.

GENITOURINARY DEFECTS

Undescended testes

About 4% of newborn boys have an undescended testis (cryptorchidism). It is more common in premature infants. In the majority, the testes descend spontaneously by 3 months of age. By 6 months, there is little likelihood of the cryptorchid testis descending spontaneously, and orchidopexy is required to fix the testis in the scrotum. Laparoscopy may be necessary to locate abdominal testes, but in some cases the testis is simply absent as the result of intra-abdominal torsion or agenesis. If the testis cannot be located, renal ultrasound should be performed as there may be associated renal agenesis.

If both testes are undescended, intersex needs to be considered (see Chapter 12, p. 151).

There is an increased risk of malignancy in undescended testes, which persists even after orchidopexy.

Hypospadias

In hypospadias, the urethral meatus opens onto the ventral shaft of the penis or scrotum, or exceptionally, the perineum. In 60% the meatus is distal (glandular or coronal hypospadias) and in 15% proximal (perineoscrotal or perineal hypospadias), with the remainder affecting the penile shaft (subcoronal or mid-penile hypospadias). Hypospadias affects the urinary stream and may be associated with bowing of the erect penis, 'chordee', which will affect sexual function in later life. Proximal hypospadias may be associated with urinary tract abnormalities, and a micturating cystogram should be performed. Hypospadias with an undescended testis may be seen in intersex states (see Chapter 12, p. 151) and genetic sex determination should be performed. Surgical correction in infancy is straightforward. The parents should be advised not to have their son circumcised as the foreskin may be used as part of the surgical repair.

Inguinal hernia and hydrocele

Inguinal hernias and hydroceles arise from a patent processus vaginalis. The processus vaginalis is a pouch of peritoneum which accompanies the testis into the scrotum, and thereafter involutes. Before birth, peritoneal fluid enters the scrotum, resulting in a hydrocele. The great majority of hydroceles resolve spontaneously by 6 months but if the processus remains patent, surgery will be necessary. Inguinal hernias and hydroceles are especially common in premature infants. Presentation of hernias is usually with a variable groin swelling, particularly seen on crying or coughing, but complications include incarceration, strangulation and bowel infarction. Treatment is surgical.

Congenital anomalies of the urinary tract

> ### Case 11.1 A baby with a congenital anomaly
>
> Routine antenatal ultrasound scanning at 20 weeks' gestation had shown bilateral renal pelvic dilatation in an apparently normal male infant. The dilatation persisted on a repeat scan at 32 weeks' gestation. After birth, he was nursed with his nappy unfastened so that the urinary stream could be seen. His urinary stream was poor. He underwent ultrasound and MCUG to exclude obstruction of the urinary tract and was found to have severe bilateral hydronephrosis secondary to posterior urethral valves. He was catheterized to decompress the urinary tract and subsequently underwent surgery.

Congenital anomalies of the urinary tract may affect the kidney, urinary collecting system, bladder or urine outflow tract (as in Case 11.1).

Renal agenesis or dysplasia affecting both kidneys may produce ante-natal oligohydramnios with lethal pulmonary hypoplasia (Potter's syndrome) as fetal urine is essential for lung development. Unilateral agenesis or dysplasia may be associated with other congenital abnormalities such as contralateral vesico-ureteric reflux. The remaining kidney undergoes compensatory hypertrophy in post-natal life.

Abnormalities of the ureter include obstruction at the level of the renal pelvis (pelvi-ureteric junction obstruction) or bladder, normally due to a ureterocele – a cystic dilatation of the terminal ureter with a pinhole ureteral orifice. These result in proximal dilatation and predispose to infection and renal injury. Treatment is surgical. Occasionally, the ureter may be partially or completely duplicated. Typically, the ureter draining the upper pole inserts ectopically and is commonly obstructed, whereas the lower pole ureter inserts non-obliquely into the bladder, predisposing to reflux. In girls, an ectopic ureter commonly empties into the vagina leading to constant dribbling incontinence. In boys, the insertion is commonly into the prostatic utricle, seminal vesicle or vas deferens and thus leads to obstruction (see Figure 11.1).

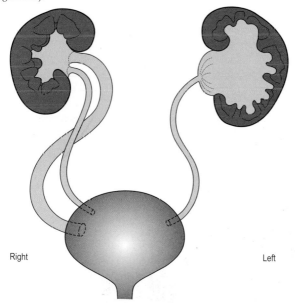

Right

Left

Figure 11.1 Left pelvi-ureteric junction obstruction with resultant dilatation of the renal pelvis (hydronephrosis). The right kidney is duplex, with two pelvicalyceal systems, in this case, each supplied by its own ureter. The lower moiety of duplex systems is commonly affected by vesico-ureteric reflux (70%) due to its more lateral and less oblique course. The upper pole ureter is more susceptible to obstruction from a ureterocoele (ballooning of the distal ureter as it enters the bladder), producing vesico-ureteric junction obstruction, as in the illustration. The insertion of the upper pole ureter is usually inferior and medial to the normal position, and may be associated with dysplasia of the upper pole.

Table 11.2 Congenital anomalies of the kidney and urinary tract

	Anomaly	Clinical consequence
Kidney	Agenesis or multicystic dysplasia	Bilateral: lethal pulmonary hypoplasia (Potter's syndrome) Unilateral: associated congenital abnormalities
	Infantile polycystic kidney disease	Chronic kidney disease
	Renal ectopia and horseshoe kidney	Association with other congenital anomalies
Ureter	Pelvi-ureteric junction obstruction	Hydronephrosis
	Ureterocele	Hydronephrosis and hydro-ureter
	Ectopic ureter	Hydronephrosis or dribbling incontinence
	Vesico-ureteric reflux	Risk of infection, renal scarring
	Duplex ureter	Often associated with a combination of reflux and obstruction
Bladder	Bladder or cloacal exstrophy	Major reconstructive surgery required Incontinence, chronic kidney disease
	Neuropathic bladder	Incontinence, chronic kidney disease insufficiency
Urethra	Posterior urethral valves (boys)	Chronic kidney disease, vesico-ureteric reflux

The most important congenital bladder abnormality is neuropathic bladder, in which the nerve supply to the bladder is defective, as occurs with spina bifida or spinal dysraphism. The bladder outlet fails to relax fully, leading to hydronephrosis and renal injury. Management is usually with intermittent self-catheterization.

Obstruction to the urethra occurs with posterior urethral valves in boys, in which the prostatic urethra is obstructed by abnormal tissue leaflets which impede renal flow, producing a variable degree of obstruction. The obstruction commonly results in renal injury with one-third of boys developing chronic kidney disease.

See Table 11.2 for congenital anomalies of the kidney and urinary tract.

URINARY TRACT INFECTION

The link between UTI and urinary symptoms is not always clear-cut. Even if the diagnosis seems clinically apparent (as in Case 11.2) the culture may be negative. In some cases the symptoms may be non-specific (irritability or failure-to-thrive) or severe enough, as in Case 11.3, to mimic septicaemia. Hyponatraemia due to renal salt loss may complicate urinary tract infection.

Case 11.2 A girl with urinary tract infection

Helen was a 3-year-old girl who presented with a 24-hour history of fever and vomiting. She had urinary frequency and cried on micturition. Her urine looked cloudy. She had achieved urinary continence for 2 years but had been getting spells of day- and night-time wetting for the previous 6 months. On examination she was flushed and lethargic with a high fever (39.5°C) and a tachycardia (110 beats per minutes).

Investigations showed a white blood cell count of 35 000, and a plasma sodium of 129 mmol/L. Urine showed blood, nitrites and leucocytes on dipstick testing, and organisms and white blood cells were seen on microscopy. A presumptive diagnosis of UTI was made and subsequently confirmed on urine culture.

Case 11.3 A baby with urinary tract infection

Harvey presented at the age of 9 weeks with high fever, irritability and diarrhoea. His general condition gave cause for concern so he underwent a number of investigations, including blood culture, lumbar puncture and, in view of his diarrhoea, catheterization to obtain a sterile urine sample prior to being commenced on high-dose intravenous antibiotics. Urine dipstick showed blood, leucocytes and nitrites, and Gram-negative cocci were seen on urine microscopy. Harvey remained ill with a high swinging fever and therefore had an urgent renal ultrasound. This showed the left kidney to be large and hyperechoic, suggesting pyelonephritis, associated with marked dilatation of the left renal pelvis with free reflux of urine visible on ultrasound. Harvey recovered after a 10-day course of antibiotics. A subsequent MCUG showed severe left vesico-ureteric reflux and a DMSA scan showed extensive scarring with the left kidney contributing 36% of renal function. A follow-up MAG3 scan at age 2 years showed a further decline in renal function with persistent left-sided reflux, despite apparently being free of infections, so he underwent a 'Sting' procedure in which an inert substance was injected into the ureteric orifice to abolish reflux during micturition.

UTI is very common in children, and affects 3–5% of girls and 1–2% of boys. In infancy, boys and girls are equally affected, but thereafter girls are much more commonly affected. The finding of UTI, especially in infancy, leads to a number of investigations, and it is essential to collect urine samples properly and to obtain repeat samples for confirmation prior to initiating therapy, if possible.

UTIs fall into three groups:
- Pyelonephritis
- Cystitis
- Asymptomatic bacteriuria.

The great majority of infections are due to ascending infection from faecal organisms, especially *Escherichia coli, Klebsiella* and *Proteus*. Pyelonephritis may occur secondarily to haematogenous spread, particularly in the neonatal period.

Pyelonephritis is characterized by malaise, fever, loin pain and vomiting. In infants, symptoms may be very non-specific, and a urine culture should be routinely obtained in any infant with unexplained fever. Pyelonephritis may lead to renal scarring, which, in turn, may lead to hypertension and chronic kidney disease. Scarring is most likely to accompany UTI in infancy. Infections after the age of 5 years are very unlikely to produce scarring if the kidneys were previously normal.

Cystitis is associated with bladder symptoms of urgency, frequency, dysuria, incontinence and abdominal pain, and is much more common in girls. It does not produce renal scarring. Cystitis is commonly associated with constipation.

Asymptomatic bacteriuria affects older girls and describes asymptomatic bacterial colonization of the bladder.

Investigation

The key objectives in investigating UTI are to determine the presence of congenital anomalies, scarring, or vesico-ureteric reflux. Ascending infection leading to pyelonephritis is more likely if there is vesico-ureteric reflux or anatomical abnormalities of the renal tract.

Anatomical abnormalities may predispose to pyelonephritis by producing stasis secondary to urinary obstruction, or by permitting reflux. Scarring may be visualized on ultrasound as obvious anatomical deformity or discrepancy in the size of the kidneys – normally length differs by less than 1 cm. More subtle scarring may be demonstrated by radio-isotope scanning with DMSA.

Vesico-ureteric reflux describes the backflow of urine from the bladder up the ureter due to a failure of the functional valve where the ureter penetrates the bladder wall. Reflux can be severe enough to distend the renal pelvis and produce backflow into the renal collecting ducts. It is a worrying finding in infants as it may be associated with renal scarring (see Figure 11.2).

An MCUG is used in young children to determine the presence of reflux, whereas in older children MAG3 scanning is used. MCUG is often very distressing, and should not be used after infancy, with rare exceptions. It has the advantage of demonstrating abnormalities of the bladder or ureters such as the presence of bladder diverticula, ectopic ureters and duplex systems, not readily apparent by other imaging modalities. Antibiotic cover is required following MCUG to prevent ascending infection. MAG3 scanning is useful to differentiate reflux from obstruction and to determine the anatomical site of obstruction (see Figure 11.3).

Treatment

Treatment is directed to reducing the risk of renal injury. This requires prompt recognition and treatment of UTIs, with an appropriate antibiotic. High rates of resistance to trimethoprim and amoxicillin make these

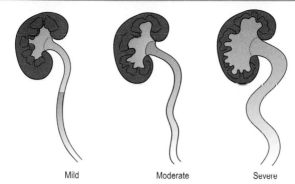

Mild   Moderate   Severe

Figure 11.2 Grades of vesico-ureteric reflux.

unsuitable choices, unless antibiotic susceptibility has been confirmed. Good first-line choices are co-amoxiclav or a cephalosporin such as cefalexin. Prophylaxis of UTI is no longer recommended. Urinary tract obstruction requires surgery. If vesico-ureteric reflux is severe, and renal function declines, then a 'Sting' procedure (as in Case 11.3) is usually performed, in which an inert substance, such as Deflux™), is injected just below the ureteral orifice. This usually alleviates reflux. If the Sting procedure fails, ureteric reimplantation may be effective. New scarring after the age of 2 years is uncommon and extremely rare after the age of 5 years.

Older girls with recurrent cystitis and/or bladder instability – *voiding dysfunction* – in which there may be dysuria, frequency, urgency and urge incontinence, are treated with antibiotics if appropriate. A regime of regular voiding, adequate fluid intake, good perineal hygiene and, if necessary, use of anticholinergic drugs such as oxybutynin or tolterodine, will assist in resolving symptoms. Concurrent constipation is common and should be treated, but may be exacerbated by use of anticholinergic medication. Very frequent infections may be ameliorated by antibiotic prophylaxis.

HAEMATURIA

Often the clinical context will help in discovering the cause of haematuria. Otherwise the haematuria may be an isolated or chance finding (see Table 11.3).

Incidental haematuria

Polycystic kidney disease (PKD) has two forms – autosomal recessive or infantile, and autosomal dominant (as in Case 11.4). The infantile form may be detected by antenatal ultrasound. The kidneys are enlarged with innumerable cysts, and some degree of renal impairment is usually present at birth. Stage IV chronic kidney disease affects over 50% by the age of 10 years. Autosomal dominant PKD usually presents in adult life but presentation with frank or microscopic haematuria, UTI or hypertension may occur in affected children. Wilms' tumour may present with haematuria (as in Case 7.14, Chapter 7), usually with a palpable flank mass.

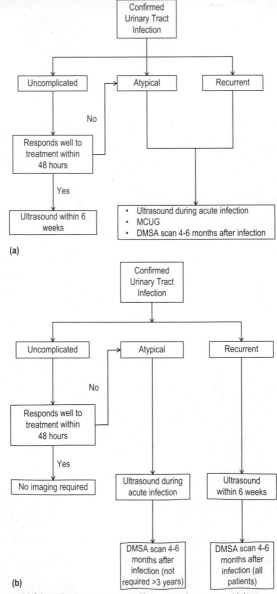

Figure 11.3 Investigations in children with confirmed urinary tract infection. (a) Infants under 6 months; (b) children over 6 months.

Definition of atypical UTI
- Seriously ill at diagnosis (includes septicaemia, elevated creatinine)
- Poor urine flow
- Abdominal or bladder mass
- Non-coliform UTI
- Failure to respond well to treatment within 48 hours

Figure 11.3, cont'd.

Table 11.3 Causes of haematuria

Diagnosis	Other clinical features
Wilms' tumour	Palpable abdominal mass
Acute glomerulonephritis	Oliguria, proteinuria, raised blood urea
Henoch–Schönlein purpura	Vasculitic non-blanching rash on legs, arthropathy, abdominal pain
Haemolytic-uraemic syndrome	Preceding gastroenteritis, haemolytic anaemia, renal failure
Pyelonephritis	Fever, rigors, back pain
Renal or ureteric calculi	Renal colic
Sickle-cell disease	Anaemia, painful crises
Subacute bacterial endocarditis	Congenital heart disease, fever, changing heart murmurs
Haemorrhagic cystitis	Heavy haematuria with dysuria
Urinary tract infection	Fever, dysuria, irritability

Case 11.4 A boy with microscopic haematuria

Darren, a 9-year-old boy of Jamaican parents, was seen in the outpatient department with a history of enuresis. A routine urine dipstick test showed 3+ blood. This persisted on follow-up urine specimens. He had no abdominal pain, examination was normal and he was normotensive. The presence of red blood cells was confirmed by urine microscopy. Urine culture was negative and renal function was normal, with normal complement levels and a negative sickle screen. Renal ultrasound showed multiple renal cysts affecting both kidneys, confirming autosomal dominant polycystic kidney disease. His father, who was markedly hypertensive, was also found to be affected.

Incidental microscopic haematuria also occurs with subclinical nephritis, Alport's syndrome, renal calculi and IgA nephropathy.

Alport's syndrome is an X-linked dominant condition causing glomerulonephritis starting in childhood, and deafness in later life.

IgA nephropathy causes brief bouts of haematuria (microscopic, or frank haematuria) usually precipitated by an upper respiratory tract infection. Some of these children will develop chronic kidney disease in adult life.

Urinary calculi are uncommon. They may complicate UTI, particularly if there is urinary stasis. The stones may remain in the kidney or enter the ureter with sometimes excruciating renal colic which radiates from loin to groin.

Management of haematuria

A clinical assessment and urinalysis will suggest the diagnosis in most cases. Haematuria should always be investigated with at least an ultrasound examination. Persistent haematuria may indicate the need for cystoscopy, particularly if symptomatic.

Children with persistent or recurrent microscopic haematuria (e.g. following Henoch–Schönlein purpura, or for suspected IgA nephropathy) require monitoring until resolution occurs, with periodic urinalysis and measurements of blood pressure and renal function.

GLOMERULAR DISORDERS

Nephrotic syndrome

> **Case 11.5** A boy with generalized oedema
>
> Michael, a 5-year-old boy, was referred to hospital with facial oedema and abdominal distension. Symptoms had been emerging for 5 days but he did not feel particularly unwell. He had obvious facial and ankle oedema with ascites and enlargement of the scrotum. A urine dipstick showed heavy proteinuria, and his serum albumin was low (18 g/dL). Twenty-four hour urine protein excretion exceeded 40 mg/m^2.

Nephrotic syndrome describes the triad of oedema, proteinuria (>40 mg/m^2/day) and hypoalbuminaemia (as in Case 11.5). Glomerular protein leak leads to loss of albumin and other plasma proteins. The low plasma oncotic pressure reduces capillary reabsorption of tissue fluid leading to oedema. Reduced plasma volume stimulates antidiuretic hormone (ADH) secretion and the renin–angiotensin system, producing sodium and water retention, compounding the pre-existing oedema.

Nephrotic syndrome is commoner in boys (male to female ratio 2:1), and about 85% of cases arise from minimal change glomerulonephritis. Most cases respond to high-dose prednisolone 60 mg/m^2/day for 4–6 weeks, followed by a reducing course of steroids over 1–2 months.

The initial steroid treatment takes about 10 days to work. This can leave a child with uncomfortable and potentially dangerous oedema whilst waiting for a response. Fluid balance should be monitored. Both circulatory collapse and overload can complicate this condition. If the oedema becomes too uncomfortable, diuretics may be used. The effect can be potentiated by the combination of intravenous replacement albumin and diuretics, although this may precipitate pulmonary oedema.

The combination of ascites with loss of circulating immunoglobulins leaves the risk of acute pneumococcal peritonitis and prophylactic penicillin should be given. Thrombotic complications are rare – but do not forget the possibility of renal vein thrombosis if haematuria or renal failure supervenes.

Whilst some children have a single episode, some move on to chronic relapsing nephrotic syndrome when other immunosuppressants such as cyclophosphamide or ciclosporin may be used. Children who are not varicella immune should be immunized when remission is achieved. If a child who is not immune is exposed to varicella, they should receive zoster immune globulin and aciclovir, to reduce the risk of disseminated chicken pox, which may be fatal.

Nephritis

> ### Case 11.6 A girl with oedema and cola-coloured urine
>
> Casey, a 7-year-old girl, presented with malaise, headaches and abdominal pain with dark urine 2 weeks after a sore throat. On examination, she was hypertensive – 150/95 mmHg, miserable, and had a gallop rhythm and basal crepitations. Her urine was cola-coloured and strongly positive for blood and protein. Urine microscopy showed granular casts. Urea and creatinine were significantly elevated (urea 17.7 mmol/L, creatinine 242 µmol/L), but with normal electrolytes. Her C3 levels were depressed. She had an elevated DNase B antigen and ASO (anti-streptolysin O) titre, indicating recent streptococcal infection, confirming the diagnosis of post-streptococcal glomerulonephritis complicated by hypertensive heart failure.

Post-streptococcal glomerulonephritis is an immune-complex-mediated glomerulonephritis, which follows cutaneous or pharyngeal streptococcal infection (as in Case 11.6). It typically affects children aged 5–12 years. It is very common worldwide, but in developed countries it is less frequent and viral aetiology is as common as streptococcal disease. The severity of renal involvement determines prognosis, with presentations ranging from asymptomatic haematuria to acute renal failure. Greater degrees of renal impairment are associated with hypertension, which, if severe, may lead to hypertensive encephalopathy and heart failure.

Treatment is directed at eradicating streptococcal carriage and treating hypertension and oedema. Over 95% of children make a full recovery, although haematuria may persist for 1–2 years. If the symptoms do not remit, and haematuria and proteinuria persist, a renal biopsy should be performed to exclude other causes of nephritis such as membranous or membranoproliferative glomerulonephritis, sometimes secondary to connective tissue diseases, notably systemic lupus erythematosus (SLE).

Henoch–Schönlein purpura (see Chapter 6, p. 55) is associated with glomerulonephritis in 50% of cases. Children with this condition should have regular urine testing, and renal function and blood pressure checks until resolution. A minority of children develop aggressive glomerulonephritis with a mixed picture of nephritis and nephrotic syndrome, and usually progress to stage IV chronic kidney disease.

See Box 11.1 for the causes of glomerulonephritis.

Box 11.1 Causes of glomerulonephritis

- Hereditary
- IgA nephropathy
- Alport syndrome
- Post-infectious
- Post-streptococcal
- Hepatitis B and C
- Infective endocarditis
- Parasite infection
- Immune-mediated
- Henoch–Schönlein nephritis
- Systemic lupus erythematosus
- Goodpasture disease
- Membranous and membranoproliferative glomerulonephritis
- Polyarteritis nodosa
- Wegener's granulomatosis

RENAL TUBULAR DISORDERS

Renal tubulo-interstitial disease may be conveniently divided into disorders of tubular function, such as renal tubular acidosis (usually inherited) or inflammatory diseases of the renal interstitium with sparing of glomeruli – interstitial nephritis. Interstitial nephritis may present acutely, with fever, urticaria and arthralgia, or with eosinophilia and renal impairment. Analgesics are an important cause. Chronic interstitial nephritis most usually occurs secondarily to chronic obstructive uropathy or vesico-ureteric reflux (see above).

The boy in Case 11.7 has generalized proximal tubular dysfunction – known as renal Fanconi syndrome. Measurement of leucocyte cystine content confirmed cystinosis as the cause. In cystinosis, cystine accumulates in lysosomes and causes progressive renal tubular dysfunction, culminating

---

Case 11.7 An infant with failure-to-thrive and glycosuria

Irfan, a 14-month-old male infant of Turkish parents, was referred with severe failure-to-thrive. His weight was far below the 0.4th centile. His length was also below the 0.4th centile and his head circumference was on the 2nd centile. His parents reported that he always seemed thirsty, but preferred water to milk. He vomited frequently. He also appeared to dislike light. A urine dipstick showed 1+ glycosuria. Preliminary investigations showed hypophosphataemia with markedly elevated alkaline phosphatase suggestive of rickets, coupled with a metabolic acidosis, but a normal anion gap (Na – [HCO_3 + Cl] < 12). His urine was inappropriately alkaline, given his underlying metabolic acidosis, indicating renal tubular acidosis. A urine amino acid profile showed generalized aminoaciduria.

Box 11.2 Disorders of renal tubular function

- Renal tubular acidosis
- X-linked hypophosphataemic rickets
- Specific amino acid transport disorders, e.g. cystinuria, Hartnup disease
- Fanconi syndrome
- Cystinosis
- Lower syndrome
- Galactosaemia
- Tyrosinosis type I
- Lead poisoning
- Mitochondrial diseases
- Nephrogenic diabetes insipidus
- Bartter's syndrome

---

in renal failure. Cystine accumulation in the cornea causes photophobia. Hypothyroidism, central nervous system (CNS) abnormalities and myopathy occur in later life.

Renal tubular dysfunction may be specific, when just one element of tubular function is impaired, or part of a generalized disorder – renal Fanconi syndrome – of which cystinosis is the commonest cause (see Box 11.2).

WATER HOMEOSTASIS

Water homeostasis is achieved using the twin controls, thirst and antidiuretic hormone (ADH, also known as vasopressin). ADH is secreted from the posterior pituitary in response to increasing plasma osmolality. It acts by increasing the permeability of the collecting ducts and allowing the urine to become more concentrated as it flows through the hyperosmolar regions of the renal medulla. ADH is regulated by plasma osmolality and plasma volume. Plasma osmolality is exquisitely regulated by hypothalamic osmoreceptors, and ADH secretion is completely inhibited at plasma osmolalities below 282 mOsmol/kg. In contrast, low-pressure baroreceptors, which detect volume depletion, in the heart, pulmonary vessels and great veins stimulate ADH secretion only when volume depletion is significant (>8–10% dehydration or volume loss, such as haemorrhage). The latter mechanism stimulates ADH secretion regardless of osmolality. Sodium balance is regulated in the renal tubules by aldosterone produced in the adrenal gland under the control of the renin–angiotensin system. The juxtaglomerular apparatus within the kidney senses sodium concentration and renal blood flow. Low sodium or impaired perfusion leads to secretion of renin, which cleaves the plasma protein angiotensinogen to angiotensin I. This is converted, in the pulmonary vasculature and elsewhere, to angiotensin II. Angiotensin II stimulates thirst, and aldosterone and ADH secretion, in addition to direct pressor effects on the vasculature. These mechanisms stimulate sodium and water retention and increase blood pressure, thus restoring water and sodium balance. Hyperkalaemia also stimulates aldosterone production directly. Drugs that act on the renin–angiotensin system, such as angiotensin-converting enzyme (ACE) inhibitors, are very useful for regulation of blood pressure and volume overload states such as cardiac failure.

This complex control system is tested by various pathologies that may overwhelm the capacity of the kidney to maintain homeostasis. Fluid-losing conditions such as gastroenteritis may result in water loss or as salt loss. A mixed picture of water and salt loss may occur.

If homeostasis is overwhelmed this may result in hypernatraemic or hyponatraemic dehydration (see Chapter 13, p. 166).

Primary failure of the control systems is less common but includes inappropriate ADH secretion, diabetes insipidus and aldosterone deficiency (see Chapter 12).

Syndrome of inappropriate ADH secretion

Inappropriate ADH secretion occurs in certain pathological states, notably the post-operative period, chest infections and CNS disorders. The hallmark is a low sodium with oliguria. Rarely, mainly in the intensive care situation, cerebral salt-wasting may occur. In this condition, sodium depletion leads to hyponatraemia, but oliguria is not usually present, unless there is coexisting volume depletion.

Treatment of the syndrome of inappropriate ADH secretion is with volume restriction and diuretics if necessary. Tolvaptan, an ADH receptor antagonist (not licensed for children), may be appropriate in the intensive care situation. Cerebral salt-wasting requires cautious sodium replacement, with close monitoring of urine output, weight and cardiovascular parameters.

Polyuria

Damage to the hypothalamus or pituitary caused by tumours, trauma or infection may prevent release of ADH, causing diabetes insipidus. This leads to the production of large volumes of dilute urine. Congenital diabetes insipidus may also occur, usually in boys due to defective V2 ADH receptors (the X-linked disorder, nephrogenic diabetes insipidus).

Diabetes insipidus must be distinguished from habitual or psychogenic polydipsia, which is much commoner. Some toddlers appreciate the comfort of having some juice to hand and may consume several litres each day. They can usually be discouraged by offering smaller volumes and increasing dilutions. Habitual drinkers will seldom drink water. If simple measures to restrict fluid intake are ineffective, habit polydipsia and diabetes insipidus may be distinguished by a water-deprivation test. This may rapidly result in severe dehydration in diabetes insipidus so must be carefully managed in hospital. Children with habit polydipsia will produce concentrated urine within a few hours. Children with ADH deficiency continue to pass large volumes of dilute urine and rapidly lose weight. The water deprivation test is onerous, and potentially hazardous, and should be carried out under the supervision of a paediatric endocrinologist.

KIDNEY FAILURE

Introduction

In renal failure of whatever cause, there is a progressive breakdown of renal homeostatic mechanisms. In acute renal failure, the progression is rapid, with the principal clinical manifestations being oliguria, hypertension and oedema. This is accompanied by elevated urea and creatinine and derangement of electrolyte, calcium and acid–base balance with resulting hyperkalaemia, hypocalcaemia and acidosis. Acute renal failure may be temporary, depending on the cause, or may progress to chronic kidney disease. In chronic kidney disease, the same derangements occur progressively as renal function declines from early chronic kidney disease to stage IV chronic kidney disease, requiring renal replacement therapy (dialysis or transplantation). Failure to eliminate toxins may result in uraemic encephalopathy, which may be compounded by hypertension, acidosis and electrolyte imbalance.

Chronic kidney disease is also associated with:

- Anaemia from chronic disease and erythropoietin deficiency
- Growth failure from several causes
- Renal bone disease from hyperparathyroidism secondary to chronic hypocalcaemia and hyperphosphataemia
- Uraemic toxins leading to impaired cellular immunity
- Bleeding and easy bruising secondary to impaired platelet function.

See Table 11.4 for the causes of acute and chronic kidney disease.

Management of renal failure

Treatment is directed at alleviating the cause, if possible, and to mitigating the consequences of loss of renal function.

In acute renal failure, it is essential to determine whether it is of renal or prerenal origin. This may be apparent from the clinical situation. Useful clues may be obtained from the composition of urine. In prerenal failure, oliguria is associated with the passage of concentrated urine (osmolality >500 mOsmol/kg) with little sodium (<20 mmol/L), whereas intrinsic renal failure is suggested by the passage of dilute urine (osmolality <350 mOsmol/kg) with high sodium concentration (>40 mmol/L). In prerenal uraemia, cautious volume loading coupled with a diuretic may prevent progression to acute tubular necrosis.

Table 11.4 Causes of acute and chronic kidney disease

	Acute	Chronic
Prerenal	Shock, e.g. haemorrhage dehydration, burns, sepsis	
Renal	Glomerulonephritis Haemolytic-uraemic syndrome Renal vein thrombosis Liver failure (hepatorenal syndrome)	Congenital cystic or dysplastic diseases, e.g. medullary cystic kidney Chronic reflux nephropa Glomerulonephritis Metabolic disease, e cystinosis
Post-renal	Acute urinary tract obstruction	Posterior urethral Bilateral pelvi-ur vesico-ureteric Renal calculi Neurogenic spina bifid

Table 11.5 Treatment of renal failure

Problem	Treatment
Hyperkalaemia	Calcium polystyrene sulphonate enemas Intravenous or inhaled salbutamol Intravenous calcium gluconate Insulin and glucose infusion Dialysis
Hypertension and/or oedema	Loop diuretics, e.g. furosemide ACE inhibitor Calcium-channel blocker Beta-blocker
Acidosis	Sodium citrate or bicarbonate
Hypocalcaemia	Phosphate binders, e.g. calcium carbonate Parenteral calcium for severe hypocalcaemia 1α vitamin D, calcium supplements
Hyponatraemia	Sodium supplements
Anaemia	Blood transfusion B_{12} and folate supplementation Erythropoietin
Growth failure/failure-to-thrive	Optimal nutrition Treatment of anaemia and acidosis Growth hormone Renal transplantation
Uraemic encephalopathy	Treatment of hypertension Correction of metabolic abnormalities Renal transplantation

Obstructive renal failure usually responds well to relief of the obstruction, e.g. catheterization in the child with a neurogenic bladder or percutaneous nephrostomy in a child with pelvi-ureteric junction obstruction.

See Table 11.5 for the treatment of renal failure.

Dialysis and transplantation

allows correction of metabolic abnormalities by allowing plasma rate with an appropriately constituted dialysate across a permembrane. This may be achieved through haemodialysis, or by tient's peritoneum as a dialysis membrane via peritoneal dialysis al dialysis takes longer, and is less efficient, so it must be y, but can be done at home, whereas haemodialysis, usually is done three times weekly.

Dialysis is necessary in acute renal failure if there is severe volume overload with hypertension refractory to diuretics, severe hyperkalaemia, acidosis or hypocalcaemia, or inexorable progression of the underlying renal failure.

In the child with stage IV chronic kidney disease, it is preferable to proceed to renal transplantation to avoid the necessity for dialysis as this gives a much better quality of life, with the least disruption to the child's life.

GASTROENTERITIS AND RENAL FAILURE

Haemolytic-uraemic syndrome

> **Case 11.8** A girl with acute renal failure
>
> Katie, a 3-year-old girl, presented with a 12-hour history of severe gastroenteritis. She was pale and febrile, with abdominal pain, severe vomiting and bloody diarrhoea. Initial investigations showed severe anaemia and thrombocytopenia with a coagulopathy and markedly elevated urea and creatinine with hyperkalaemia, confirming haemolytic-uraemic syndrome. Stool cultures subsequently grew *Escherichia coli* O157:H7. Katie quickly deteriorated and was transferred to a specialist renal unit for dialysis. She recovered after 24 days of intensive care, but unfortunately her renal failure did not improve and she remained dialysis-dependent. Katie was one of six children and four adults who were infected following ingestion of contaminated hamburgers from a local fast-food restaurant.

Haemolytic-uraemic syndrome (HUS) is the commonest cause of acute renal failure in children. Eighty per cent of cases result from infection with Shiga-toxin-producing *Escherichia coli* O157:H7 (as in Case 11.8). The infection results from contact with infected domestic animals or ingestion of under-cooked or contaminated meat. The toxin induces widespread endothelial injury with resultant haemolytic anaemia with platelet consumption and renal failure. One in ten children with HUS die, and a further 10% develop stage IV chronic kidney disease.

REGULATING CALCIUM AND BONE METABOLISM

Introduction

Ionized calcium is very tightly maintained within the normal ...
parathyroid hormone (PTH). PTH mobilizes calcium from ...
activates 1α-hydroxylase in the kidney, thus facilitating ...
of 1,25-dihydroxycholecalciferol, the active form of vitami...
D increases calcium and phosphate absorption by the s...
and the kidney. Vitamin D is essential for bone turnover a...

Hypocalcaemia

> **Case 11.9** A baby with low blood calcium
>
> A baby born at 32 weeks' gestation and small for gestational age was very irritable on the second day of life and had a brief seizure. The blood glucose was normal (4.2 mmol/L) but the serum calcium was only 1.32 mmol/L.

Acute hypocalcaemia leads to neuromuscular excitability, which may manifest with seizures (as in Case 11.9), tetany and laryngeal spasm. Chronic hypocalcaemia leads to psychomotor retardation, sometimes with raised intracranial pressure, cataracts and photophobia. Low calcium may occur due to deficiency (hypoparathyroidism) or end-organ resistance to PTH (pseudohypoparathyroidism), or due to vitamin D deficiency. Low magnesium commonly accompanies hypocalcaemia.

In the sick neonate, transient hypoparathyroidism may lead to severe hypocalcaemia, as in Case 11.9. This may also be observed in infants born to mothers with hyperparathyroidism, due to suppression of fetal PTH secretion by maternal hypercalcaemia. Hypoplasia of the parathyroid glands occurs to a variable extent in Di George syndrome (see Chapter 18, p. 272), although in most infants hypocalcaemia is transient. In pseudo-hypoparathyroidism the PTH receptor is defective. It is associated with a characteristic appearance and mental retardation in some cases. Hypoparathyroidism also occurs as an autoimmune disease, classically in association with chronic mucocutaneous candidiasis and adrenal insufficiency, and other autoimmune disorders, and is inherited in an autosomal dominant manner (polyglandular endocrinopathy).

Vitamin D deficiency sufficient to cause hypocalcaemia and rickets is rare. In the UK, it is most commonly seen in children from ethnic minorities with restricted diets. Renal tubular loss of calcium may occur in renal Fanconi syndrome (see below). Chronic renal failure leads to progressive impairment of vitamin D activation, and may lead to hypocalcaemia.

Acute treatment of hypocalcaemia for tetany or seizures is with intravenous calcium and, if appropriate, magnesium. Hypoparathyroidism is most conveniently treated with supraphysiological doses of vitamin D, adjusted according to the serum calcium.

Hypercalcaemia

nic hypercalcaemia, if severe, leads to irritability, muscular weakness, ria, constipation, polyuria and nephrocalcinosis. Hypercalcaemia 'hood results from excess parathyroid hormone (from parathy-·oma or hyperplasia) or vitamin D intoxication, and is also seen 's' syndrome (see Chapter 18, p. 278), although the cause is /ild hypercalcaemia may also occur in adrenal insufficiency ·cosis.

Endocrinology and metabolism 12

(Nandu Thalange, Richard Beach)

CHAPTER CONTENTS

INTRODUCTION

The body maintains stability of its many functions by means of a complex network of control systems. Such controls are present in every system controlling e.g. heart rate, respiration and body temperature. This chapter is concerned with the systems that regulate the body's endocrine and metabolic functions, and how they are affected by disease.

REGULATING BLOOD GLUCOSE

Glucose is a key energy-providing substrate for the body's metabolism – especially the brain. Insulin produced by the pancreatic beta cells controls the flow of glucose into cells and is produced in response to hyperglycaemia.

Hypoglycaemia results in release of glucagon, cortisol and adrenaline (epinephrine) with resultant gluconeogenesis and release of glucose from glycogen stores.

Glucose measurement is conveniently performed at the bedside on a capillary blood sample using a blood glucose meter. These meters greatly simplify assessment of children with suspected hypo- or hyperglycaemia.

HYPOGLYCAEMIA

Significant hypoglycaemia – defined as blood glucose <2.6 mmol/L (as in Case 12.1) – is rare outside the neonatal period. The symptoms of altered consciousness, pallor and sweatiness are secondary to impaired cerebral metabolism (*neuroglycopenia*) and adrenaline (epinephrine) release. After a period of fasting, blood glucose levels fall, insulin secretion is suppressed and lipolysis leads to ketone body production. Thus, ketosis during fasting is a normal physiological response. This response is exaggerated in *ketotic hypoglycaemia*, and ketones rise to toxic levels causing severe acidosis, in addition to the presence of hypoglycaemia, as in Case 12.1. Affected children may have recurrent episodes during illness or after exercise. Treatment is with additional high-energy snacks and carbohydrate-containing drinks at bedtimes and during illness.

Case 12.1 A boy with hypoglycaemia

A 4-year-old boy presented with a 12-hour history of drowsiness, vomiting and sighing respiration. He was pale, sweaty and confused but circulation was normal with no evidence of shock or dehydration. His blood glucose was 1.0 mmol/L and blood ketones (beta-hydroxybutyrate) 5.6 mmol/L (normal <1.0). After treatment with 5 mL/kg of 10% dextrose he recovered to an alert, albeit irritable, state. The vomiting and ketosis resolved over a few hours of intravenous dextrose therapy. His parents recalled repeated episodes of vomiting and lethargy in the past.

Hypoglycaemia with ketosis also occurs with hypopituitarism and primary and secondary adrenal insufficiency secondary to growth hormone and/or cortisol deficiency. Metabolic causes include glycogen storage diseases, fatty acid disorders, galactosaemia and fructose intolerance. Absence of ketones with hypoglycaemia implies the presence of insulin; this occurs with dysregulated insulin secretion as occurs in persistent hyperinsulinaemic hypoglycaemia of infancy, or insulinoma, or exogenous insulin administration as in diabetes.

DIABETES

Type 1 diabetes mellitus results from progressive immune-mediated destruction of insulin-producing pancreatic beta cells, as in Case 12.2. It is increasingly common in children (0.2% of children under 16 years), and the mean age of diagnosis is falling. Insulin deficiency results in progressive hyperglycaemia, weight loss, polydipsia and polyuria (as in Case 12.2). Rapid lipolysis results in production of acidic ketone bodies (ketosis), and ultimately diabetic ketoacidosis, if the symptoms of diabetes are not recognised. For management of diabetic ketoacidosis, see Appendix I, p. 290.

When diabetes is suspected, it is imperative to measure blood glucose. If diabetes is confirmed (random glucose >11.1 mmol/L), then prompt referral to the local diabetes team is indicated, even if the child seems well, as deterioration may be rapid.

Case 12.2 A girl with hyperglycaemia

A 7-year-old girl had been lacking in energy for a month or so and losing weight. For a week she seemed thirsty all the time and was awake at night, drinking and passing large amounts of urine. On the day of admission she had abdominal pain and had vomited once. On examination she had clearly lost some weight but there was no circulatory compromise. Her blood glucose was 19.6 mmol/L with blood ketones of 0.5 mmol/L, thus excluding diabetic ketoacidosis. Islet cell antibodies were found on investigation, confirming type 1 diabetes.

In hospital, it is now routine to assess blood ketones (beta-hydroxybutyrate) using a rapid bedside test. This is very helpful in identifying the child with ketoacidosis and gives a result within minutes. Blood ketones above 3.0 mmol/L indicate the potential for ketoacidosis, which is confirmed by blood gas testing. Particularly in the very young, symptoms of diabetes may be difficult to spot. Ketosis may induce abdominal pain and vomiting which may be mistaken for gastroenteritis, and hyperventilation secondary to metabolic acidosis ('Kussmaul respiration') may be mistaken for asthma or pneumonia.

After diagnosis, the key goals are to teach the child and parents to administer insulin and to perform blood glucose testing. Insulin administration is facilitated by modern insulin pens and, in the younger child, pens which can administer insulin in ½ unit increments. Blood glucose monitoring should be made integral to insulin therapy, and parents and children should be encouraged to adjust insulin doses from the outset. With conventional 'human' insulins, it is necessary to wait 20–30 minutes before eating, but with newer rapid-acting insulin analogues this is unnecessary. Modern intensive insulin regimes use a once-daily injection of long-acting 'basal' insulin and mealtime boluses of quick-acting insulin ('basal-bolus'). This allows flexible mealtimes and insulin dosing adjusted to carbohydrate intake, and is particularly suitable for older children and teenagers with diabetes. Insulin infusion pumps are a refinement of the basal-bolus technique, and are increasingly being used in the UK.

Diet

Dietary management of diabetes boils down to a healthy diet, with low sugar choices, comprising regular meals and appropriate snacks before exercise. Ideally, carbohydrate should contribute 45–60% of energy needs, primarily as unrefined complex carbohydrate. Fat intake should be moderated to a maximum of 35% of energy intake. Dietetic help is vital in managing the child at diagnosis.

Control

The management of diabetes requires a team approach using the skills of the paediatrician, diabetes specialist nurse, dietitian, psychologist, and of course the parents and child, to achieve the best results. The quality of diabetes control may be judged from home blood glucose measurements and measurement of glycated haemoglobin A_1 (HbA_{1C}). HbA_{1C} provides an integrated measure of glycaemic control over 2 to 3 months. Above the target of 48–58 mmol/mol (6.5–7.5%) for each 10–15 mmol/mol rise in HbA_{1C} complication risk increases by 30%. Good glycaemic control reduces the long-term risk of microvascular complications of diabetes: nephropathy, retinopathy and neuropathy, and macrovascular disease – ischaemic heart disease, strokes and peripheral vascular disease. Management is geared to attaining the lowest practicable HbA_{1C} for each individual, taking into account what is realistic and achievable for them.

Complications and co-morbidity

Hypoglycaemia is part of life for children with diabetes. Mild hypoglycaemia in which the patient feels 'low' occurs commonly in a well-controlled diabetic, but moderate and severe hypoglycaemia should be avoided if possible. Moderate hypoglycaemia induces irritability and autonomic symptoms: sweating, pallor, tachycardia. Recurrent episodes of hypoglycaemia cause loss of hypoglycaemic awareness and greatly increase the risk of severe hypoglycaemia. Severe hypoglycaemia, characterized by collapse, coma or seizures secondary to neuroglycopenia, requires third-party assistance. Treatment of mild and moderate hypoglycaemia is with glucose in the form of food, drink or dextrose tablets or oral glucose gel. Severe hypoglycaemia requires prompt administration of oral glucose gel (not in unconscious or fitting patients), intramuscular glucagon, or, if practicable, intravenous glucose.

Screening for microalbuminuria and elevated blood pressure should be undertaken at least annually from diagnosis. Microalbuminuria is an early marker of diabetic nephropathy. Screening for diabetic retinopathy should commence annually from 12 years of age, ideally with retinal photography. In adults, it is recognized that blood pressure and lipid levels also contribute to complication risk. Trials of therapy are under way to determine whether adolescents may benefit from antihypertensive and lipid-lowering therapies.

Growth may be impaired, particularly if there is marked non-compliance with therapy, and height and weight should be plotted at each visit to the clinic.

Annual thyroid function testing is recommended for all children with diabetes, due to the high incidence of autoimmune thyroid disease. Coeliac screening is recommended at diagnosis. Some centres continue to screen for coeliac disease 3-yearly, but this falls outside current NICE guidance on screening for coeliac disease. The value of lipid screening in children with type 1 diabetes is unclear. Elevated cholesterol and/or triglycerides are commonly seen with poor glycaemic control.

Diabetes in adolescence

Teenage years are challenging – especially so for the teenager with diabetes. It is essential to have a non-judgemental approach that focuses on realistic shared goals. Threats of future complications are counterproductive and should be avoided. There needs to be effective preparation for adult life, including advice on sexual health, pregnancy and contraception, driving, employment, living away from home, alcohol and drugs. Eating disorders and depression are very common in older teenagers and require specialist input.

Good hand-over arrangements to the adult diabetes service are also essential, as many young people fall by the wayside at this stage.

Type 2 diabetes and MODY

Type 2 diabetes is increasingly evident in obese adolescents, particularly those from ethnic minorities. Management is aimed at weight control through healthy eating, exercise and the use of metformin to maximum tolerated doses. Other oral hypoglycaemic agents are added as necessary. Ultimately, all individuals with type 2 diabetes will required insulin therapy (on average after about 6–7 years).

Maturity-onset diabetes of the young (MODY) is a form of non-insulin-dependent diabetes due to specific genetic defects of beta cell function, the commonest being mutations affecting hepatic nuclear factor 1α. MODY may present similarly to type 1 diabetes. It is dominantly inherited, therefore a parent is usually affected. Specific genetic tests are available. Treatment with a sulfonylurea such as glibenclamide is effective.

Secondary diabetes

Diabetes or glucose intolerance may occur secondarily to steroid excess, as in Cushing's syndrome, or from high-dose steroid therapy.

THE HYPOTHALAMUS AND PITUITARY

The hypothalamus and pituitary gland are together the principal command centre of the endocrine system. Pituitary hormones regulate metabolism (TSH), growth (growth hormone) and sexual development (follicle-stimulating hormone and luteinizing hormone – see 'Sexual development' later in the chapter), the adrenal gland (ACTH), water balance (antidiuretic hormone; see Chapter 11, p. 131) and lactation (prolactin and oxytocin). Structural lesions of the hypothalamus and pituitary include congenital malformations and tumours, e.g. craniopharyngioma (see Chapter 7, p. 74), and result in deficiency of some or all of the pituitary hormones – known as hypopituitarism.

The pituitary gland may be congenitally absent or hypoplastic. This may be associated with other midline congenital anomalies such as cleft palate. Congenital hypopituitarism of hypothalamic or pituitary origin may be associated with the development of neonatal hypoglycaemia and, less commonly, cholestatic jaundice secondary to neonatal hepatitis (see also Chapter 13, p. 175).

CUSHING'S SYNDROME

Cushing's syndrome in children is almost always iatrogenic. The principal clinical features are growth impairment, central obesity, moon face, buffalo hump, hypertension and glucose intolerance or frank diabetes. After iatrogenic steroid exposure, ACTH-secreting pituitary adenomas (Cushing's disease) are the commonest cause of Cushing's syndrome in childhood, albeit still very rare. Adrenocortical tumours may also cause Cushing's syndrome. Investigation is aimed at confirming glucocorticoid excess and determining if it is ACTH-dependent. Imaging is then used to localize the lesion, preparatory to surgery.

ADRENAL INSUFFICIENCY

The adrenal glands, named for their position at the superior pole of each kidney, comprise an inner medulla and an outer cortex. The medulla secretes the vasoactive catecholamines adrenaline (epinephrine), noradrenaline (norepinephrine) and dopamine. The adrenal cortex secretes the steroids cortisol and aldosterone and a modest quantity of androgens. Cortisol production is stimulated by the pituitary hormone, adrenocorticotrophic hormone (ACTH).

Cortisol is essential for survival and has diverse effects on metabolism, immunity and cardiovascular and renal function. These effects are most apparent as mediators of the body's response to stress, such as illness, through its ability to mobilize glucose stores, improve myocardial and skeletal muscle contractility, and to enhance the pressor action of catecholamines.

Aldosterone has a key role in maintaining electrolyte balance and blood pressure by causing sodium retention and potassium excretion by the kidney. Retention of sodium leads to elevation of blood pressure.

Adrenal insufficiency most often occurs due to congenital adrenal hyperplasia (see p. 152) or secondary to hypopituitarism (as in Case 12.3). Primary adrenal insufficiency is extremely rare. It may be congenital, but it most commonly arises from autoimmune destruction of the adrenal gland, often in association with other autoimmune diseases, notably mucocutaneous candidiasis, hypoparathyroidism, hypothyroidism and diabetes mellitus (polyglandular endocrinopathy), in which case there is often a positive family history. It manifests with insidious malaise, weakness and weight loss and orthostatic hypotension. Hyperpigmentation may occur, classically affecting the buccal mucosa, scars and skin creases.

Case 12.3 A boy with adrenal insufficiency

Freddie, aged 7 years, was admitted with gastroenteritis. He had congenital hypopituitarism requiring multiple pituitary hormone replacement therapy. His oral hydrocortisone treatment was doubled, but the following morning he was found to be hypotensive and drowsy. His blood glucose was 2.9 mmol/L, and his serum sodium was 128 mmol/L. A diagnosis of adrenal crisis was made, and he was promptly treated with parenteral glucose, intravenous hydrocortisone and 20 mL/kg of normal saline. Within a few hours, he was much better.

Physiological steroid replacement with hydrocortisone is essential. This must be doubled or trebled with intercurrent illness, and in severe illness the parenteral route must be used. Failure to give adequate steroid therapy results in adrenal crisis, as in case 12.3, when the patient presents with refractory hypotension, hypoglycaemia, hyponatraemia and variable hyperkalaemia. Prompt treatment with intravenous fluids, glucose and hydrocortisone is essential.

Adrenal crisis may also occur with surgery or intercurrent illness in patients on chronic steroid therapy, or following abrupt cessation of high-dose steroid therapy. Patients at particular risk include those with asthma on high-dose inhaled steroids, notably fluticasone preparations, or those who have recently completed high-dose steroid therapy, such as children with leukaemia or inflammatory bowel disease.

THYROID GLAND

The thyroid gland primarily secretes thyroxine (T_4) – a ubiquitous regulator of cell function. The active hormone, tri-iodothyronine (T_3),

Table 12.1 Clinical assessment of thyroid function

	Congenital hypothyroidism	Congenital hyperthyroidism
Neonatal onset	Lethargy	Goitre
	Poor feeding	Low birth weight
	Prolonged jaundice	Irritability
	Coarse features	Tachycardia
	Hoarse cry	Tachypnoea
	Umbilical hernia	Hypertension
	Mental retardation	Failure to thrive
	Juvenile hypothyroidism	**Graves' disease**
Childhood onset	Growth failure	Emotional lability
	Dry skin and hair	Insomnia
	Yellow pigmentation	Tremor
	(carotenaemia)	Voracious appetite
	Intellectual impairment	Goitre
	Goitre	Tachycardia
	Constipation	Muscle weakness
	Cold intolerance	Proptosis
	Early puberty (girls)	

is created by de-iodination of thyroxine in target tissues. Thyroxine secretion is regulated by the hypothalamus and pituitary glands through secretion of thyrotrophin-releasing hormone and consequently thyroid-stimulating hormone (TSH). TSH secretion increases thyroxine production and may produce enlargement of the thyroid gland – goitre. Excess thyroxine inhibits TSH secretion. See Table 12.1 for the clinical assessment of thyroid function.

Thyrotoxicosis

Hyperthyroidism in older children – usually girls (as in Case 12.4) – is an autoimmune condition. These children make thyroid-stimulating

Case 12.4 A girl with high metabolic rate

Anna, aged 12 years, presented with a 4-month history of weight loss despite a huge appetite. She had been more irritable of late and was not sleeping. She complained of a tremor. On examination she had warm hands and a tachycardia (100 beats per minute at rest). There was a marked tremor of her outstretched hands. She had an evident goitre with an easily heard vascular bruit.

antibodies, which mimic the action of TSH. Although Graves' disease seems obvious it may be subtle. Irritability, poor exercise tolerance and some thyroid enlargement can be normal in adolescence. The weight loss may be ascribed to anorexia!

Hyperthyroidism is treated with anti-thyroid drugs such as carbimazole or propylthiouracil in combination with symptomatic relief with beta-blockers. A proportion of patients with Graves' disease develop thyroid eye disease with exophthalmos. Such patients need joint management with an ophthalmologist. Eye protection such as patching, and use of artificial tears, is needed in the initial phase of management. The therapeutic goal is suppression of thyroxine synthesis. Two different therapeutic strategies may be employed: dose titration, in which the dose of carbimazole or propylthiouracil is adjusted to maintain thyroxine in the upper normal range, or 'block and replace' in which endogenous thyroxine synthesis is completely suppressed, and thyroxine is given to maintain the euthyroid state. If relapse occurs after cessation of maintenance therapy, then radioiodine therapy or thyroidectomy is normally undertaken. Most clinicians advise radio-iodine therapy as this avoids the risks of surgery and the cosmetic distress of a prominent neck scar. Radioiodine is safe in children and adolescents. Nevertheless, some families prefer the option of surgery.

Neonatal thyrotoxicosis affects 1–2% of infants born to mothers with a history of autoimmune hyperthyroidism due to transplacental passage of maternal thyroid-stimulating antibodies. It is important to advise girls who have had Graves' disease of the potential risk to future children, due to transplacental passage of thyroid receptor antibodies, so that the infant may be appropriately monitored.

Hypothyroidism

Congenital hypothyroidism is a relatively common disorder affecting about 1 in 3500 births. If undetected in early infancy, irreversible mental handicap results. The full syndrome, as described in Case 12.5, is rarely seen, as most developed countries have instituted screening for neonatal hypothyroidism. Occasionally, hypothyroidism detected at birth is temporary, but normally it is a life-long condition. If diagnosed promptly on screening, the progress for growth and intellectual development is good.

Hypothyroidism can also present later in childhood with growth failure, constipation, lethargy, dry skin and hair and poor school progress. *Juvenile hypothyroidism* is typically of gradual onset, and goitre is not readily evident. It is almost always an autoimmune disease and consequently more

Case 12.5 A baby with slow metabolic rate

A 3-month-old baby, a refugee from Kosovo, presented with failure-to-thrive. The facial features were rather coarse and the skin was dry. The tongue tended to protrude and there was an umbilical hernia. There was a tinge of jaundice. The baby seemed apathetic and was not smiling or interacting with the carers. Blood testing showed a low thyroxine but very high TSH levels.

common in children with diabetes and coeliac disease. Hypothyroidism also occurs more commonly in children with chromosomal abnormalities, notably Down syndrome. Hypothyroidism is treated with thyroxine replacement.

NEONATAL SCREENING

The advent of neonatal screening for congenital hypothyroidism and phenylketonuria has allowed effective treatment for affected children. Treatment at an early stage is completely effective at preventing the poor neurodevelopmental outcomes seen in the past. In the UK, hard-to-reach groups such as travelling families, or newly arrived refugees, may slip through the net, and these diagnoses must be considered. Screening for cystic fibrosis, haemoglobinopathy and medium-chain acyl-CoA dehydrogenase deficiency (MCADD) is also part of the neonatal screening test (see Chapter 17, p. 250).

Phenylketonuria

Phenylketonuria (PKU) is normally detected by the neonatal screening test, which is performed once a child is established on feeds at 5 to 9 days old. In Case 12.6, early treatment with dietary restriction of phenylalanine would have prevented its toxic effect on the brain, which is largely irreversible. PKU is caused by deficiency of phenylalanine hydroxylase, which prevents phenylalanine (an essential amino acid) being converted to tyrosine, and toxic metabolites accumulate.

> **Case 12.6** An infant with impaired metabolism
>
> A travelling family attended clinic with their only child, Davie, who was 10 months old. They described episodes of arching his back with crying, as if distressed. He was not able to sit by himself or crawl and had blonde hair and blue eyes despite his parents' dark hair. There was a musty smell to his urine and his head circumference was below the 0.4th centile. He had not been brought for his neonatal screening and was lost to follow-up. Phenylketonuria was suspected, and confirmed on plasma amino-acid analysis.

After diagnosis, dietary treatment with a very low protein diet is commenced. Small amounts of phenylalanine are required in the diet for normal growth and development, given as 'exchanges'. Vitamin and mineral supplements are given to prevent micronutrient deficiencies. Monitoring of phenylalanine levels is used to adjust the number of exchanges. Poor compliance with diet leads to poor concentration, lethargy and deteriorating school performance.

Children born to mothers with PKU are at risk of mental retardation if the diet is not very strictly observed from before conception and throughout pregnancy (see Chapter 18, p. 265).

GROWTH

Paediatrics is practised against a moving baseline. Children grow and develop through fetal life, infancy, childhood and on into adolescence when the upheavals of puberty herald sexual maturity, after which linear growth ceases. This natural progression is one of the joys and fascinations of child health. 'Has it affected growth?' is an important question for any complaint – poor growth signifying significant constitutional disease.

History

As growth continues through childhood we need information about past growth to comment on any abnormality. It also helps to compare children with their peers and with other family members. 'He is the smallest in his class' tells us something. 'He used to be average but now he's the smallest' tells us more. 'She's tiny, but her Mum is only 142 cm' is useful, but remember that her mum may have an undiagnosed cause for her short stature. Parents often keep records of children's height and weight, and any available past medical records should be reviewed. Ask about diet, especially if weight change is a concern. Make careful enquiries about any other symptoms. Perinatal events may impair long-term growth so collect information about conditions such as preterm delivery and low birth weight. Severe illnesses or impaired nutrition in early life may also impair growth.

Examination

Children's growth can be conveniently compared with population norms using a growth chart. These show the average height for age and sex – the 50th centile – and other centiles above and below. Always plot the height and weight and, in young children, the head circumference and add any available historical measurements.

It is useful to consider parents' heights; short but normal children usually have short parents. The mid-parental target height may be calculated by averaging the parents' heights and either adding 7 cm for boys, or subtracting 7 cm for girls. The resultant value ± 8.5 cm (girls) or ± 10.0 cm (boys) is the target height ± 95% confidence interval.

Children's growth potential is influenced by perinatal events and early illnesses.

Always perform a careful general examination, looking for any systemic disease that might cause growth failure.

Look at the body proportions. Are the arms and fingers unusually long or unusually short? Are there any dysmorphic features? Ask if the parents have difficulty obtaining clothes – this is a clue to unusual proportions.

Finally, remember that pituitary abnormalities might affect vision as well as growth or puberty. Test visual acuity (finger counting), pupil reactions, visual fields by confrontation, and ophthalmoscopy, looking in particular for the pale optic disc of optic atrophy. Remember that these clinical tests are rather crude. Accurate tests of visual acuity and visual field measurement should be considered.

Physical examination of progress through puberty demands careful recording of the extent of breast development, the nature and distribution of pubic hair, the volume of the testes and the development of the penis and scrotum. These examinations can be embarrassing for the adolescent and should be carried out by those competent to make a sensible assessment. Guidance on the staging of puberty is included on growth charts.

Investigations

Bone age

A radiograph of the non-dominant hand and wrist is compared with reference standards to give a bone age – the age equivalent to the degree of bone maturation.

PHASES OF GROWTH

Growth may be conveniently considered as four phases: fetal, infant, childhood and adolescent. At each stage, optimal growth requires a normal capacity to grow, an unrestricted nutrient supply, appropriate hormonal stimuli and emotional well-being. To these, may be added the absence of significant constitutional illness.

Fetal growth

The fetus depends for its nutrition on the mother via the placenta. Maternal intake may be compromised by poor diet, by hyperemesis gravidarum, and by poor maternal health. Impaired placental function, as with maternal hypertension, will progressively compromise the fetus. Nutrient supply to the fetus may be limited by competition from other siblings in multiple pregnancy. The fetus itself may have a reduced capacity to grow, due to chromosomal disorders such as Down syndrome or other genetic anomalies such as skeletal dysplasia, or from congenital infection.

In the absence of maternal or fetal compromise, birth weight is primarily a reflection of the intrauterine environment, and may not correspond to the child's growth potential after birth. The child with intrauterine growth retardation typically shows rapid 'catch-up' growth, whereas a big baby may show the reverse phenomenon – 'catch-down' growth. It is helpful to look at length and head circumference in deciding if such a growth pattern is abnormal. If development is normal, and a thorough physical examination is unrevealing, watchful waiting will normally suffice.

Intrauterine growth retardation

Poor maternal nutrition and impaired placental function exert progressive effects on the fetus as the nutrient requirement increases through pregnancy. Such infants show marked asymmetry at birth, with low birth weight but preservation of head circumference and, to a lesser extent, length – so called asymmetrical intrauterine growth restriction (IUGR). In contrast, fetal causes of growth impairment usually produce symmetrical IUGR.

Large birth weight (macrosomia)

In the mother with poorly controlled diabetes, there may be excessive nutrient supply to the fetus. Maternal hyperglycaemia results in compensatory fetal hyperinsulinism and excessive fetal growth. After birth, the fetus continues to secrete insulin to excess and is at risk of severe hypoglycaemia. More rarely, the fetus produces excessive fetal growth factors – as with Beckwith syndrome, resulting in excessive fetal growth and neonatal hypoglycaemia, associated with other congenital abnormalities.

Infant growth

After birth, growth in weight, length and head circumference is rapid. Impaired growth in infancy – failure-to-thrive, as in the fetus – may signify nutrient lack, impaired growth potential, underlying illness or emotional deprivation. Several factors may work in combination.

Faltering growth (failure-to-thrive)

> **Case 12.7** An infant who is failing to thrive
>
> Michael was born to a 17-year-old mother after a concealed pregnancy. He was born significantly growth-retarded with a birth weight of 2.2 kg. He had persistent vomiting with feeds and poor weight gain and was admitted to hospital for investigation at 4 weeks of age weighing 2.4 kg. His feeding was observed, and it was noted that his mother did not appear to interact with him or respond to his crying until prompted by the nursing staff. She handled him roughly. She admitted to very mixed feelings about having a baby, and felt she was unable to cope with the responsibility. She appeared depressed.
>
> Michael's vomiting improved with a milk thickener, and his weight gain also improved. Michael temporarily went into the care of his maternal grandparents. His mother was advised to seek treatment for her depression, and parenting classes were arranged for her. Michael later returned to his mother's care, where he continued to thrive.

Case 12.7 highlights the importance of a nurturing environment, and adequate food intake in infant growth. Hormone imbalance is very rare as a cause of faltering growth in infancy. Relevant considerations when seeing a baby with failure-to-thrive are:

- Is there an underlying pathological cause for growth failure, or is the baby constitutionally small?
- Does poor weight gain reflect poor food supply and intake or nutrient loss through vomiting?
- Could faltering growth reflect emotional neglect?

A careful history should suggest the cause of low birth weight. Physical examination and some investigations will determine if the baby is ill. An admission to observe the mother and child together, and to assess the baby's food intake, can be useful. Maternal post-natal depression is common and needs appropriate management.

See Table 12.2 for the principal causes of failure-to-thrive.

Growth in childhood

Short stature

For practical purposes in the UK, short stature is defined as height less than the 2nd centile; however, this definition includes 1 in 50 normal, healthy children. The 0.4th centile includes only 1 in 250 normal but short children, and the likelihood of an underlying pathological cause for short stature is much higher. An individual height measurement is a 'snapshot' of growth,

Table 12.2 Principal causes of failure-to-thrive

Classification	Diagnosis	Investigation
Inadequate intake	Neglect Failure of breast-feeding Cleft palate	Observation
Vomiting	Gastrooesophageal reflux Pyloric stenosis	Observation, upper gastrointestinal barium study, abdominal ultrasound
Malabsorption	Cystic fibrosis, coeliac disease Milk intolerance	Sweat test Coeliac antibodies, upper small bowel biopsy Stool sugar chromatography, urine reducing substances, trial of alternative milk
Renal	Urinary tract infection	Urine culture
Cardiac	Congenital heart disease	Echocardiogram
Respiratory	Infection	Nasopharyngeal aspirate, chest X-ray
Constitutional	Chromosomal disorders Congenital syndromes Inborn errors of metabolism Perinatal infections	As appropriate

and previous height measurements are extremely helpful. The child who has always been short is more likely to be normal, whereas the child who has shown poor growth and is crossing centiles should provoke concern, even if still within the normal range. Only a small number (<10%) of short children have an endocrine cause for short stature. See Table 12.3 for the causes of short stature.

Psychosocial growth failure

In contrast to organic causes of growth failure, the effects of emotional deprivation on growth are hard to define and to diagnose. Case 12.8 is fairly cut and dried but the diagnosis must always be considered.

In Case 12.9, the severity of the boy's short stature, his physical characteristics and the history of neonatal hypoglycaemia were strongly suggestive of growth hormone deficiency, which was confirmed by a growth hormone test. Subsequently, an MRI scan showed an empty pituitary fossa due to congenital absence of the anterior pituitary. In these cases the posterior pituitary is often abnormally placed (ectopic).

Use of growth hormone in children

Growth hormone is available for treatment of short stature due to several causes. It must be administered by a daily subcutaneous injection,

Table 12.3 Causes of short stature

	Cause	Diagnostic factors
Constitutional		Parental heights Growth follows centile line
Emotional		History of deprivation Withdrawn or disturbed behaviour
Syndromes	Turner syndrome	Girls Dysmorphic features Delayed puberty
	Achondroplasia	Abnormal body proportions Short limbs
	Russell–Silver syndrome	Low birth weight Triangular facies
Loss of growth potential	IUGR Severe early illness	Low birth weight For example, extreme prematurity or malnutrition
Chronic illness		Evidence of the illness Remember the effect of steroids
Endocrine	Growth hormone deficiency	Growth crossing centile lines Obesity Dysmorphic features

---

Case 12.8 A short and underweight boy

Michael was referred at the age of 5 years, following an adoption medical, because he was short and underweight. He had been taken into local authority care a year previously, after concerns about physical and emotional abuse. On examination, he was reserved, and did not play with the toys in the consulting room, preferring to sit under a table. On examination his height and weight were in proportion, although he was small, and no physical abnormalities were found. Routine investigations were normal. A diagnosis of probable psychosocial growth failure was made and his growth observed. After adoption, his growth progressively improved, confirming the diagnosis.

---

normally given at night. Side-effects are rare, but include headaches, arthralgia, oedema and benign intracranial hypertension.

Current indications for growth hormone treatment in the UK include:
- Growth hormone deficiency
- Turner syndrome (see Chapter 18, p. 278)
- Prepubertal children with chronic renal failure
- Short children >3 years, born small for gestational age

Kieran, aged 5 years, was noted to be extremely short at school entry. He was born by vaginal breech delivery after induction of labour at 38 weeks' gestation. His birth weight was 3.06 kg. He was admitted to special care at 6 hours of age with hypoglycaemia which resolved with nasogastric tube feeding. Thereafter, he had put on weight satisfactorily, but had always been small and his 3-year-old brother was as tall as Kieran. On examination he had a prominent forehead with delicate facial features. His hands and feet were small and he was relatively fat.

- Prader-Willi syndrome (see Chapter 18, p. 276).
- SHOX deficiency – the SHOX gene (short stature homeobox gene on X) is present on the X and Y chromosomes. Deficiency of SHOX contributes the majority of the growth failure seen in Turner's syndrome. SHOX deficiency also occurs as an isolated condition due to genetic mutations affecting SHOX.

SEXUAL DEVELOPMENT

Disorders of sexual development

The first phase of sexual development occurs in the fetus, with genetically determined male or female sexual differentiation occurring in early fetal life. Occasionally, this process is perturbed, resulting in disorders of sex development.

The birth of a child of uncertain sex is a harrowing experience for parents and presents a major diagnostic challenge. The fetus is programmed to develop as a female in the absence of masculinizing signals – testosterone and anti-müllerian hormone from the fetal testes. Accordingly, a genetically female infant will only have disorders of sexual development (DSD) following fetal androgen exposure – normally due to congenital adrenal hyperplasia (CAH).

DSD in a genetically male infant potentially has many causes, the commonest being androgen insensitivity. In 60% of males with DSD no cause is identified.

Diagnosis of the cause of DSD requires a systematic approach. Ambiguous genitalia may be associated with other congenital abnormalities, and these may point to the diagnosis. Physical examination may reveal palpable testes, indicating male DSD. An abdominal ultrasound will determine the presence or otherwise of the uterus and ovaries, and may show adrenal enlargement in CAH. Blood and urine tests for CAH should not be done before 72 hours of age as placental steroids will affect the result, making interpretation difficult or impossible.

Congenital adrenal hyperplasia

Congenital adrenal hyperplasia is the commonest cause of impaired adrenal steroid secretion in childhood. This results from inborn errors affecting steroidogenic pathways – principally 21-hydroxylase, which accounts for over 95% of CAH. The inability to synthesize cortisol leads to hypersecretion of ACTH, which in turn produces adrenal hyperplasia. As 21-hydroxylase also mediates aldosterone synthesis, severe enzyme deficiency leads to loss of aldosterone also, and results in salt-losing CAH. The block in cortisol synthesis results in cortisol precursors being converted into androgens. The diagnosis is confirmed by the finding of elevated 17-alpha-hydroxyprogesterone (as in Case 12.10).

Case 12.10 A baby of indeterminate sex

A baby born after an uneventful pregnancy was found to have ambiguous genitalia. There was a small but distinct phallus. Doctors could not determine if there was labial fusion or an underdeveloped scrotum. There were no gonads palpable. Investigation revealed normal female chromosomes and normal vagina, uterus and ovaries on ultrasound. On the 8th day of life the baby's potassium rose to 7.8 mmol/L, with a sodium of 129 mmol/L. The 17-alpha-hydroxyprogesterone level was raised, confirming salt-losing congenital adrenal hyperplasia due to 21-hydroxylase deficiency.

In female infants, androgen exposure causes virilization with clitoral hypertrophy and variable fusion of the labia minora. The male infant with 21-hydroxylase deficiency appears normal, and commonly the first manifestation is with a salt-losing adrenal crisis, typically in the 2nd week of life. The baby may present in extremis with shock, hyponatraemia, hypoglycaemia and severe hyperkalaemia.

Once the diagnosis of CAH is made, hydrocortisone is used to replace cortisol, restoring negative feedback to the hypothalamus and pituitary. ACTH secretion falls to normal levels, switching off androgen production. Salt-losing children require mineralocorticoid replacement with fludrocortisone and, in infancy, additional sodium chloride.

Corrective surgery of the virilized female infant is complex, and presents significant ethical and practical dilemmas. In the first instance, examination under anaesthesia is required to delineate the perineal anatomy. Severe degrees of virilization result in the urethra entering the vagina in a common urogenital sinus. It is necessary to restore the normal position of the urethra to achieve continence in later life. Surgery is best performed in infancy, when excellent healing may be achieved. In the past, clitoral reduction surgery ('cliteroplasty') was also routinely performed, but this is purely a cosmetic procedure, and may result in loss of clitoral sensation, with detrimental sexual functioning in adult life. Accordingly, most surgeons prefer to defer clitoral reduction until the girl herself wishes to have it done, usually in the early teenage years. With severe degrees of virilization, where the clitoris has formed into a well-developed phallus, this is impractical, and early surgery is needed. Exposure to androgens also results in vaginal stenosis. In the past, it was routine to perform vaginoplasty in infancy, but this requires the daily use of vaginal dilators to prevent re-stenosis, which is painful and psychologically distressing to child and parents alike. Accordingly, vaginoplasty is normally deferred until the girl is in puberty, at which point endogenous oestrogen will normally greatly reduce re-stenosis, thus minimizing the need for use of dilators. The desire to delay corrective surgery may be at variance with the parents' wishes. The parents often want a normal appearance to be achieved without delay, even when this may conflict with the advice of the medical team as to the child's best interests.

The ongoing care of the girl and her family with CAH requires the input of a multi-disciplinary team, including an endocrinologist, urologist, clinical psychologist and specialist nurse. In the UK such services are based at specialist supra-regional centres.

PUBERTY

Puberty – the transition from childhood to sexual maturity – is a complex, hormonally regulated process. Gonadotrophin-releasing hormone (GnRH), secreted by the hypothalamus, stimulates secretion of the gonadotrophins: follicle-stimulating hormone (FSH) and luteinizing hormone (LH) by the pituitary. FSH acts on the ovary and testis to induce gametogenesis – the production of eggs or sperm – whilst LH stimulates oestrogen and testosterone production, respectively. Oestrogen and testosterone levels rise progressively as puberty progresses until attaining adult levels. Oestrogen and testosterone stimulate growth and development of secondary sexual characteristics. Oestrogen and testosterone are inter-convertible through the action of the enzyme aromatase, particularly found in adipose tissue – thus boys make small amounts of oestradiol, and girls make small amounts of testosterone and androstenedione. Through poorly understood mechanisms, the adrenal cortex also secretes androgens (adrenarche), contributing as much as 50% of total androgens in girls.

In girls, normal puberty is signalled by breast development known as thelarche, and is normally followed within 6–12 months by the appearance of pubic hair – pubarche. The attainment of fertility is signalled by the onset of menstruation – menarche. Onset of puberty in girls normally occurs between the ages of 9 and 13 years, with menarche occurring about 2 years later. Onset of puberty in girls is associated with rapid growth. After menarche, growth progressively declines until epiphyseal fusion marks the end of growth, typically about 18 months later.

In boys, puberty is signalled by testicular enlargement. Testicle size may be assessed with an orchidometer (see Figure 12.1). Puberty starts when testicular size reaches 4 mL, progressing through puberty to 15–25 mL in adulthood. In boys, puberty normally starts between 10 and 14 years. The first visible sign of puberty is the appearance of pubic hair, followed by growth of the penis. Testicular size of 12 mL is attained by mid-puberty, when nocturnal FSH secretion reaches adult levels. This corresponds both to the timing of the first ejaculation and the peak of the adolescent growth spurt. Growth continues until epiphyseal fusion occurs in the mid to late teens.

There are a number of normal variants of puberty:

1. *Premature thelarche* describes the appearance of breast tissue, sometimes unilateral, in female infants and young girls. The breast size fluctuates, and prolactin and oestrogen levels are in the normal prepubertal range. It remits spontaneously by 2 or 3 years of age.
2. *Premature adrenarche* is a result of the secretion of adrenal androgens by the adrenal cortex. It typically occurs in girls in mid childhood and may result in the development of body odour, acne, and axillary and pubic

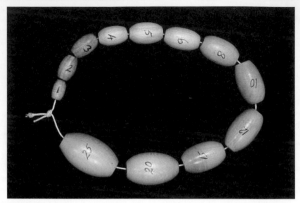

Figure 12.1 Orchidometer for assessment of testicular size in boys. The numbers indicate size in millilitres.

hair. Oestrogen levels are prepubertal. Measurement of the exclusive adrenal androgen dehydroepiandrosterone or its sulphate confirms the diagnosis.

3. *Gynaecomastia* is breast development in boys. It occurs to some degree in all boys in early to mid puberty, but may be pronounced, particularly in obese boys. Where gynaecomastia leads to social difficulties, such as severe embarrassment or school refusal, surgery may be appropriate.

Precocious puberty

When puberty occurs before 8 years in girls or 9 years in boys, it is said to be precocious. Normal, but early puberty is described as central precocious puberty, whereas puberty arising from autonomous oestrogen or androgen secretion is described as gonadotrophin-independent precocious puberty.

In central precocious puberty, as in Case 12.11, gonadotrophin levels are elevated to pubertal levels, with elevated oestrogen or testosterone. Central precocious puberty is relatively common in girls, and is usually idiopathic, but in a small number there is an underlying cause such as a hypothalamic hamartoma or hydrocephalus. In contrast, central precocious puberty in

---

Case 12.11 A girl with precocious puberty

Katie presented with rapid growth, breast development and pubic hair at the age of 4 years. She had spastic diplegic cerebral palsy secondary to hydrocephalus and prematurity at birth. Investigation showed elevated gonadotrophins and oestradiol, confirming central precocious puberty. Her hydrocephalus was felt to be the likely cause. MRI scan confirmed that her hydrocephalus was stable, and showed no other abnormality.

boys is nearly always abnormal. Severe hypothyroidism may cause precocious puberty in girls, but unlike other causes of early puberty, there is no accompanying growth spurt. In boys, testicular enlargement, but not true puberty, is seen.

Gonadotrophin-independent precocious puberty is always abnormal; gonadotrophins are suppressed, or even undetectable with high oestrogen or androgens. In boys, testicular examination reveals prepubertal testes (<4 mL), or unilateral enlargement associated with a functional testicular tumour. If the testes are small, an androgen-secreting tumour, usually adrenal, or previously undiagnosed CAH, are the most likely causes. Some boys have familial, male-limited precocious puberty due to activating mutations of the LH receptor – testotoxicosis.

In girls, ovarian ultrasound will usually show unilateral ovarian enlargement, either from a functional ovarian tumour or McCune–Albright syndrome. In girls with McCune–Albright syndrome, gonadotrophin-independent precocious puberty is common due to an activating mutation affecting a number of endocrine and other systems.

Girls with androgen excess from CAH or androgen-secreting tumours show virilization – excessive development of facial and body hair with clitoral enlargement and other symptoms such as deepening of the voice or frontal recession.

Some tumours such as hepatoblastomas and teratomas may secrete human chorionic gonadotrophin (hCG), thus inducing gonadotrophin-independent precocious puberty. hCG and alpha-fetoprotein are markedly elevated.

The great majority of children with precocious puberty are girls in mid-to-late childhood with idiopathic central precocious puberty. Precocious puberty after age 7 is unlikely to affect final adult height, and is not physically harmful. Accordingly, the main indication for treatment is behavioural or emotional problems associated with sexual development.

Treatment of central precocious puberty is with GnRH super-analogues, which, after initial stimulation of the pituitary, down-regulate gonadotrophin secretion and thus switch off oestrogen or testosterone synthesis. Treatment of gonadotrophin-independent precocious puberty is directed towards treating the underlying cause, if possible, and using specific inhibitors of sex hormone synthesis and/or action.

Delayed puberty

Puberty is said to be delayed if onset occurs after 13 years in girls or 14 years in boys. Delayed puberty is not normally pathological. Delayed puberty is very common in boys, and there is often a family history of delay affecting either parent or other relatives. Delayed puberty is usually associated with short stature and delayed bone age – constitutional delay in growth and adolescence. In a short prepubertal boy, with a family history of delay, minimal investigation is required. If desired, a course of testosterone therapy (or oestrogen in girls) will induce puberty and an accompanying growth spurt, success being determined by a rise in testicular volumes to pubertal size. A boy with normal or tall stature and delayed puberty is more likely to have an underlying cause.

Pathological causes of delayed puberty can result from abnormalities in pituitary production of gonadotrophins or disorders of the testis or ovary. Measuring gonadotrophin levels (FSH and LH) in the blood will

> ### *Case 12.12* A girl with short stature and delayed puberty
>
> Gemma was referred at the age of 13 years with short stature
> and delayed puberty. She was born at term with a birth weight
> of 3.66 kg. She had problems with glue ear, requiring insertion
> of grommets at the age of 4 years, but there was otherwise no
> medical history of note. She was making generally satisfactory
> school progress, but was poor at mathematics. She was below
> her parental target height, and previous measurements showed a
> progressive decline from the 25th centile in early childhood to well
> below the 0.4th centile at presentation. On examination, she had
> slightly low ears, a high palate and small in-curved little fingers
> (clinodactyly), with ridged, brittle nails. There were no secondary
> sexual characteristics. Turner's syndrome was suspected, and
> confirmed by chromosome analysis which showed a mosaic
> 45XO/46XX karyotype.

distinguish these. Investigation will also include chromosomal analysis as
Turner syndrome (see Chapter 18, p. 278) in girls (as in Case 12.12) and
Klinefelter syndrome in boys (XXY karyotype; see Chapter 18, p. 274) each
cause gonadal failure and pubertal delay. In contrast to Turner syndrome,
boys with Klinefelter syndrome are tall. Lack of pubertal development
with absent sense of smell (anosmia) occurs in Kalman syndrome.

Digestion and nutrition 13

(Mary-Anne Morris, Lisa Jackson)

CHAPTER CONTENTS

HISTORY

Where growth or nutrition problems are suspected, take a careful feeding history (Table 13.1). Ask the parent to tell you everything the child has eaten and drunk in the last 24 hours, talking them through the meal times and asking about snacks and drinks between meals. Ask specifically how much milk and fruit juice drink (squash) is consumed and how many portions of fruit and vegetables are eaten daily. Are there battles over the child's eating? Does the child eat alone or with other family members? A food diary kept by the parents over a 3- or 4-day period is sometimes useful.

Key symptoms of gastrointestinal problems in children are vomiting, diarrhoea and abdominal pain (Table 13.2).

Table 13.1 Infant feeding history

History	Comments
Which milk?	Breast or formula? If formula, note which one and details of reconstitution
How much feed?	In breast-fed infants, does the mother have a good milk supply? In formula-fed infants, note volumes offered and taken
How often?	Note the times of feeds in the previous 24 hours
How long does the feed take to complete?	
Characteristics of feeding?	Hungry, windy, apathetic, slow, sleepy, etc.

Table 13.2 Symptoms of gastrointestinal problems

Symptoms	Enquire about
Vomiting	Volume: dribble onto clothes or a full stomach Nature: effortless, forceful (onto child or parent), projectile (several feet away), single vomit or run of vomits Frequency Relationship to feeds and posture Presence of blood or bile in vomit
Diarrhoea	How often: a bowel action after each feed is common if breast-fed Consistency: pure liquid, porridgey or mixed texture, undigested food Colour Presence of blood or mucus
Constipation	How often; is wind passed between times How difficult: straining to go or withhold, painful Soiling Child's attitude to the problem
Abdominal pain	Site/radiation Pattern of onset and relationship to food, stress, medication Colicky or constant duration Waking the child at night (this implies an organic cause)

EXAMINATION

Start by looking generally at the child and their nutrition. Does the child look thin? Are there loose folds of skin in the groin or around the buttocks? Note the health of hair, skin, nails and teeth and look for jaundice and pallor.

Gently examine the abdomen. Explain what you are going to do and get the child to tell you if it hurts. Watch the child's face for signs of discomfort as you examine. Do not forget to examine hernial orifices and the genitalia in boys with acute abdominal pain. The following scheme is recommended.

General points

- Assess the child's growth – is there poor weight gain?
- Look for jaundice or anaemia
- Assess the child's muscle bulk – wasting of the gluteal muscles is seen in coeliac disease
- Is there any finger clubbing (see Table 10.3, p. 101)?
- Is there any evidence of assisted feeding such as a nasogastric tube or a gastrostomy?

Inspection

- Look for abdominal distension. If present, is it symmetrical?
- Are there any operative scars?
- Look for hernias
- Inspect the genitalia. Do they look normal? Are there any signs of puberty?

Palpation

Look at the child's face while palpating the abdomen. Start palpating at a point furthest away from any tenderness (see Figure 13.1). A reluctant child may be put at ease if their own hand is used, with the examiner 's hand overlying.

Feel for any tenderness. Is there any rebound tenderness or guarding?

Identify any enlargement of the liver, kidneys or spleen. The liver should be felt for along a path from the right iliac fossa to the right hypochondrium. The spleen should be felt for on a path from the right iliac fossa to the left hypochondrium. It is common to feel the liver edge and the tip of the spleen in younger children. Many children have a more prominent liver edge with concurrent respiratory disease as hyperinflation pushes the liver down.

The lower pole of each kidney may be felt by palpating with both hands – one behind the flank pressing forwards towards the other.

Feel for other masses. Commonly, faeces are palpable in the left iliac fossa. Constipation is common, and may be associated with tenderness over the caecum due to gaseous distension. In severe constipation the whole lower abdomen may be distended.

Percussion

Percussion can be useful in delineating the edge of the liver or spleen and in examining for ascites.

Auscultation

Listen for bowel sounds in the acutely unwell child.

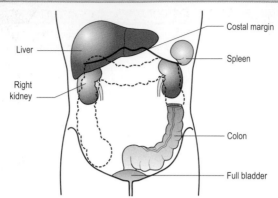

Figure 13.1 Anatomical landmarks on abdominal palpation.

Rectal examination in childhood

This is never a routine examination and is rarely helpful. Careful thought must be given to undertaking this examination in any child.

Assessment of growth

Well infants are often weighed regularly to reassure parents and professionals. Results are recorded in the Personal Child Health Record – usually a red book in the United Kingdom.

Failure to gain weight is a cause of stress and anxiety. Infants may take up to 14 days to regain their birth weight. Failure to regain birth weight by 14 days, or a loss of over 10% of birth weight, needs assessment. Birth weight usually doubles by 4 months and trebles by 12 months. Review the child's growth in length, head growth and weight gain. Failure to grow in any of the parameters is of concern, but *weight loss* needs urgent investigation at any age. A child whose weight crosses two centile lines is 'failing to thrive' and nutritional, physical or psychological causes should be sought.

INFANT FEEDING

Breast-feeding

There is no doubt that 'breast is best' and with the correct support, advice and encouragement the majority of babies will thrive on breast-feeding until at least 6 months of age. The milk is easily digested with low anti-genicity and anti-infective properties. Breast-feeding is good for mother–child bonding, is convenient and is free. Moreover, breast milk tastes different from day to day, reflecting the mother's diet, and this is associated with improved diversity of food intake, particularly vegetables, when weaning is underway.

Problems and contraindications to breast-feeding are very few (see Table 13.3).

Breast-fed babies feed 'on demand'. This will be at least every 2–3 hours for the first few weeks, gradually increasing to every 3–4 hours by day and 6–8 hours overnight by a few months of age. Babies who are getting

Table 13.3 Problems with breast-feeding

Problem	Management
Feeding difficulties	Support for mother (health visitor, midwife, support groups)
Inborn errors of metabolism	Rare, require specialist advice
Maternal drug/alcohol abuse	Careful monitoring of infant
Maternal HIV	Contraindication in developed countries
Maternal medication	Check safety in BNF (British National Formulary) or with pharmacist
Prematurity	Expressed breast milk given via nasogastric tube
Tuberculosis	Contraindicated

enough breast milk settle after feeds, have 6–8 wet nappies per day, tend to pass soft stool quite often – after every feed possibly – and exhibit satisfactory weight gain.

Breast milk is nutritionally complete for term infants until at least 6 months of age. Mothers who are unable or choose not to breast-feed directly should be actively encouraged to express. Expressing should be started as soon as possible after delivery to take advantage of the normal physiological changes that occur after the birth.

Bottle-fed infants should be fed on demand. To start with, a term infant will take 50–70 mL, 7 or 8 times per day, increasing to 180–220 mL, 5 times per day by 3 months of age. Various teats are available, different types suiting different babies.

Alternative milks

Cow's milk-based formulae are modified to resemble breast milk as closely as possible. Standard formulae are 40% casein plus 60% whey, and those marketed for the 'hungrier infant' are 80% casein plus 20% whey. Standard formulae are suitable for up to 12 months of age and the casein-based feeds have no proven benefit. Soy milks are not recommended under 6 months of age due to concern about levels of naturally occurring plant oestrogens. Furthermore, 20% of infants with cow's milk allergy show cross-reactivity with soy protein.

Goat or sheep milk is not recommended due to high solute load, similar immunogenic potential to cow's milk and concerns about sterility.

Hypoallergenic formulae are recommended for infants with milk allergy or those considered at risk of developing it. They are either highly hydrolysed cow's milk (hydrolysed feeds) or composed of amino acids (elemental feeds).

Infant weaning

Weaning should be commenced by 6 months of age, even if the baby was born prematurely. Some hungrier infants may benefit from earlier weaning, but this should not be instituted before 4 months of age. Renal and gastrointestinal immaturity means earlier weaning is inadvisable, and delaying longer may increase the risk of feeding difficulties. The World Health Organization guidelines suggest exclusive breast-feeding until 6 months, which is appropriate for developing countries where risk of infection is greater.

Weaning foods should be introduced gradually, with a new one every few days, and starting with very simple vegetable purees or baby rice. The complexity and range of tastes and textures are gradually increased. There should be no added salt or sugar; gluten and eggs may be introduced from 6 months. Cow's milk is not used as the main drink until 1 year of age but it may be incorporated into solids from 6 months. It is recommended that full-fat milk is given until at least 2 years of age. Alternative formula milks ('follow-on' milks) are available with higher levels of iron, vitamin D and protein content, but infants eating a range of solids do not need them.

DIET FOR OLDER CHILDREN

The principles of healthy eating are a diet that is roughly 40% carbohydrate, 35% fat and 15% protein, and which includes five portions of fruit and vegetables per day, plenty of fluids (ideally water rather than squash and other soft drinks), and refined carbohydrate in moderation.

Vitamins

Vitamin deficiency syndromes are uncommon in the developed world except for children with malabsorption. Vitamin A deficiency is still the most important cause of blindness in the world. Vitamin A supplementation can also reduce the risk of death from infectious disease.

Vitamin D deficiency causes rickets. Although frank rickets is rare, there has been a resurgence of vitamin D deficiency in the UK, with dark-skinned children from ethnic minorities at especially high risk. In November 2010, the US Institute of Medicine recommended routine vitamin D supplementation (200–800 units daily) throughout life for those living at northern latitudes, such as the UK. Eighty to ninety per cent of vitamin D is derived from sunlight exposure, but in Britain this is possible only between March and September, when the sun is high in the sky. Covering-up, or use of high factor sun blocks (factor 30 or more), will abolish photosynthesis of vitamin D. Dietary sources of vitamin D are oily fish (such as sardines, tuna, pilchards, etc.), eggs and fortified foods such as breakfast cereals and some margarines. Children may present with neurological features of hypocalcaemia, or with failure-to-thrive and hypotonia, or with weak bones manifesting as knock-knees or bow legs. Lassitude, bone pain and myalgia are common with less severe degrees of deficiency.

Iron deficiency

Iron deficiency is common and may have developmental, educational and growth consequences. Toddlers with iron deficiency show impaired development, relative to their peers. Iron deficiency is associated with impaired appetite, further compounding the iron deficiency through reduced dietary intake. Severe iron deficiency may be associated with *pica*, which is characterized by consumption of non-food items, such as earth.

Simple iron deficiency without significant anaemia will respond to dietary measures. Foods high in iron include meat, fish and poultry, fortified breakfast cereals and, to a lesser degree, dark green vegetables, peas and beans. Vitamin C (in foods, fruit juice or many child squash drinks) will increase iron absorption.

Iron deficiency is a feature of a range of gastrointestinal disorders, notably gastro-oesophageal reflux disease (GORD), coeliac disease and inflammatory bowel disease, due to impaired food intake, impaired iron absorption and blood loss.

Obesity

Obesity is a rapidly growing problem for children, their families and society. The 2008 Health Survey for England reported an obesity rate of 19.5% for children aged 11–15 years. Children living in poverty, from urban areas or from ethnic minority groups are especially high risk of obesity. In the vast majority there is a simple imbalance between energy ingestion and energy expenditure. Factors contributing include high-energy snacks and fast foods, tendency for larger portion sizes, decreased levels of activity amongst children at school and social and cultural pressures. Children with simple obesity are usually tall for their age. Children who are growing poorly may have an endocrine cause for their obesity (Cushing's syndrome, hypothyroidism or growth hormone deficiency – see Chapter 12).

Children with physical and/or learning disability are at increased risk of obesity. This is primarily a consequence of reduced ability to engage in physical activity, and, in some, is compounded by increased appetite. In rare instances, obesity is a characteristic of the underlying condition, notably Prader–Willi syndrome (see Chapter 18, p. 274).

Education about the short- and long-term risks of obesity, and constructive advice on diet and exercise, are important, but it needs to include other family members. Support groups may help. Drugs are rarely appropriate. The aim is to maintain weight, rather than weight loss, whilst growth in height continues.

Parenteral nutrition

Intravenous feeds containing carbohydrate, fat, protein, minerals, vitamins and trace elements are used primarily as an adjunct to enteral feeds or short-term replacement for those who cannot tolerate enteral feeds, e.g. after bowel surgery. Five to ten per cent of children will have complications from the intravenous feeding line, including sepsis, blockage and embolism. Progressive impairment of liver function may occur with long-term parenteral nutrition, and may culminate in cirrhosis and liver failure.

THE VOMITING INFANT

Vomiting in infancy is a fact of life. Almost every baby will posset, bringing up a small amount of milk after a feed, often with wind. It is necessary to distinguish mild gastro-oesophageal reflux from GORD, or vomiting due to obstruction, or from neurological causes (such as hydrocephalus). The following cases describe some characteristic histories and their causes.

Gastro-oesophageal reflux

> ### Case 13.1 An infant with a history of vomiting since birth
>
> Anna, a 6-month-old infant, presented with a history of vomiting since birth. What had initially seemed to be harmless posseting of small amounts after feeds had progressed to bother the whole family. The vomiting was worse after feeds, or if she was being moved or carried, but could occur at any time. It seemed effortless, with enough produced to stain everyone's clothes and the floor in the vicinity. The vomit contained partly digested milk. The clinical picture of a fraught family with a cheerful well-nourished thriving baby was characteristic.

Simple gastro-oesophageal reflux (as in Case 13.1) is usually a benign disorder which resolves spontaneously between 6 and 12 months of age as infants spend more time upright, solids are introduced, and natural anti-reflux mechanisms develop. Reassurance is the mainstay of treatment. Parents can try smaller volumes of milk, given more frequently, and positioning the infant with head elevated after feeds. Feed thickeners may help.

Less commonly, reflux is severe – GORD – and infants may fail to thrive. Oesophagitis is characteristic. Reflux is commonly troublesome in infants with cerebral palsy, bronchopulmonary dysplasia and milk intolerance.

Investigation (rarely indicated)

- A barium swallow and meal will often confirm reflux and may identify abnormalities of oesophageal motility, strictures or hiatus hernias
- Endoscopy will enable confirmation of oesophagitis, and stricture formation. It is useful for diagnosis of oesophagitis associated with allergy (eosinophilic oesophagitis) which may not be associated with significant acid reflux
- A pH or impedance study will confirm the severity of acid reflux by demonstrating the duration of acid reflux into the lower oesophagus. This involves placing a pH probe just above the cardiac sphincter, in the lower oesophagus. It is vital to discontinue acid-blocking drugs (H_2 receptor blockers or proton-pump inhibitors – PPIs) prior to the procedure.

Treatment options include dietary substitution, simple antacids, acid blockade with H_2 receptor blockers or PPIs, therapy, prokinetic drugs such as domperidone, or surgery (fundoplication).

Pyloric stenosis

> ### Case 13.2 An infant with progressive and dramatic vomiting
>
> Adam, a 6-week-old infant, presented with a 5-day history of progressive and dramatic vomiting which did not contain bile. This occurred during or after meals, and the vomit was projected across the room so that carers learned to keep their distance. Despite the vomiting, the baby seemed hungry, feeding avidly until the vomiting occurred. On examination, the baby had lost weight, was constipated and mildly dehydrated.

Pyloric stenosis (Case 13.2) describes a pathological thickening of the pyloric sphincter, which hypertrophies over the first few weeks of age. This causes obstruction of the gastric outlet. It affects 1 in 150 males and 1 in 750 female infants. It is more common in first-born children and in those with an affected parent.

Diagnosis can be made by a 'test feed'. The hypertrophied muscle is palpable during a feed. Visible gastric peristalsis may be seen through the abdominal wall. Ultrasound (or less commonly now, barium examination) will confirm the diagnosis. The loss of large amounts of hydrochloric acid from the stomach leads to high plasma bicarbonate and chloride deficiency (hypochloraemic alkalosis).

Restoration of fluid and electrolyte balance is needed before pyloric stenosis is corrected by Ramstedt's pyloromyotomy. This involves longitudinally dividing the pyloric muscle, but *not* the mucosa, under general anaesthetic. Infants usually tolerate milk within a few hours of the operation.

Bilious vomiting in infancy

Case 13.3 A baby with bile-stained vomit

Jade, a 6-day-old baby, presented with bile-stained vomiting. She was not feeding and her bowels had not been open for 48 hours. The abdomen was soft, with minimal distension. There was minimal tenderness, and no evidence of a hernia.

Feeding was stopped, a nasogastric tube sited, and intravenous fluids commenced. As she had previously passed meconium, an intestinal atresia was excluded. She had an urgent abdominal X-ray which showed a paucity of bowel gas, suggesting upper small bowel obstruction. She was transferred urgently to a paediatric surgery centre, where, after a diagnostic contrast study showed malrotation, she underwent urgent surgery with fixation of the caecum to the posterior abdominal wall, and appendicectomy.

Bile-stained vomiting, as in Case 13.3, is an indicator of serious surgical pathology, and requires urgent assessment. Abdominal X-rays may reveal evidence of obstruction with fluid levels and dilated small or large bowel, or may show a displaced caecum indicating *malrotation*, as in this case. Upper or lower gastrointestinal contrast studies will clarify the picture. This congenital anomaly results in the mid-gut twisting on its mesentery, causing a volvulus, and potentially infarction from the mid-duodenum to the mid-transverse colon.

Congenital *intestinal atresias* most commonly affect the small bowel, particularly the duodenum. A significant number of affected infants have Down syndrome. Treatment is with resection of the atretic segment (see also Chapter 17, p. 260).

Hirschsprung's disease occurs due to congenital absence of ganglion cells in the intramuscular and submucous layers of the large intestine, extending proximally from the anus. The affected bowel does not exhibit peristalsis, and proximal obstruction or enterocolitis (severe diarrhoea and abdominal distension) may occur. In the first instance, treatment is with a colostomy proximal to the aganglionic bowel (determined by intra-operative histology of 'frozen sections'), followed later by resto-ration of bowel continuity, with a 'pull-through' procedure, typically around 1 year of age. Children with Down syndrome (see Chapter 18, p. 273) are also at greatly increased risk of Hirschsprung's disease.

Rarely, if only a very short segment of aganglionic bowel is present, the main symptom is constipation (see below); however, in this case, symp-toms will be present from very early life, usually from the neonatal period.

Strangulated hernias may also produce bilious vomiting secondarily to intestinal obstruction.

Feeding problems

A careful history will usually establish the cause and exclude straightfor-ward overfeeding. Infants with nasal obstruction and palate problems may feed messily, take in excess air, and vomit. Irritable babies may gulp feeds and vomit. Milk intolerance may cause vomiting, with or without diar-rhoea and pain (see below).

Gastroenteritis

> #### Case 13.4 An infant with acute diarrhoea and vomiting
>
> Srinath, a formula-fed infant aged 11 months, developed acute diarrhoea and vomiting over a few hours. He vomited all oral fluids and had four bowel actions in as many hours. This was associated with fever and listlessness. His older brother had a similar, but less severe, attack 4 days previously. Examination revealed moderate dehydration. The abdomen was soft with active bowel sounds.

Gastroenteritis (as in Case 13.4) is a common infectious disease. Most cases are viral, and rotavirus causes over 50% of cases. Bacterial causes include *Salmonella, Campylobacter, Escherichia coli* and *Shigella,* and may cause a dys-entery-like picture, with blood and pus in the stool, and high fever, com-monly with abdominal pain. However, abdominal pain is not usually a prominent feature in viral gastroenteritis. Infection with *E. coli* O157 may lead to gastroenteritis complicated by acute renal failure (see Chapter 11, p. 135).

DEHYDRATION

Dehydration results from depletion of electrolyte-rich gastrointestinal secretions through vomiting and/or diarrhoea. In response to these losses there is redistribution of water by osmosis throughout the intra- and extra-cellular fluids. This leads to a reduction in plasma volume and stimulation of thirst. Consumption of hypotonic fluids depresses extracellular sodium concentrations, reduces plasma osmolality and ADH (antidiuretic hor-mone) secretion, and reduces thirst, even if alimentary and other losses continue. The renin–angiotensin system is stimulated, conserving sodium and maintaining blood pressure. Thus, in mild to moderate dehydration (5%), there is minimal electrolyte disturbance, but the child will have reduced skin turgor and lethargy and reduced urine output.

As losses continue, severe dehydration results, with features of shock, including tachycardia and hypotension. The extremities will feel cold. The child is obtunded through severe dehydration with accompanying hyponatraemia.

Children who cannot drink sufficiently, or who have disproportionate loss of water, e.g. febrile infants, may develop hypernatraemia in response to dehydration. Hypernatraemic dehydration is associated with irritability, and in infants a full fontanelle, but tissue turgor is maintained (the skin has a doughy consistency) and thus the severity of dehydration may not be appreciated.

In formula-fed infants a short break from milk feeds may aid recovery – breast-fed infants should continue to feed normally. If unable to breast-feed, the mother should express milk to avoid impairment of subsequent lactation. Mild and moderate dehydration is best treated with oral rehydration solutions containing glucose and sodium chloride, given little and often. These may be administered via nasogastric tube if necessary.

Severe or hypernatraemic dehydration requires prompt correction of shock and administration of glucose/saline solutions appropriate to the electrolyte status of the child. Acidosis is a common accompaniment to dehydration through a combination of lactic acidosis from impaired peripheral perfusion, and ketogenesis from rapid lipolysis. Typically this responds well to simple or intravenous rehydration, although correction with sodium bicarbonate may rarely be required.

Recovery within 48 hours is the norm. The development of a secondary cow's milk protein intolerance or lactose intolerance may lead to persistent diarrhoea which can be managed using a non-cow's milk formula, or a lactose-free formula, for 1–2 months.

Intussusception

> **Case 13.5** A screaming infant with colicky abdominal pain and pallor
>
> Casey, an infant of 6 months, presented screaming with bouts of colicky abdominal pain and pallor. The pain was so bad that she seemed transiently distant and obtunded in the aftermath. There was some vomiting followed by the passage of bloody stool with mucus, likened to redcurrant jelly. A sausage-shaped abdominal mass was palpable in the abdomen. Urgent abdominal ultrasound showed the characteristic 'target' sign of intussusception. She underwent an air-contrast enema which successfully reduced the intussusception.

Intussusception (Case 13.5), in which the bowel partly invaginates, leading to ischaemia, characteristic 'redcurrant jelly stools' and severe episodes of pain with pallor, and vomiting, often causes diagnostic confusion. The highest incidence is seen around 6–9 months of age.

It may mimic gastroenteritis, and even meningitis because of obtundation. Children may be dehydrated or shocked. Sometimes an identifiable lead point is found at the point of intussusception such as a polyp, Meckel's diverticulum, or enlarged Peyer's patch. This occurs more commonly in older children.

The infant may appear well between episodes of pain. The diagnosis might be suggested on abdominal X-ray, and has a characteristic ultrasound appearance. The intussusception may usually be reduced by a contrast enema using air or liquid contrast medium. This should be performed in a paediatric surgical centre. Surgery is indicated for failed reduction (25%), perforation or recurrence (4–10%).

Systemic disease

Almost any systemic disease can present with vomiting, including upper respiratory tract infection (URTI), raised intracranial pressure, urinary tract infection and metabolic and psychological disorders. Always examine the child carefully, and obtain a clean-catch urine sample.

ABDOMINAL PAIN

Acute appendicitis

> #### Case 13.6 A boy with right iliac fossa pain
>
> Ricky, a 7-year-old boy, had a history of vague central abdominal pain after school. He ate little supper and spent a restless night during which he vomited once and passed a small loose stool. By the morning he had significant colicky central abdominal pain and would not eat. By the time he saw a doctor 18 hours into the illness the pain had begun to localize to the right iliac fossa.
>
> On examination he looked unwell with a dry furred tongue, offensive breath, and slightly sunken eyes. His pulse was raised at 100 beats per minute and his temperature was 38.2°C. He was holding himself awkwardly, bending slightly and to one side, and complained of pain on movement. His abdomen was tense and tender all over but exquisite in the right iliac fossa, with rebound tenderness.

The boy in Case 13.6 had acute appendicitis and surgery was performed as soon as possible. Where possible, emergency surgery is avoided. Trials are under way investigating antibiotic treatment in acute appendicitis, with a view to avoiding or deferring surgery. The history described is typical but it can be difficult, especially in preschool children, or if the appendix is unusually sited. Ultrasound or CT scanning may be required. Other causes of acute abdominal pain must be considered – see Box 13.1 and Table 13.4.

> #### Box 13.1 Causes of acute abdominal pain
>
> * Appendicitis
> * Mesenteric adenitis
> * Tonsillitis/URTI
> * Constipation
> * Urinary tract infection/pyelonephritis
> * Lower lobe pneumonia
> * Cholecystitis
> * Non-organic

Table 13.4 Other causes of recurrent abdominal pain

Cause	Key clinical features
Renal or ureteric pain	Pain experienced laterally or posteriorly
Gastritis or gastro-oesophageal reflux	Epigastric or chest pain
Peptic ulceration	Night pain
Spinal or back problems	Lateral pain Signs over the spine (tenderness, limited movement)
Liver or gall bladder disease	Right hypochondrial pain Jaundice
Constipation	Usually presents with constipation rather than pain; pain better if bowels are open
Gynaecological problems	Suprapubic or iliac fossa pain Periodic pain (monthly)
Abdominal migraine	Acute attacks +/- pallor and vomiting

Infantile colic

In Case 13.7, if the history and examination reveal no worrying features it is highly likely that the baby has colic.

Case 13.7 A crying baby

Crystal, a 4-week-old infant, was taken to see her GP because she had been crying inconsolably every evening for a week. She was feeding well and thriving, with no other concerns. Her parents felt there must be something seriously wrong although she was well at other times of the day.

Colic is excessive crying in a healthy infant that starts within the first few weeks of life and lasts until around 4–5 months. Strictly speaking, this means at least 3 hours of crying a day, 3 days a week for at least 3 weeks, but is used much more loosely to cover crying that parents perceive to be unacceptable. The cause of colic is not known but painful peristalsis, trapped wind, lactose intolerance, dietary protein intolerance and parental anxiety have all been suggested. It has also been regarded as a behavioural pattern with no pathology.

There is no evidence that herbal remedies, gripe water or simeticone reduce colic. In bottle-fed babies a 1–2 week trial of a cow's milk protein-free formula may be of benefit. Reassurance is vital. Acknowledge how stressful the crying is and that it will improve with age.

Non-specific abdominal pain

Abdominal pains like those in Case 13.8 affect 10% of children and can have a variety of labels including NSAP (non-specific abdominal pain), functional abdominal pain and sensitive bowels. Many children will have no worrying features in the history, or on examination, and do not require investigations. In others, inflammatory bowel disease, food intolerances or other causes (see Table 13.4) may need to be excluded.

Case 13.8 A girl with a history of **recurrent** central abdominal pain

Libby, a 9-year-old girl, attended the outpatient department with a 9-month history of bouts of intermittent central abdominal pain. During attacks, which were common after school, she looked pale and miserable and had to lie down for 30 to 60 minutes. On other days she repeatedly complained of abdominal pain. When questioned she said she always had pain. She was missing a lot of school. Over-the-counter remedies were ineffective. Her appetite was normal and there was no weight loss, vomiting or alteration of bowel habit. She was growing normally. There were no abnormal signs on examination.

Current hypotheses suggest that there may be disordered motility or perception of motility. However, many parents accept that occasional abdominal pains are stress related. Careful history, examination and reassurance are often sufficient, and the pains may respond to simple remedies like paracetamol or hot-water bottles. Some of the children are more anxious than their more care-free (and pain-free) peers. The stresses in their lives are usually common ones, such as trying to work in a noisy classroom and arguments with friends. Do not forget to ask about bullying, but do not assume that all children with pain are facing a huge problem in their lives. About half of these abdominal pains settle within a few months. In some, the pains can be recurrent and a proportion will go on to develop typical features of irritable bowel syndrome.

Mesenteric adenitis

Central abdominal pain which is associated with tenderness occurring at the same time as a URTI is often labelled as mesenteric adenitis. It is thought to be due to inflamed mesenteric lymph nodes with a peritoneal reaction, although pathological evidence of this is often lacking. Episodes of pain may be recurrent.

CONSTIPATION

Constipation (as in Case 13.9) is common and causes much distress to children and families. There may be a genetic tendency, but poor fluid and fibre intake, fear of defecation and development of a megarectum exacerbate the problems. Megarectum develops when the rectum remains over-distended and the sensations of needing to defecate are lost. Involuntary soiling

---

Case 13.9 A girl with a fear of going to the toilet

Jemima, a 3-year-old girl, was opening her bowels every 5–7 days. She was distressed for 24 hours beforehand and was frightened to sit on the toilet. The stools were hard and very painful to pass, with fresh blood on wiping. Her appetite was poor, particularly when she had not opened her bowels for a few days. She was otherwise well. The problems started 6 months previously, after she had been ill with chicken pox.

---

may then occur as liquid stool escapes past the hard impacted stool and through a stretched anal sphincter. This is very distressing to children and their families and the risks of social isolation and school avoidance are real. Constipation is rarely due to a coeliac disease or food intolerance, endocrine causes (such as hypothyroidism) or neurological causes. In short-segment Hirschsprung's disease, symptoms date back to the neonatal period.

Constipation is manageable with enthusiastic and supportive therapy. A combination of good diet, stool softeners and osmotic laxatives will produce a soft stool. Stimulant laxatives and behavioural modification will produce regular emptying. Treatment usually needs to continue for at least 2–3 years, and sometimes much longer, depending on severity.

CHRONIC DIARRHOEA

Chronic diarrhoea in children has diverse causes, ranging from toddler diarrhoea to inflammatory bowel disease (see Table 13.5).

Toddler diarrhoea

Loose or variable texture stools may be passed 3–5 times per day in well 1–3 year olds who are unaware or untroubled by it. This is very common. Also called 'peas and carrots diarrhoea', identifiable food in the stools is a

Table 13.5 Clinical characteristics of different causes of chronic diarrhoea

	Abdominal pain	Vomiting	Mucus or blood	Growth failure
Toddler diarrhoea	−	−	Occasional mucus	−
Food allergy	+	++	+	Unusual
Coeliac disease	++	+	−	++
Crohn's disease	+++	+	+ if colon affected	+++
Ulcerative colitis	++	+/−	+++	+

characteristic that can cause alarm to parents. In some, investigations may be necessary. It is due to rapid gastrointestinal transit. Triggers may be high-fibre foods such as wheat biscuit breakfast cereals, fruit juices, and sometimes an inadequate fat intake, due to mistaken use of 'healthy' low-fat foods, which are inappropriate for young children. It is a benign condition and most children grow out of it by school age. A careful history and examination will exclude coeliac disease, food allergy and sugar intolerance in most cases.

Food intolerance

Food intolerance may be caused by allergy (e.g. cow's milk protein), immune-mediated disease (e.g. coeliac disease), enzyme deficiency (e.g. lactose intolerance), or chemical irritation (e.g. chillies).

Allergy

Cow's milk protein allergy is the most common food allergy, but allergic reactions can develop to other antigenic proteins including soya, eggs, peanuts, tree nuts, cereals and fish. Risk of allergic reactions increases if there is a strong family history of atopy. Symptoms may include urticaria, stridor, anaphylaxis, vomiting, diarrhoea, abdominal pain and behavioural changes.

Investigations are rarely of value although eosinophilia, raised food-related blood IgE levels or positive skin prick tests may be found. A therapeutic trial of food withdrawal, with symptoms recurring on subsequent challenge, is the gold standard for diagnosis.

Management is to strictly exclude offending antigens from the diet. Twenty per cent of children with cow's milk protein intolerance also develop symptoms with soya, so hypoallergenic formulae are advised. Most children will outgrow the allergy by 2–5 years, although in a very few it is lifelong. If there is a history of severe allergic reactions, particularly anaphylaxis, food challenges should be carried out in hospital.

Sugar intolerance

Sugar intolerance is due to enzyme defects, and fermentation of undigested sugars causes explosive frothy stools with flatus, with or without abdominal pain and distension. Lactase deficiency is the most common cause and is usually transient (after severe gastroenteritis or untreated coeliac disease), or is due to a progressive fall in lactase production (common in non-Caucasians who have increasing intolerance with age). Very rarely, it may be congenital, when it is inherited as an autosomal recessive trait.

Coeliac disease

Coeliac disease is a small-bowel enteropathy due to intolerance to the protein gluten in wheat, barley, rye and possibly oats. It can occur at any time after the introduction of gluten into the diet. There is a very strong genetic susceptibility. The disease affects between 1 in 300 and 1 in 1000 people. The risk is higher with a family history, autoimmune disorders, such as type 1 diabetes and in Down syndrome.

Coeliac disease may be broadly classified according to clinical presentation:
● Typical – the commonest presentation in young children
● Atypical, in which abdominal signs or symptoms are minimal, and there are extra-intestinal clinical features such as dermatitis herpetiformis

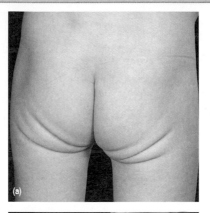

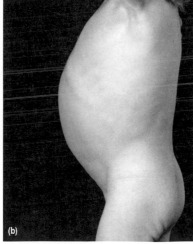

Figure 13.2 (a) Severe buttock-wasting secondary to coeliac disease. (b) Abdominal distension secondary to coeliac disease.

- Silent, in which serology is positive and biopsy findings diagnostic, but the patient is asymptomatic (often detected on screening of susceptible individuals)
- Latent, in which individuals are HLA-susceptible, may have positive serology, but biopsy is not diagnostic.

Most infants and children with coeliac disease present with typical symptoms, including diarrhoea, which is typically pale, fatty, offensive and 'porridge-like' in nature. The clinical appearance is characteristic (see Figure 13.2). Other symptoms are described in Table 13.6.

Table 13.6 Symptoms of coeliac disease

Type of presentation	Signs and symptoms
Classical presentation (9–18 months)	Pale, irritable, failure-to-thrive, abdominal distension, buttock wasting
Early presentation (<9 months)	Vomiting or constipation
Late presentation (childhood–adult)	Iron deficiency anaemia, short stature, fatigue, abdominal pain
Screening (in patients with insulin-dependent diabetes or a strong family history)	Subtle symptoms or none at all

Coeliac disease is a permanent condition and should not be confused with transient wheat or gluten intolerance, which may occur in children under 2 years, especially after gastroenteritis.

According to new European guidelines published in January 2012, a typical presentation, in conjunction with a strongly positive coeliac screen (IgA anti-tissue transglutaminase greater than 10 times the upper normal limit, with positive anti-endomysial antibodies and HLA-DQ2 or DQ8 heterodimers), coupled with a clinical and biochemical response to a gluten-free diet, is taken to be diagnostic of coeliac disease. Where the clinical picture is less clear-cut, an upper small bowel biopsy is required for confirmation. Typical histology shows subtotal villous atrophy with increased lymphocytes in the lamina propria and epithelium.

The management of coeliac disease is with a strict gluten-free diet, excluding all wheat, rye and barley. Oats may be tolerated later but are usually excluded to begin with. Staple foods can be prescribed by GPs. Support of a paediatric dietitian is essential, and the Coeliac Society is an invaluable source of up-to-date information on gluten-free products. Non-compliance with diet risks malabsorption, with growth stunting, and loss of key micronutrients, osteoporosis, female infertility and small bowel lymphoma.

Crohn's disease

Crohn's disease affects 1 in 1000 adults, 1 in 4 of whom present in adolescence. It causes an inflammation of the whole bowel wall (transmural involvement), anywhere from mouth to anus, with the terminal ileum being most often affected. It is believed that Crohn's disease arises from an abnormal immune response to bacterial antigens in the intestine, in a susceptible patient. Over 30 genetic susceptibility loci have been identified for Crohn's disease. These loci encode genes involved in lymphocyte differentiation, maintenance of epithelial barrier integrity, autophagy and the secondary immune response. The NOD2/CARD15 gene on chromosome 16q12 is one of the most important. This gene encodes an intracellular monocyte protein important in recognition and processing bacterial antigens ('innate pattern recognition'). Mutations in this gene are present in approximately 30% of individuals with Crohn's disease.

The presentation is often delayed with non-specific symptoms such as growth failure, delayed puberty, anorexia, poor concentration, lethargy, malaise and deteriorating school or sport performance. If colitis is present, diarrhoea and abdominal pain may be a feature. Examination may show evidence of malnutrition, linear mouth ulcers and perianal skin tags. Tenderness or abdominal masses are variable. Inflammatory markers such as ESR (erythrocyte sedimentation rate) or CRP (C-reactive protein) usually parallel disease activity, but the nature and extent of inflammation need to be demonstrated. This requires upper gastrointestinal endoscopy and colonoscopy with biopsy.

Management begins with induction of remission using nutritional therapy (elemental or hydrolysed feed and food exclusion) or systemic steroids. On-going maintenance treatment with 5-aminosalicylate derivatives (Salazopyrin [sulfasalazine], mesalazine), immunosuppression (azathioprine, methotrexate) or biological therapy (monoclonal anti-TNF-α) may be needed. Surgery should be avoided whenever possible but may be needed for complications such as obstruction, fistulas or failed medical treatment. Typically, the course is relapsing into and throughout adult life, and ultimately 80% of Crohn's patients require surgery.

Ulcerative colitis

Ulcerative colitis is rarer than Crohn's disease in children, but the disease is more likely to be a pan-colitis, in contrast to adults. Ulcerative colitis typically presents with cramping abdominal pain with diarrhoea containing blood and/or mucus. Urgency of stool is often a feature and may be very distressing. Anorexia, weight loss or extra-intestinal manifestations may be present such as erythema nodosa, arthritis, liver disease or eye lesions. Upper gastrointestinal endoscopy and colonoscopy and biopsy are required to confirm the diagnosis and exclude Crohn's disease. Typical colonic histology shows mucosal inflammation with crypt abscesses and goblet cell depletion.

Treatment involves the induction of remission with systemic steroids. This is followed by maintenance treatment with 5-aminosalicylate derivatives, low-dose steroids or immunosuppression (azathioprine, methotrexate). Total colectomy may be needed for complications such as toxic megacolon, haemorrhage or failed medical treatment. Surveillance colonoscopy is performed annually when disease has been active for 10 or more years to reduce the very real risk of colorectal carcinoma.

JAUNDICE IN CHILDREN

Jaundice arises from elevation of serum bilirubin. Haemolytic disorders cause jaundice (see Chapter 7, p. 60), or it may arise from impaired clearance of bilirubin in hepatocellular dysfunction, as occurs with hepatitis, or from biliary obstruction such as biliary atresia.

Congenital causes of jaundice

Bilirubin arises from breakdown of haem. It is metabolized in the liver by the glucuronyl transferase enzyme system to the conjugated form that is excreted in bile. Defects of this enzyme system result in unconjugated hyperbilirubinaemia. Severe defects, due to autosomal recessive inheritance, result in *Crigler–Najjar syndrome* with extremely severe jaundice occurring at birth, and often resulting in choreo-athetoid cerebral palsy (kernicterus) (see Chapter 14, p. 197). *Gilbert's syndrome* arises from a mild conjugation defect, resulting in intermittent mild jaundice with fatigue, usually triggered by illness. It is relatively common, and harmless. Conjugated hyperbilirubinaemia occurs in *Dubin–Johnson* and *Rotor* syndromes, which are due to defective hepatic excretion of conjugated bilirubin. Aside from jaundice, patients are usually asymptomatic.

The infant with obstructive jaundice

The young infant with obstructive jaundice (as in Case 13.10) requires urgent evaluation to exclude *biliary atresia*. In biliary atresia there is progressive obliteration of the extra- and intra-hepatic bile ducts, leading to hepatocellular injury, with cirrhosis and portal hypertension. Surgery to construct a bile conduit (Kasai procedure) is performed as soon as possible. If surgery is unsuccessful, then liver failure results, requiring liver transplantation. If bile drainage is achieved, then the progression of liver disease may be slowed, although ascending cholangitis, malnutrition due to fat malabsorption, and portal hypertension leading to oesophageal varices and consequent gastrointestinal haemorrhage are common complications.

The differential diagnosis of obstructive jaundice includes congenital *choledochal cyst* affecting the extrahepatic biliary tree, and *neonatal hepatitis*. Neonatal hepatitis presents with prolonged obstructive jaundice and evidence of hepatocellular dysfunction. It is usually idiopathic, but infective, endocrine and metabolic causes – notably galactosaemia and alpha-1-antitrypsin deficiency – must be excluded.

Galactosaemia (Case 13.11) results from an inability to metabolize galactose. Toxic metabolites accumulate with resultant hepatic and renal toxicity and cataracts. High levels of galactose-1-phosphate provide an ideal

---

Case 13.10 A baby with lingering jaundice

Peter was referred by his GP at 25 days of age, after his health visitor noticed that he was still jaundiced. His weight gain was poor, and he had dark urine with putty-coloured stools. Urine testing was positive for bilirubin, but negative for urobilinogen. His bilirubin level was 148 pmol/L, the majority of which was conjugated. He had abnormal coagulation. Biliary atresia was suspected and he was urgently referred to a tertiary specialist centre. Biliary atresia was subsequently confirmed, and he underwent surgery.

Case 13.11 A baby with prolonged jaundice

Bridget was a term baby who had difficulty establishing feeds. She presented with sepsis at 16 days of age. She had vomiting, diarrhoea and hypoglycaemia, and was lethargic and jaundiced. Examination revealed hepatomegaly. The liver enzymes were elevated, with an elevated conjugated bilirubin and abnormal coagulation studies. Blood cultures were positive for *Escherichia coli*. Reducing substances were present in the urine, and Bridget was found to have reduced levels of galactose-1-phosphate uridyl transferase, confirming the diagnosis of galactosaemia.

substrate for *E. coli* sepsis, which complicates half of cases. It is treated by elimination of all sources of lactose and galactose, which includes breast and bottled milks. This rare condition is inherited in an autosomal recessive manner. Despite early treatment, learning difficulties are common, notably verbal dyspraxia (see Chapter 4, p. 30). Girls are almost always infertile due to premature ovarian failure. Cataracts may occur, due to accumulation of the galactose metabolite, galactitol, in the lens of the eyes, and ophthalmological surveillance is required.

Hepatitis

Acute hepatitis

Acute hepatitis is characterized by elevation of transaminases, sometimes with other features of hepatocellular dysfunction, and often jaundice with dark urine containing bilirubin and urobilinogen. Other common symptoms include:

- Fatigue
- Abdominal pain
- Loss of appetite, nausea and vomiting
- Diarrhoea
- Low-grade fever
- Headache.

However, infection is commonly asymptomatic or subclinical.

Drug reactions, paracetamol poisoning and a range of infections, most commonly viral, can cause hepatitis. The principal causes of viral hepatitis are summarized in Table 13.7. *Hepatitis A* is by far the most common cause of viral hepatitis. The maximum period of infectivity occurs in the 2 weeks prior to onset of jaundice. There is little systemic upset but often abdominal pain, vomiting and loss of appetite, which may last several weeks. Travellers to endemic areas, or exposed contacts, such as other family members at risk of infection, should receive hepatitis A immunization.

Chronic hepatitis

Chronic hepatitis may result from infection with hepatitis virus B or C and, less commonly, from metabolic disorders such as Wilson's disease and alpha-1-antitrypsin deficiency. Chronic hepatitis may result in cirrhosis and liver failure, and the risk of hepatocellular carcinoma is greatly increased.

The risk of chronic hepatitis B infection is very high (90%) with congenital infection (vertical transmission from mother to child), hence the importance of screening at-risk mothers and, where necessary, offering immunization to the infant. Interferon alpha and lamivudine have been used to treat childhood hepatitis virus B infection. Concurrent infection with hepatitis virus D also makes chronic hepatitis virus B infection more likely. Vertical transmission rates with hepatis C are low (7%). Response to treatment with interferon alpha and ribavirin is dependent on genotype, with response rates varying between 50% and 90%. A poor response is associated with the development of chronic hepatitis.

Autoimmune hepatitis and *sclerosing cholangitis* are often associated with inflammatory bowel disease. The liver problems may be the first manifestation of this. Autoimmune hepatitis is characterized by elevated autoantibodies, particularly antinuclear, and liver-kidney

Table 13.7 Transmission, prevention and complications of viral hepatitis

Virus	Transmission	Prevention	Complications	Notes
Epstein–Barr virus	Oral secretions		Other features of glandular fever may be present	Usually subclinical infection
Hepatitis A	Faeco-oral	Hygiene measures[1] Immunization post-exposure immunoglobulin	Prolonged/relapsing illness lasting 6–9 months in 15%	
Hepatitis B	Congenital Blood Sexual Body secretions	Immunization of at-risk groups Blood precautions[2]	Chronic carriage Chronic hepatitis Cirrhosis Hepatocellular carcinoma	May be complicated by immune complex disease
Hepatitis C	Blood Sexual (uncommon) Congenital (rare)	Blood precautions[2]	Chronic hepatitis (70–80%) Chronic carriage Cirrhosis Hepatocellular carcinoma	
Hepatitis D	Blood Sexual	Hepatitis B immunization Blood precautions[2]	Chronic carriage Cirrhosis Hepatocellular carcinoma Fulminant hepatic failure	Not pathogenic unless active infection with hepatitis B

Hepatitis E	Faeco-oral	Hygiene measures[1]	Severe infection in pregnancy (15–20% mortality)	
Hepatitis G	Blood Sexual (uncommon) Congenital (rare)	Blood precautions[2]	Chronic infection common but does not cause liver disease or cirrhosis	Delays progression of concurrent HIV infection

[1]Hygiene measures:
• Hand-washing
• When travelling in areas where the water supply may be subject to faecal contamination:
• Drink sealed bottled water or other bottled drinks
• Avoid ice in drinks
• Avoid uncooked shellfish
• Avoid uncooked vegetables, salads or fruits.

[2]Blood precautions:
• Use of condoms
• Avoidance of exposure to:
• Infected blood and blood products
• Contaminated needles
• Infected person's personal items (toothbrush, razor, nail clippers, etc.).

microsomal antibodies. Cirrhosis is often present at diagnosis, and indicates a poorer prognosis. Treatment is with aggressive immune-suppressive therapy.

Obstructive jaundice in childhood

Obstructive jaundice in older children is seen with choledochal cyst (see above), and gall stones secondary to chronic haemolysis or hypercholesterolaemia. Children requiring long-term parenteral nutrition are at high risk of progressive liver disease and resultant liver failure.

Fulminant hepatic failure

Fulminant hepatic failure (FHF) is fortunately rare, and manifests with encephalopathy, hepatocellular dysfunction (impaired coagulation, hypoalbuminaemia with oedema, acidosis, hypoglycaemia), renal failure and sepsis. The commonest cause in the UK is *paracetamol poisoning* (see Appendix I, p. 299), followed by fulminant viral infections. Other causes include metabolic diseases such as Wilson's disease, Reye's syndrome and disorders of fatty acid metabolism.

Wilson's disease is an autosomal recessive disorder presenting with severe liver disease, typically FHF, or in teenagers with neurological manifestations.

Reye's syndrome is an idiopathic acute encephalitis with liver failure and renal damage. Aspirin and salicylate-containing medication increases risk, and should not be given to children under the age of 16 years.

Further reading

Husby, S., et al., 2012. Guidelines for the diagnosis of coeliac disease. Journal of Paediatric Gastroenterology and Nutrition 54, 154–160.

Neurology and the senses 14

(Richard Beach, Nandu Thalange)

CHAPTER CONTENTS

INTRODUCTION

The nervous system determines how we interact with the world around us. The developing child is learning these interactions while maturing and learning. The impact of illness or injury on the nervous system will depend on age, maturity of the nervous system and developmental level. Interpreting the child's responses against this moving background is the challenge of paediatric neurology.

HISTORY

Remember to ask if the child can run, jump, climb, speak and communicate, and use toys like other children. Ask about sociability and development in the younger child, and behaviour and school progress in the older child. Take note of personality changes, particularly if they coincide with other symptoms such as headache or clumsinesss. Establish the natural history. Has the problem always been present? Did it come on suddenly or slowly? Is the child losing skills over time?

EXAMINATION

Formal neurological examination is difficult in young children. You can learn a lot by watching the child playing, moving around and interacting with carers. The examination may be opportunistic and haphazard but must be thorough. It should include pupil reflexes, fundoscopy, cranial nerve examination, arms and legs – power, tone, coordination, reflexes and sensation. With careful observation, gentle coaxing, patience and parental support it is surprising how far it is possible to get.

Keep to the schemes you know for examining the nervous system in adults and use observation and imagination to overcome the difficulties!

Neck stiffness

Neck stiffness ('meningism') in an acutely unwell child is a sign of meningitis or, rarely, a subarachnoid haemorrhage. Meningism may occur with other infections such as tonsillitis. Neck stiffness may also indicate a subarachnoid tumour in the posterior cranial fossa, or an orthopaedic problem. It should be possible to flex their chin onto their chest, or to touch their knees with their nose.

In toddlers, getting them to look up or down following a toy is helpful. When formal examination is possible lay the child flat. Cradle the head in both your hands and gently flex the neck. It is said that having the head over the edge of the bed while you support it in your hands is helpful but few children trust you that much!

Movement and coordination

- Observe the gait as children walk and run
- What are their arms doing?
- Look at their shoes for uneven wear
- Can they stand on one leg?
- Can they hop?
- Ask them to stand from lying down.

Children with Duchenne's muscular dystrophy turn themselves prone, get up on to all fours then, climbing up their legs, rise to a standing position – Gower's sign.

Limb examination

The key to this group of examinations is communicating to children what you want them to do. Use age-appropriate language and description. Demonstration helps.

Tone

Take the weight of the whole limb and gently manipulate it through a full range of movement. It may take a minute or so of movement before the child relaxes enough to make an accurate assessment.

Power

- Make this enjoyable
- 'Try and squash my fingers!'
- Compare sides
- It is difficult to assess limb power in babies and toddlers.

Reflexes

Attempt to elicit all limb reflexes and planter response. Hold the tendon hammer like a pen, relax and tap gently. A tendon hammer may be a frightening object. Percussion with the index or middle finger is satisfactory for eliciting reflexes in babies.

Muscle bulk

Wasting – this is seen in cerebral palsy and, very rarely in neuropathies and myopathies.

Hypertrophy of the calves, forearms and jaw muscles is seen in Duchenne's muscular dystrophy.

Cranial nerve examination

I – Olfactory nerve

● Ask whether the child can smell their mother's cooking or perfume. Formal examination requires use of a panel of different scents but is rarely necessary. Note that very pungent smells like ammonia can still be detected in olfactory nerve dysfunction as the trigeminal nerve also conveys olfactory fibres that detect noxious substances.

II – Optic nerve

● Check pupillary responses to light and accommodation
● Visual acuity – use finger counting or object recognition in young children and a Snellen (Visual Acuity) chart in older children.

III, IV and VI – Occulomotor, trochlear and abducens nerves

● Place one hand gently on the child's head and ask the child to follow your finger through a range of movements. Look for conjugate eye movements and any nystagmus. Does the child have a squint (Figure 14.1)?

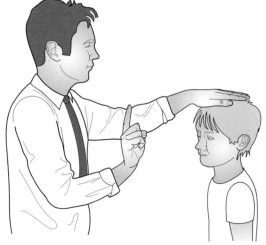

Figure 14.1 Testing the ocular muscles.

V – Trigeminal nerve
- Ask children to close their eyes and say 'yes' when you touch their forehead, cheek and chin on both sides of the face (ophthalmic, maxillary and mandibular divisions of the trigeminal nerve)
- Can they clench the teeth (palpate over the angles of the mandible) and open their mouth against resistance (deviation to the weaker side)? This tests the muscles of mastication.

VII – Facial nerve
- 'Smile please. Screw your eyes up tight. Can I see your teeth?'

VIII – Auditory or vestibulocochlear nerve
- How well do the parents think their child can hear?
- Can the child hear your wrist watch, or fingers gently rubbing? Formal hearing tests require special equipment and expertise
- A tuning fork may help diagnose conductive hearing loss (Rinne and Weber's test, Figure 14.2), but an age-appropriate hearing assessment and tympanometry (to look for normal movement of the tympanic membrane) is essential if there is any significant concen regarding hearing.

IX–Glossopharyngeal nerve
- 'Say AAAHH.' Look for uvular deviation.

X – Vagus nerve
- Is the voice hoarse?
- Is the gag reflex present? (Only do this in unconscious or poorly responsive patients.)

XI – Accessory nerve
- 'Can you turn your head and look over your shoulder?'
- 'Can you shrug your shoulders?'

XII – Hypoglossal nerve
- 'Stick your tongue out and wave it from side to side.'

Neurological investigations

All the following investigations may be alarming for children who, in any case, find it difficult to lie still. In babies and toddlers, sedation or anaesthetic may be needed. Careful preparation with parents and a play therapist is helpful.

MRI scan
This is now the investigation of choice to detect structural abnormalities in the brain or spinal cord. The scanner may be claustrophobic and frighteningly noisy for some children. The help of a play specialist, combined with sedation, is usually effective, but, in some, general anaesthesia is required.

CT scan
CT scan is largely reserved for emergency situations where a quick answer is needed, e.g. to detect brain trauma, haemorrhage, tumours and hydrocephalus. The scanner is less enclosed than the MRI, and modern scanners acquire images very rapidly. CT is more sensitive for bony lesions or intracranial calcification, but nevertheless exposes the child to significant ionizing radiation.

EEG
EEG is an important test in the diagnosis and classification of seizures but may be overused.

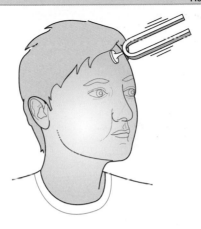

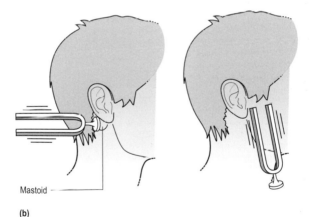

Figure 14.2 Rinne and Weber's tests for hearing loss. (a) Weber's test. (b) Rinne's test positive: air conduction louder than bone conduction (normal).

HEADACHES

Causes of headache in children are summarized in Box 14.1.

Tension headache

Case 14.1 gives an example of tension headache which is the commonest cause of headache in children. The key features are:

● Headache is present 'all the time'

Box 14.1 Causes of headache in children

- Tension headache
- Migraine
- Raised intracranial pressure (ICP)
- Referred pain from neck, ears, eyes or teeth

Case 14.1 A girl with headache

Jennifer, aged 8 years, was having headaches on a daily basis, particularly when she was at school. The headaches tended to come on after lunch, and were not associated with vomiting or visual symptoms. They improved with paracetamol and a period of rest. Jennifer described the headaches as a dull ache like a tight band around her head. Clinical examination was normal. On exploring the family circumstances more fully, it transpired that Jennifer's grandmother had been disabled after a stroke 6 months previously, and that Jennifer was frightened of visiting her grandmother, which she often used to do after school.

- Frontal or occipital headaches are described as 'like a tight band round the head'
- Long (though commonly intermittent) history
- Poor response to analgesia
- Pain worse as the day goes by
- Tearful and listless at times
- No abnormal physical signs.

The headache appears to arise secondarily to muscle tension in the neck, face and scalp which, in turn, relates to stress, anxiety and worry. The exact mechanism is unclear. Dental problems or short sight may contribute.

Teasing or bullying in school and family stress at home are common causes but children of an anxious disposition may suffer tension headache simply as a result of the stresses and strains of everyday life. With reassurance, explanation of the cause of the pain, and relief where possible of aggravating factors, spontaneous improvement is the norm.

Migraine

Migraine has been described in children as young as 2 years. The most widely accepted hypothesis is the trigemino-vascular theory. Migraineurs are hypothesized to have a hyperexcitable cerebral cortex. Focal neurological excitation is followed by cortical depression, with reflex changes in cortical blood flow; oligaemia is followed by reactive hyperaemia. Serotonin (5-HT) is a key neurotransmitter implicated in migraine pathogenesis. The migraine preventers, pizotifen and propranolol, block 5-HT_2 receptors, whereas triptans (e.g. sumatriptan), used in acute migraine treatment, are 5-HT_1 receptor agonists. The key features are:

- An episodic disorder with defined attacks
- Attacks may occur in clusters

- Visual disturbance ('aura'), prior to onset in about 30%. Sparkling lights, coloured lines, hemianopia and micropsia are typical. They precede the headache, and typically last for 5–20 minutes. Sensory symptoms such as loss of sensation, and focal motor deficits such as hemiplegia occur uncommonly.
- Incapacitating throbbing headache which may be localized to one side. In young children, headache may be absent or minor, with abdominal pain and vomiting being the most prominent symptoms ('abdominal migraine')
- Nausea, vomiting and abdominal pain
- Prostration often leading to sleep
- No abnormal physical signs after resolution.

The acute attack is best managed with rest and analgesia. Analgesia is most effective if taken very quickly after symptom onset. The earlier treatment is given, the more effective it is. In those with recurrent episodes, a food diary is helpful in identifying dietary triggers. A trigger is implicated in at least 20% of cases of chronic migraine. Triggers include prostaglandin E and the vasoactive amines, tyramine and phenylethylamine, found in chocolate, cheese and red wine. Caffeine and nitrates/nitrites (found in processed meats) are important triggers.

Medication, particularly the oral contraceptive pill, may also be a migraine trigger.

If attacks are frequent – more than once or twice a month – a prophylactic such as propranolol or pizotifen will usually reduce their frequency. Propranolol must not be used if there is a history of asthma. Treatment should be combined with avoidance of known triggers, and a good sleep routine.

In the acute situation, prompt use of simple analgesia (e.g. ibuprofen, paracetamol) at symptom onset is often effective. In those with severe symptoms, refractory to simple analgesia, triptans are appropriate.

In *status migrainosus*, in which severe migraine persists for more than 72 hours, treatment consists of rehydration and anti-emetics (e.g. parenteral metoclopramide). Triptans may be used in refractory cases.

Migraine variants

- **Complicated migraine** – neurological symptoms persist beyond the duration of headache, e.g. hemiplegic migraine
- **Basilar migraine** – most commonly seen in adolescent girls, occipital headache is associated with brain stem, occipital and/or cerebellar dysfunction (e.g. altered consciousness, vertigo or ataxia)
- **Confusional migraine** – typically in children and young adults (10–20 years), and often triggered by minor head trauma. Attacks are associated with rapid onset of confusion and agitation, but not usually headache. There is usually no recall of the period of confusion. Typical migraines later develop.

Raised intracranial pressure

Once the skull sutures have fused at about 1 year of age, any obstruction to the flow of cerebrospinal fluid (CSF) will produce increased intracranial pressure (ICP) and consequent dilatation of the cerebral ventricles. The key features are:

- Often a short history (less than 3 months)
- Morning or nocturnal headache
- Headache on moving and bending. A degree of neck stiffness may be present
- Vomiting

> ### Case 14.2 A young boy with morning headaches and unsteadiness
>
> Ben, aged 4 years, had started to complain of headaches about
> 2 months previously. He would often wake up with a headache, but
> would feel better as the morning went on. On occasion, he would
> vomit his breakfast. His parents said he was wobbly, but that he
> had always been clumsy. On examination, he had a broad-based
> gait and was mildly ataxic. There was slight neck stiffness. An
> urgent CT scan showed hydrocephalus secondary to a tumour, later
> confirmed as medulloblastoma, in the posterior cranial fossa.

- Behavioural change – irritability, lack of energy, lethargy
- Large head circumference, especially in those under 2 years of age
- Impaired visual acuity or other visual impairment
- Papilloedema – note that this is a comparatively late sign
- Sixth nerve palsy
- Abnormal head posture or head tilt
- Ataxia or nystagmus
- Poor growth.

In children over 1 year of age, the commonest cause is a tumour (as in
Case 14.2). Brain tumours are collectively the second commonest malignancy in childhood, although still rare (see Chapter 7, pp. 72–74). Other
intracranial space-occupying lesions may cause raised pressure, including
head injury resulting in subdural bleeding or effusion, particularly in infants
and young children, when non-accidental injury must be considered (see
also Chapter 5). Infectious causes include postmeningitic hydrocephalus and
brain abscess. Cerebral oedema may also cause acutely raised pressure, typically after severe head injury or encephalitis. These conditions frequently
present with altered consciousness rather than headache. An example of
raised ICP secondary to a medulloblastoma is shown in Figure 14.3.

Untreated raised ICP leads to loss of vision due to retinal damage and
eventually to unconsciousness, and finally to unstable vital signs as the
mid-brain is pushed through the foramen magnum (coning). Children
with headache and abnormal neurological signs require urgent intracranial imaging and, if necessary, neurosurgical referral.

In infants with open sutures, obstruction to CSF flow will cause rapid
head growth. This prevents very high ICPs but brain injury may still result
if this is left untreated. These children are too young to complain of headache. It is very important to monitor the head circumference, and consult
an appropriate centile chart.

Management of raised intracranial pressure

In cases of raised ICP where CSF flow is obstructed within the brain (e.g. by
congenital aqueduct stenosis in an infant or a posterior fossa tumour in an
older child) a ventriculoperitoneal shunt is usually required to relieve the
obstruction and prevent brain or retinal damage. In other cases, caused, for
example, by meningitis or haemorrhage, the obstruction is within the basal
cisterns (as in Case 14.3), the subarachnoid space or the arachnoid villi.
These blockages are commonly transient. Repeated CSF drainage by lumbar puncture will reduce CSF protein and may control CSF pressure and
head growth for a few days while the blockage resolves spontaneously.

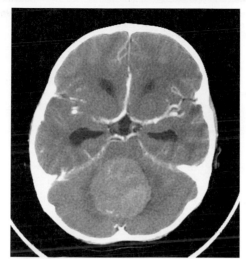

Figure 14.3 MRI scan showing medulloblastoma. A scan of a 6-year-old child presenting with a 6-week history of headache and vomiting. There is a large tumour in the posterior fossa. Medulloblastoma was the most likely diagnosis (subsequently confirmed at surgery). The ventricular system is starting to enlarge as the intracranial pressure rises.

> **Case 14.3** A girl with rapidly increasing head circumference following meningitis
>
> Lacy was admitted to hospital at 7 months of age with pneumococcal meningitis. She was treated with high-dose antibiotics and her head circumference measured daily. She remained very irritable, fed poorly, and her head circumference increased by 1.8 cm in 10 days. A CT scan carried out as a prelude to a repeat lumbar puncture showed communicating hydrocephalus. All the cerebral ventricles and basal cisterns were distended with cerebrospinal fluid. Lacy was referred to the regional neurosurgical unit, and eventually had a ventriculoperitoneal shunt inserted to relieve the raised pressure.

A ventriculoperitoneal shunt consists of a catheter which sits in a lateral ventricle, with a non-return valve located under the scalp, and a peritoneal catheter which is tunnelled under the skin to lie in the right hypochondrium. Shunts may become blocked. Children then present with headache, irritability, altered consciousness and sometimes seizures. Urgent referral for shunt revision is required. Subacute symptoms such as fever and irritability may represent shunt blockage, shunt infection or an incidental viral illness.

Epileptic and non-epileptic seizures

For management of the child with status epilepticus, see Appendix I, p. 291.

In Case 14.4 the diagnosis of day-dreaming was made because the turns were indistinct with a gradual onset and lasted a long time if the boy was not stimulated. The first-hand account is vital and can avoid the need for investigation.

Like Adam, most children presenting with seizures or turns do not have epilepsy. Indeed, children present with a rich variety of seizures and non-epileptic turns and making a diagnosis depends crucially on a careful history of the event.

Case 14.4 A day-dreaming boy

Adam was referred with possible 'petit mal' epilepsy after his teachers expressed concerns about his lack of attention in class. He would appear distant and unaware of his environment. His schoolwork was said to be falling behind. A detailed history was obtained from his classroom helper. She described 'trance-like' episodes where he seemed oblivious to his classwork. There were no abnormal movements or unconsciousness. No one saw them start – he just seemed to drift away. He could be distracted from his trance by being spoken to or nudged. A maternal uncle had a history of 'petit mal' epilepsy in childhood. Adam's neurological examination was normal.

History

It is helpful to ask the family to recall one particular seizure in detail. Use the following guide (ACOPEA) in taking a seizure history:

● **Antecedents.** What happened in the hours before the attack? Was the child well or ill, excited or calm, tired or alert?
● **Context.** What happened immediately before the attack? What was the child doing? Were there any provoking factors?
● **Onset.** How did the fit start? Was there an aura? What was the first thing the child or witnesses noticed?
● **Progression.** What was noted during the attack? Ask about colour, breathing, stiffness or floppiness, movements – what sort and where: mouth, eye, facial, limbs, etc.
● **Ending.** How did the seizure end? How long did it last?
● **Aftermath.** Drowsy? Headache? Confusion? How long before getting back to normal?

This detailed description of the episode can then be compared with the seizures and turns of childhood described in Tables 14.1 and 14.2.

Diagnosis

It should now be possible to work through the following logical sequence in the diagnosis of childhood seizures.

1. *Is it really an epileptic seizure?* Common patterns of seizures and non-epileptic events at different ages are illustrated in Tables 14.2 and 14.3. Most non-epileptic events can be managed with simple explanation and reassurance.
2. *Is it an acute symptomatic seizure?* These are seizures caused by an acute insult to a previously normal brain, such as encephalitis, hypoglycaemia or fever. Febrile seizures are a special category of symptomatic seizures (see below). Look for evidence of acute illness. If the child is unconscious see Appendix I, pp. 291–292. Check blood glucose in all children presenting with a seizure. (See Table 14.3 for the causes of acute symptomatic seizures.)

Table 14.1 Common epileptic seizure types

Seizure type	Clinical features
Tonic-clonic seizure	Rapidly unconscious. Initial tonic (stiff) phase followed by irregular jerking movements (clonic)
Focal motor seizure	Clonic movements starting in one limb or one side of the body. May spread and become generalized
Absence	Abrupt onset of altered consciousness with postural control maintained. Usually brief (less than 10 seconds) and with no motor features
Focal seizures with temporal lobe automatisms	Onset with disturbing or indescribable sensations. Children often announce the onset ('I've got my funny feelings') and seek the support of a carer. Symptoms include lip smacking, mouthing, repetitive hand movements or stereotyped behaviours
Atonic or drop attacks	Abrupt loss of postural tone leading to falls, often with facial injury
Myoclonic jerks	Sudden, brief involuntary single or multiple contractions of muscles or muscle groups

Table 14.2 Non-epileptic seizures

Seizure type	Clinical features
Infants	
Apnoea	Includes benign sleep apnoea, apnoea of prematurity and apnoea associated with illness, e.g. RSV (respiratory syncytial virus) infection
Laryngeal spasm	Reflex closure of vocal cords as a response to trivial aspiration or reflux
Benign sleep	Rhythmic symmetrical jerking of limbs, myoclonus during sleep
Preschool children	
Reflex anoxic seizure	Vagally mediated bradycardia in response to painful or shocking stimuli. Typically a fall is followed within a few seconds by pallor and collapse, usually with stiffening followed by hypotonia. There may be a few rhythmic limb jerks before recovery, which is rapid and complete
Self-gratification (masturbation)	Rhythmic movements of trunk often with limb flexion. Often flushed. Occurs when bored. Can be distracted

Continued

Pocket Essentials of Paediatrics

***Table 14.2** Non-epileptic seizures—cont'd*

Seizure type	Clinical features
Tantrums	Need no description
Blue breath holding	Starts to cry and gets respiratory arrest at full expiration. Goes blue and stiff or floppy. May suffer an anoxic seizure
Night terrors	Children disturbed at night and seem disorientated and confused. Children have no recall the next day
Nightmares	Bad dreams. May still be frightened the next day
School children	
Reflex anoxic seizures	May be precipitated by disgust or revulsion as well as painful stimuli
Vasovagal syncope	Typically, tall thin girls in hot school assemblies have these attacks, but they can occur at any age. Key features are pallor and an aura of light-headedness. There may be some jerking while unconscious
Day-dreaming	Gradual onset of vague distant behaviour with a vacant stare. May last several minutes. Associated with boredom
Non-epileptic attacks	These children are able to mimic an epileptic seizure, producing with variable accuracy the clinical features but the EEG is normal

***Table 14.3** Causes of acute symptomatic seizures*

Classification	Cause
Infections	Meningitis, encephalitis, cerebral abscess
Trauma	Head injury, non-accidental injury, post-traumatic intracerebral bleeding
Metabolic	Hypoglycaemia, hyponatraemia, hypocalcaemia usually complicating an acute illness
Vascular	Spontaneous intracerebral bleeding and stroke Hypertension

3. *Is it a febrile seizure?* In young children (6 months to 6 years) seizures may be precipitated by fever alone. Five per cent of children are affected. Typically the child has a brief, generalized, tonic-clonic seizure early in the course of an illness as the temperature is rising rapidly. It is important to exclude meningitis clinically – a lumbar puncture is rarely needed except in those under 1 year. Half of children will have a further

febrile seizure but only 10% have three or more. The risk of future epilepsy is 3%. Anticonvulsants are of limited value. Traditionally families have been advised to use paracetamol early in the course of subsequent febrile illnesses. NICE guidance in 2009 made it clear that there is no evidence to support this advice. Tepid sponging is largely impractical and may do more harm than good.

4. *Is it an isolated epileptic seizure?* Single unprovoked seizures are not uncommon in mid-childhood. They carry a 50% risk of developing epilepsy characterized by further seizures. Normally isolated seizures do not demand investigation, treatment or follow-up.

5. *Does the child have epilepsy?*

Epilepsy

Epilepsy is defined by the tendency to suffer recurrent unprovoked seizures. Epilepsy is not one condition but a wide variety of clinical syndromes from the transient and benign to those characterized by intractable seizures with neurological deterioration.

Such a complex condition demands classification to define clinically important syndromes. The broadest classification is between generalized and partial epilepsies. Generalized epilepsies typically produce seizures such as absences, drop attacks and myoclonic jerks which are associated with a generalized disturbance of brainwave activity. Focal epilepsies on the other hand are characterized by an irritable focus in one part of the brain from which abnormal brainwaves may spread to produce secondary generalization. Either pattern of EEG abnormality can produce a tonic-clonic seizure. If the cause of the epilepsy is unknown, it is described as idiopathic, but if the cause can be defined, e.g. scarring from an old head injury, it is said to be a symptomatic epilepsy. Certain patterns of epilepsy have been defined within this basic classification. These epilepsy syndromes define the aetiology, natural history, EEG appearance and therapy for many childhood epilepsies (see Table 14.4).

Table 14.4 Important epilepsy syndromes

	Syndrome	Clinical features
Generalized	Infantile spasms	See Case 14.5
	Childhood absence	See Case 14.6
	Juvenile myoclonic	Adolescents with early morning myoclonus and tonic-clonic seizures after late nights or alcohol excess
Partial	Temporal lobe epilepsy	See Case 14.7
	Symptomatic focal	Epilepsy following a brain insult, e.g. brain injury or meningitis
	Benign childhood epilepsy with centrotemporal spikes	Infrequent nocturnal partial seizures in mid-childhood Temporal spikes on EEG

Infantile spasms (Case 14.5) are the clinical manifestation of a severe epileptic encephalopathy characterized by a grossly disordered EEG – hypsarrhythmia (Figure 14.4). The syndrome is treated with steroids, unless there is coexisting tuberous sclerosis (see p. 204), in which case vigabatrin is usually more effective. Lack of response indicates a poor neurodevelopmental outcome, as in this case. Infantile spasms may occur secondary to an underlying congenital or metabolic disorder.

The boy in Case 14.6 has childhood absence epilepsy – an idiopathic generalized epilepsy. Simple absence seizures develop between 5 and 10 years. The treatment of choice would be sodium valproate, lamotrigine or ethosuximide and the condition often resolves in later childhood.

The girl in Case 14.7 is having focal seizures with temporal lobe automatisms (semi-purposeful, repetitive movements like fumbling with buttons). Her awareness at the onset and subsequent tonic-clonic seizure illustrate the progression of the EEG abnormality across the brain. There is an epileptic EEG focus in the right temporal area and an MRI scan shows right-sided temporal lobe changes (mesial temporal sclerosis affecting the right hippocampus). If these seizures fail to respond promptly to anti-epilepsy medications then a referral for epilepsy surgery should be considered.

Case 14.5 A baby with funny movements and developmental arrest

Hannah was seen in the outpatient department at 10 months of age after concerns from her health visitor about her lack of developmental progress. Her mother reported that Hannah also had frequent jerks. For example, on awakening from sleep on her mother's knee, she might without warning throw her head forwards and jerk her arms out. She would slowly relax and start to cry before a second spasm occurred. There could be seven or eight such spasms over 2 minutes. An urgent EEG was arranged and showed a chaotic EEG ('hypsarrhythmia') confirming the clinical diagnosis of infantile spasms. A follow-up MRI scan showed multiple hamartomas, typical of tuberous sclerosis (see 'Neurocutaneous syndromes', later in the chapter). Hannah responded poorly to treatment and subsequently had intractable seizures with profound developmental delay.

Case 14.6 A boy with blank spells

Joshua, a 7-year-old boy, presented after his teacher expressed concern about his concentration. Parents described absence attacks. The onset was abrupt. He stopped what he was doing and stared blankly. The turns lasted about 5 seconds and there was instant recovery. There were no abnormal movements. It was possible to trigger an attack in clinic on getting Joshua to hyperventilate. The EEG demonstrated bursts of 3 per second spike wave activity (see Figure 14.5).

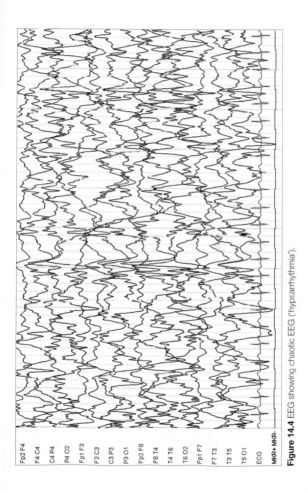

Fp2 F4
F4 C4
C4 P4
P4 O2
Fp1 F3
F3 C3
C3 P3
P3 O1
Fp2 F8
F8 T4
T4 T6
T6 O2
Fp1 F7
F7 T3
T3 T5
T5 O1
ECG
MKR+ MKR-

Figure 14.4 EEG showing chaotic EEG ('hypsarrhythmia').

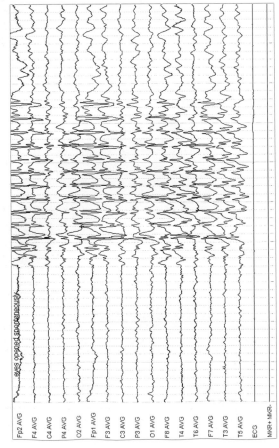

Figure 14.5 EEG showing generalized 3 Hz 'spike and wave' activity.

> **Case 14.7** A girl with abnormal movements and confusion
>
> Emily, a 9-year-old girl, experienced disturbing attacks. She would often announce their onset: 'I am having one of my heads'. She clutched her mother or father, then seemed vague and distant with mouthing and swallowing movements and confused semi-purposeful hand movements. Sometimes the seizure moved on to a tonic-clonic phase. In the past she had suffered febrile seizures, two of which were prolonged, but she had been seizure-free for 4 years before these attacks.

Management of epilepsy

After accurate diagnosis the family will need plenty of information both on the epilepsy and on the likely effects on the child's lifestyle. Safety and first aid advice are important but it should be possible to maintain relatively unrestricted activities. Liaison with the school is necessary and an epilepsy care plan should be arranged. Drug therapy will be advised when the morbidity from seizures seems to outweigh the possible side-effects of medication.

The prognosis of epilepsy depends on the syndrome diagnosis or the underlying cause. Childhood absence epilepsy usually resolves during childhood. Juvenile myoclonic epilepsy usually requires lifelong treatment. Sudden unexpected death in epilepsy (SUDEP) is rare. The risk from accidents and drowning can be reduced by sensible safety advice. SUDEP can occur even in young people with mild epilepsy but it is commoner in those with poor control and multiple seizures.

Families and professionals can find out more about epilepsy on the epilepsy action web site at: http://www. epilepsy.org.uk.

CHRONIC NEUROLOGICAL DISABILITY

Introduction

Neurological disability affects 1% of children. These children can be divided into two groups – those who deteriorate with time and those who do not. Most of these children have an unchanging neurological problem such as cerebral palsy or learning difficulties. It is essential to distinguish those children with progressive disorders. Children generally get more able as time passes. Be alert to any suggestion of children losing skills. Key symptoms are:

- Difficulty moving
- Slow development (see Chapter 8)
- Sensory impairment (see 'Hearing' and 'Vision' later in the chapter).

Difficulties with movement

Difficulties in control of movement may arise in the brain (upper motor neurone) or peripheral nervous system (lower motor neurone) (Figure 14.6). These can usually be distinguished clinically (Table 14.5). In either case, deteriorating conditions must be detected by careful history taking and investigation if necessary.

Abnormalities of central motor control – cerebral palsy

The motor control systems within the brain are complex and susceptible to malfunction caused by congenital brain abnormalities or acquired damage

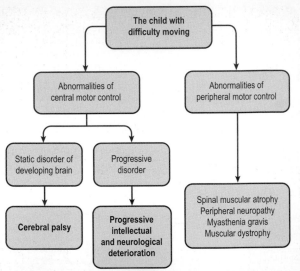

Figure 14.6 Classification of motor disability.

Table 14.5 Clinical features of motor disorders		
	Upper motor neurone	**Lower motor neurone**
Power	Normal or reduced	Reduced
Tone	Typically increased but can be normal or may reduce with repetition	Reduced
Reflexes	Increased	Reduced or absent
Plantar responses	Usually up-going	Down-going or absent
Chorea or athetosis	Sometimes present	Never present
Ataxia	Occasional	Never – but may be confused with weakness

to the developing brain. The various patterns of movement that result are described as cerebral palsy. Cerebral palsy (CP) is defined as a persistent, although not unchanging, disorder of movement caused by abnormalities arising early in life affecting the motor control systems in the brain.

Cerebral palsy is classified by the type of motor abnormality observed (spasticity, chorea, athetosis, dystonia, ataxia) and, if relevant, the parts of the body involved, e.g. spastic diplegia (see Table 14.6).

There are four major types of cerebral palsy as illustrated in Cases 14.8 to 14.11.

Case 14.8 An infant with spastic hemiplegia

George presented at 9 months because his parents were worried about his right arm. The limb was held stiffly and largely unused. Pregnancy and birth history were unremarkable and general development normal. On examination the hand stayed fisted and the elbow flexed. He ignored the right arm and reached past with the left hand to grasp toys. Sitting balance was normal but the tone and reflexes were increased in the right leg and he went up onto his right toes on standing.

Table 14.6 Classification of cerebral palsy

By type of movement disorder	
Spasticity	Stiff muscles with high tone
Athetosis	Unwanted writhing movements
Chorea	Unwanted jerky movements
Dystonia	Variable tone associated with athetosis
Ataxia	Shaky uncoordinated movements
By parts of the body involved	
Hemiplegia	Involves the arm and leg on one side
Quadriplegia	Also called whole-body cerebral palsy
Diplegia	Involves four limbs but legs are more severely affected
Monoplegia	Rare – look carefully for abnormalities in the other limbs

Hemiplegia (65% of CP) typically presents between 6 and 10 months. Birth history is usually normal – it is thought the unilateral brain abnormality develops in early pregnancy, perhaps as a result of a vascular occlusion. In Case 14.8, George will learn to walk – even if this is a little delayed. Associated problems, including learning difficulties, seizures and behaviour problems affect about a third of children and may result in complex disability.

Spastic quadriplegia (10% of CP), or whole-body cerebral palsy (Case 14.9), may result from birth events, although severe congenital brain

Case 14.9 A baby with whole-body cerebral palsy

Helen suffered a severe neonatal encephalopathy with seizures and was ventilated for 4 days. Although the encephalopathy resolved she had never been neurologically normal. At 1 year of age she struggled to achieve useful head control. Her arms and legs were stiff and she was unable to feed. She had spasms of her back muscles when she was upset (extensor spasms) which made it difficult to get her into a seat or chair. She continued to suffer seizures.

Case 14.10 A toddler with spastic diplegia

Timothy was being followed up after a spell on a neonatal intensive care unit following delivery at 29 weeks' gestation. Initially all was well, but at about 6 months corrected age, parents and professionals noticed some odd postures of the trunk, poor head control and delayed sitting. By 2 years the diagnosis was clear, with high tone in the legs and only minor impairment of arm function. He walked on his toes with feet turned in.

---

anomalies cause a similar clinical picture. The associated problems of learning difficulties and epilepsy affect most children when the disability is profound. Long-term complications include a 'windswept posture', hip dislocation, scoliosis, gastro-oesophageal reflux and recurrent chest infections.

Spastic diplegia (20% of CP) is the classic abnormality after preterm delivery (Case 14.10), although most children with diplegia have an unknown cause. Inherited forms (X-linked and dominant) are recognized.

Choreoathetoid, or dystonic cerebral palsy (as in Case 14.11) (5% of CP), is rare. Neonatal bilirubin encephalopathy is the classic cause of this type of cerebral palsy but many cases are idiopathic and a few are familial. Deafness is a common association. Intelligence is often normal.

Case 14.11 A boy with choreoathetosis

Ahmed was a 10-year-old boy with choreoathetoid (dystonic) cerebral palsy. Voluntary movement was difficult for him because of continuous writhing and jerking movements of the limbs and trunk which got worse when he was excited or attempted a task. The same movement problem reduced speech to poorly articulated sounds and hindered chewing and swallowing. He was supported in a purpose-built chair and harness. Careful attention to support and switching allowed him to drive his own electric chair. The same switch-gear enabled an electric communicator and access to a computer for schoolwork. Feeding difficulties were overcome by use of a gastrostomy tube.

Progressive intellectual and neurological deterioration

The child who is losing skills presents a worrying clinical picture. Causes include space-occupying lesions and severe epilepsies, and children with severe emotional and physical neglect, as well as a host of extremely rare metabolic disorders.

Progressive central nervous system disease may present in infancy (as in Case 14.12), childhood or adolescence. Earlier presentations are more severe. Intellect, motor skills, vision and behavioural control may all be lost. Seizures may occur. The cause is often a metabolic or storage disease but some are idiopathic. The prion disease, new variant Creutzfeldt–Jakob disease, remains very rare.

Case 14.12 An infant with loss of motor milestones

Jacob was referred aged 15 months with declining motor skills. He initially developed normally, but having learned to sit, crawl and pull to stand by 10 months of age, he was now unable to do any of these things. On examination he had marked truncal hypotonia with spasticity of his limbs. He did not babble or interact, and did not appear to fix his gaze, although his pupils were reactive to light. The combination of progressive developmental decline with spasticity suggested a central degenerative disorder. White cell enzyme studies showed a severe deficiency of arylsulphatase A, confirming the diagnosis of metachromatic leukodystrophy. Jacob continued to decline, and died of an intercurrent chest infection aged 4 years.

While the progression of intellectual and neurological deterioration can rarely be halted, referral to a specialist centre is vital. Specific enzyme replacement therapy is available for some conditions, and others are amenable to bone-marrow or stem-cell transplantation.

Abnormalities of peripheral motor control – the weak and floppy child

When the pathology of a movement disorder lies in the muscles, the peripheral nerves, the motor end plate or the anterior horn cell within the spinal cord, the resultant clinical picture is of weakness and low tone. The key clinical features in these cases are weakness, which is often progressive, and absence of limb reflexes. Many cases are inherited (see Figure 14.7).

In Case 14.13 the diagnosis of *infantile-onset spinal muscular atrophy*, also known as Werdnig–Hoffman disease (a recessive condition), was made on DNA analysis. It is incurable and invariably fatal in the first 3 years of life, with the majority dying before their first birthday. Caitlyn quickly deteriorated and died less than a month later of respiratory failure. There may be a 1 in 4 recurrence risk, and genetic counselling is essential. Note that cervical fracture secondary to non-accidental injury may present similar clinical features.

Case 14.13 A baby with severe weakness and respiratory distress

Caitlyn, a 5-month-old baby, presented with poor head control and lack of arm movement. She appeared alert. Delivery was normal and a 6-week check raised no concerns. On examination she had profound hypotonia and slipped through the examiner's hands like a rag doll. She was unable to move her arms or legs against gravity. Intercostal muscle weakness resulted in abdominal breathing. On close inspection her tongue was fasciculating. The limb reflexes were absent.

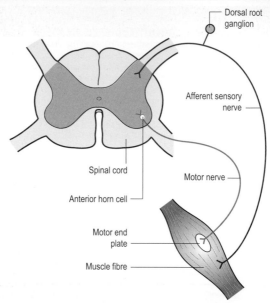

Figure 14.7 Schematic illustration of site of peripheral motor abnormalities.

Duchenne muscular dystrophy (Case 14.14) is a slowly and inexorably progressive condition. It is an X-linked recessive condition due to large mutations in the dystrophin gene and so only affects boys. Presentation is typically between 3 and 7 years of age, with lordosis, waddling gait and Gower's sign. Calf muscle hypertrophy follows within 1–2 years. The majority of boys need a wheelchair by 12 years. About 1 in 3500 boys are affected, worldwide, with 20% of cases arising as de novo mutations. Diagnosis can be quickly obtained by measuring creatine kinase (CK) which is hugely elevated. Genetic confirmation and counselling is necessary for carrier females. Twenty per cent of boys have associated learning difficulties. Careful physical therapy and support is needed to prevent postural deformity and maintain function. Oral steroids have been shown to significantly slow the progression of muscle weakness, and maintain ambulation, on average by an additional 2–3 years.

Trials of novel gene therapies are in the very early stages.

Cardiac surveillance with annual echocardiography is needed, as progressive cardiomyopathy develops in the teenage years. ACE (angiotensin-converting enzyme) inhibitors are usually effective in relieving symptoms. Life expectancy is markedly shortened, with death usually in the third decade from cardiac or respiratory failure.

While some neuromuscular conditions can now be diagnosed by DNA analysis a muscle biopsy may still be necessary for accurate diagnosis. This procedure demands highly specialized pathological analysis and should be carried out in a specialist centre.

Freddie, a 4-year-old boy, presented because of frequent falls. Early motor development was normal but in recent months he had been more reluctant to climb stairs or walk over uneven ground. The family were alarmed because he was finding it difficult to get up after falling. On examination he had absent reflexes and bulky calf muscles. Weakness of proximal muscles was illustrated by his difficulty in flexing his hips to ascend stairs and his use of Gower's manoeuvre in rising from the floor. The CPK (creatine phosphokinase) was very high at 5342 IU (normal range 50–150 IU), suggesting Duchenne muscular dystrophy. This was subsequently confirmed on genetic analysis of the dystrophin gene. Sadly, Freddie's younger brother was also affected.

Myasthenia gravis (Case 14.15) is rare. Think of it when weakness is variable, with deterioration during the day, especially with intermittent diplopia and difficulty chewing or swallowing. It is often associated with other autoimmune diseases.

Acetylycholine receptor antibodies are present in 80–90%. Seronegative patients often have antibodies to muscle specific kinase. Those with striated muscle antibodies are more likely to have an associated thymoma.

The mainstays of treatment are acetylcholinesterase inhibitors (most commonly pyridostigmine) and immunomodulatory therapy (prednisolone – usually combined with steroid sparing agents such as azathioprine or cyclosporin; intravenous immunoglobulin, anti-CD20 monoclonal antibody, plasmapheresis, thymectomy).

Infants born to affected mothers are at increased risk of postural deformities (arthrogryposis multiplex) and congenital myasthenia gravis.

Neurocutaneous syndromes

There are a number of neurological conditions associated with cutaneous manifestations. Two disorders account for the majority of presentations: neurofibromatosis and tuberous sclerosis. These conditions are dominant but show variable penetrance. The subtle diagnosis in a parent may not be made until a more severe clinical picture is diagnosed in the child.

Case 14.15 A teenager with diabetes and progressive weakness

Chris, aged 14 years, had suffered from diabetes for 8 years. At his annual review, he complained of variable muscle weakness, which was gradually getting worse. The hallmark was that he was well in the morning but his symptoms of weakness progressed through the day. Physical examination showed rapid fatigue but he was otherwise normal. His acetylcholine receptor antibody level was found to be markedly elevated, and the diagnosis of myasthenia gravis was made by electromyography.

In *tuberous sclerosis,* hamartomas occur throughout the brain and also commonly occur in the heart and kidney. Epilepsy and variable mental retardation may result. Infantile spasms (see p. 194) carry an especially poor neurodevelopmental prognosis. Cutaneous signs include small oval depigmented patches, *ash-leaf macules,* which fluoresce under ultraviolet light, hard leathery *Shagreen patches* in the lumbosacral region, and acne-like lesions, *adenoma sebaceum* on the face.

Two types of *neurofibromatosis* are recognized. Both are inherited in an autosomal dominant fashion.

Type 1 neurofibromatosis (NF1) results from mutations in the NF1 gene on chromosome 17 (>95%). The gene product, neurofibromin, is a tumour suppressor. Reduced levels of neurofibromin predispose to myriad different features. Mutations in SPRED1 also give rise to a phenotype of neurofibromatosis with café-au-lait patches and axillary or inguinal freckling, but other features do not develop. Incidence is estimated at about 1 in 3000 individuals, but milder cases are not recognized, and this is undoubtedly an underestimate.

NF1 is characterized by progressive development of café-au-lait patches (greater than 5 mm in children under 10 years, or >15 mm in children over 10 years, satisfies one of the major criteria for clinical diagnosis), axillary or inguinal freckling and cutaneous neurofibromas. Characteristically, children have relative macrocephaly. Learning difficulties (40%), hyperactivity and seizures may occur. There is remarkable phenotypic heterogeneity, even in the same family. Children with this condition are prone to tumours of the nervous system and other organs.

Neurofibromas are less common in childhood, often appearing at adolescence. Plexiform neurofibromas are problematic, and may grow to huge proportions. If complete resection is feasible, this is the preferred option, but radical debulking is an alternative. Malignant peripheral nerve sheath tumours and neurosarcomas may also arise in teenagers. These are often very difficult to treat, but newer agents such as sorafenib which target the Ras pathway have shown promising results.

Children require annual opthalmological review in early childhood, as optic gliomas may affect vision, and are most likely to develop before age 6–7 years.

Annual blood pressure screening is also recommended, as hypertension may result from renal artery stenosis or phaeochromocytoma.

Orthopaedic abnormalities are common, including scoliosis, pseudo-arthroses and pathological fractures. Scoliosis is usually mild, but there is a subset of children with early-onset scoliosis in whom aggressive treatment is necessary.

Type 2 neurofibromatosis (NF2) is less common (about 1 in 35 000–40 000) and cutaneous manifestations such as café-au-lait patches and neurofibromas are unusual. Commonly, the diagnosis is not made until late teenage years or adulthood. The principal manifestation is with bilateral acoustic neuromas, and other brain and spinal cord tumours. Acoustic neuromas typically present with tinnitus, vestibular symptoms and hearing loss. In contrast to NF1, cataracts often occur. It arises from mutations in NF2 on chromosome 22. The gene product, merlin, is a tumour suppressor. Half of all cases arise de novo.

Sturge–Weber syndrome describes the association of a facial angioma ('port-wine stain') in the ophthalmic division of the trigeminal nerve with an ipsilateral leptomeningeal angioma, most commonly parietal or occipital, resulting in epilepsy (70–90%) and sometimes stroke-like episodes or permanent hemiplegia. Low-dose aspirin may reduce the frequency of stroke-like episodes. Congenital glaucoma (buphthalmos) affects over 30%.

An isolated port-wine stain without an underlying intracranial vascular malformation or glaucoma is not uncommon, particularly if the opthalmic division of the trigeminal nerve is spared. Mental retardation affects 50–75%. Although the lesions are static, the neurological sequelae may be progressive, with cerebral atrophy on the affected side. Effective seizure control improves outcome. Epilepsy surgery may be indicated.

In older children, migraine-type headaches are commonly reported (40–50%), and may be severe. Scoliosis and body asymmetry are commonly seen in older children.

Laser therapy may be used for port-wine stains, and is more effective when started at an early age (ideally in infancy). Skin camouflage is very effective in disguising lesions and may help self-confidence and self-esteem. The British Red Cross offer a free skin camouflage service.

Bell's palsy

Children present with an acute unilateral lower motor neurone facial weakness – the onset is rapid, often over a few hours or overnight. The hallmark is unilateral lower motor neurone facial paralysis, affecting the entire side of the face. The involvement of the forehead distinguishes Bell's palsy from upper motor neurone facial palsy, in which the forehead (frontalis) and eye (orbicularis oculi) are spared. The right side is affected in over 60% of cases. It is uncommon in children (10–15 per 100 000 per year). It may cause weeping of the eye due to lack of blinking, or dribbling due to failed lip closure. It is believed to arise from nerve injury arising from compression secondary to inflammation and oedema, as the nerve traverses the facial canal in the petrous temporal bone. There is growing evidence for an infectious aetiology, with herpes simplex and varicella most commonly implicated.

In the first instance, careful examination is required to exclude other neurological features. Swelling of the parotid may indicate inflammation or tumour affecting the facial nerve. The presence of contralateral limb weakness or diplopia may suggest a stroke or other central cause. Diabetes and hypertension are recognized associations. A history of tick bite may suggest Lyme disease, particularly if the facial palsy is bilateral.

Treatment with steroids (prednisolone 1 mg/kg, maximum 60 mg for 6 days) to reduce postulated facial nerve swelling is most effective if started within 3 days of onset. Evidence from randomized trials in adults suggests that use of antivirals (e.g. aciclovir) either alone, or in combination with steroids, is no better than placebo treatment in improving outcome. There is some evidence that specific facial exercises may be beneficial. It is important to protect the cornea by eye-patching at night and with the use of artificial tears. Eighty to ninety per cent make a spontaneous complete recovery within 6 weeks to 3 months. Patients not showing some recovery by 2 weeks should be referred for specialist evaluation.

Guillain–Barré syndrome

Guillain–Barré syndrome is an acute demyelinating polyradiculoneuropathy. In its classic form, it presents as an ascending flaccid paralysis of arms and legs with areflexia. However, a subset of patients (~30%) have *increased* reflexes. Pain and dysaesthesia are commonly reported, but objective sensory loss does not occur. Autonomic neuropathy may develop, with resultant tachycardia, and less commonly tachyarrhythmias. Urinary retention affects 10–15%. The majority of cases of Guillain–Barré syndrome are in boys (60–70%).

Since the demise of polio, Guillain–Barré syndrome is the commonest form of acute motor paralysis in children. It follows a respiratory or gastrointestinal infection in two-thirds. *Mycoplasma pneumoniae* and *Campylobacter jejuni* are most consistently associated with Guillain–Barré syndrome. Serology for *C. jejuni* is positive in 50% of paediatric cases. Immunization may be a trigger of Guillain–Barré syndrome, and has been reported with a range of vaccines, notably certain types of influenza vaccine used in Europe.

Guillain–Barré syndrome is believed to arise from aberrant T-cell targeting of neural antigens. *C. jejuni* is particularly strongly associated with the Miller–Fischer variant of Guillain–Barré syndrome in which cranial nerve palsies and ataxia also feature, and antibodies to GQ1b ganglioside are typically found.

Inflammation of spinal roots leads to disruption of the blood–brain barrier, with a resultant increase in CSF protein, used as a diagnostic test. CSF protein may be normal at onset, but is elevated in the great majority by 10 days into the illness. Lumbosacral MRI with gadolinium enhancement shows abnormal enhancement of the nerve roots. Electromyographic studies are similarly best left to the second week of illness, when they will be diagnostic. Antibody tests may be helpful in Guillain–Barré syndrome variants when diagnosis is more problematic.

Treatment consists of supportive measures, including ventilation if respiratory failure supervenes. Thromboprophylaxis is advisable for non-ambulant children. Children more commonly develop respiratory failure than adults, but respond better to immunomodulatory therapy with immunoglobulin infusion being the mainstay of treatment. Plasmapheresis may be used in refractory cases. Full recovery is the norm, but it is a lengthy process, taking 6–12 months.

Spinal cord tumours

Spinal cord tumours are mercifully rare, but difficult to diagnose. They arise from either the spinal cord itself (medullary tumours) or its sheath, the dura mater. Progressive sensory and motor dysfunction arises from spinal cord compression. Precise symptoms depend on the location of the tumour. Pain is a prominent feature due to venous engorgement in the region of the tumour. Medullary neoplasms (most commonly, astrocytomas, ependymomas or haemangioblastomas) account for 10% of paediatric CNS tumours. Lumbar puncture may be associated with severe deterioration, and should only be undertaken under expert guidance for specific diagnostic purposes. Surgery is necessary for diagnosis and treatment. Radiotherapy may be useful for metastatic or inoperable tumours.

HEARING

Hearing is important for normal development. Impaired hearing presents at different ages and with different causes. Hearing loss may be conductive – due to impaired middle-ear function – usually glue ear, or sensorineural due to impaired cochlear or acoustic nerve function.

Causes of permanent hearing loss

- **Genetic causes.** These account for about half of permanent deafness. Some genetic causes are progressive, and only become apparent postnatally. Usually, deafness is non-syndromal, but in about 40–45% it is part of a wider syndrome. The range of conditions affecting hearing is very diverse, they are individually very rare.

- **Antenatal causes (10–15%).** These include exposure to teratogens (e.g. alcohol, cocaine) and congenital viral infections, notably cytomegalovirus (CMV).
- **Perinatal causes (10–15%).** Prematurity, need for intensive care, significant jaundice and exposure to aminoglycoside antibiotics are all risk factors for deafness.
- **Postnatal causes (10–20%).** Postnatal deafness is primarily a consequence of infection (notably meningitis) or trauma. Rarely, ototoxic medication such as furosemide or aminoglycosides is implicated.

The baby

Universal screening of all newborn babies in the UK was implemented in March 2006. The screen uses oto-acoustic emission screening, with brainstem audiometry used to confirm permanent sensorineural hearing impairment (PSNI). Treatment in the first instance is with hearing aiding, but cochlear implants are necessary if hearing loss is severe. Previous targeted screening missed 50% of cases, with resultant poor outcomes. Groups at high risk of PSNI include premature infants, particularly those who were given aminoglycoside antibiotics, infants with craniofacial abnormalities and babies born to a family with a family history of hearing impairment.

The infant

Hearing loss in this age group is usually identified by the parent. The child may not turn to sounds, or, at an older age, respond to their name being called. Their language development is delayed. Since the advent of universal hearing screening, the health visitor distraction test (7–9 months of age) is no longer performed.

The child at school

Poor school performance or behaviour may indicate a problem. Speech delay is another common presentation. Screening at school entry picks up some cases. See Table 14.7 for assessment and diagnosis of hearing loss.

Table 14.7 Hearing loss and testing		
Age	**Diagnosis**	**Assessment**
Neonate	Aminoglycoside toxicity Congenital infection – CMV, rubella Hypoxia associated with birth or prematurity Genetic	Otoacoustic emission Brain stem evoked potential
Child	Otitis media/chronic secretory otitis media (glue ear) Trauma Meningitis	Parental questionnaire Visual reinforcement audiometry Pure tone audiometry Speech discrimination test

Chronic secretory otitis media (glue ear)

Glue ear is the commonest cause of a conductive hearing loss in childhood. The child's Eustachian tube is less vertical than in an adult, so it drains less readily. This causes a middle-ear effusion. If chronic, this fluid becomes thick and tenacious like glue.

For many, glue ear is a self-limiting condition that requires no management, other than explanation and reassurance to the family. Steroid nasal sprays may be beneficial in improving symptoms. In children with a persistent hearing, ventilation tubes ('grommets') may be appropriate. Grommets are small tubes sited in the tympanic membrane. They equalize the pressure between the middle and outer ear. This allows aeration of the middle ear, and resolution of the effusion with resultant improvement in hearing. Adenoidectomy is often performed at the same time as the insertion of grommets. Adenoidal hypertrophy is common. Large adenoids narrow the posterior nasal space. This may affect the functioning of the Eustachian tube.

The grommets remain in situ until they fall out as the tympanic membrane grows. Children are able to go swimming with grommets, but should be discouraged from submerging their heads or diving. Ear plugs are useful for baths or showers, to prevent ingress of dirty or soapy water.

Deafness (as in Case 14.16) is classified according to the level of impairment (Table 14.8). The impact of this loss on a child is not always easily determined.

Supporting deaf children

The goal of supporting the deaf child is to ensure they are functionally integrated into their family, school and the wider world. This requires an approach tailored to the individual needs of the child and family.

Hearing aids

Hearing aids help many deaf children. However, some children find them intrusive and are reluctant to wear them. Cochlear implants are increasingly used for severe PSNI.

School-age children struggle within the noisy environment of a classroom and special provision may be necessary. Specialist teachers working within a sensory support service are invaluable. Speech and language therapy input to assist communication is vital. Learning to sign is appropriate for some.

Table 14.8 Classification of deafness

Diagnosis	dB loss
Mild	30–50
Moderate	50–70
Severe	70–90
Profound	>90

Case 14.16 A boy with deafness after meningitis

Liam, aged 2 years, was admitted to hospital 3 weeks previously with bacterial meningitis due to *Streptococcus pneumoniae*. Shortly after admission, his mother noticed that he seemed unable to hear her voice. Liam recovered from his meningitis and went home, but there was no recovery in his hearing. Testing revealed that Liam had profound deafness. He subsequently received a cochlear implant.

VISION

Most visual defects in childhood are correctable. Serious defects in vision are rare. Parents are usually good judges of their child's visual acuity but referral to an orthoptist or ophthalmologist is necessary for accurate diagnosis.

Refractive errors

Myopia (short-sightedness)

This usually presents in school-age children. It is uncommon in the younger age group. Glasses may be necessary for significant defects.

Hypermetropia (long-sightedness)

This is commonly diagnosed as a result of investigation for a squint. Children struggle to visualize near objects and compensate by converging their eyes to accommodate.

Astigmatism

This refers to a difference in the optical power of the cornea in different planes. It results in a distorted image. Glasses correct the defect.

Squint

Squints are common. They can be divided into paralytic and non-paralytic types.

Paralytic

These squints are caused by nerve palsy. Rapid evolution suggests sinister pathology. The clinical appearance depends on the cranial nerve involved. Management focuses on identifying where and why that nerve has been affected.

Non-paralytic

Aetiology of these squints varies:
- When associated with ocular disease, it may be the result of:
  - Refractive error
  - Corneal or lens opacities
  - Retinal abnormality
  - Hypermetropia
- Normal eyes – the acquisition of a squint in children with normal eyes is not well understood.

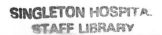

Diagnosing squints

Referral to an orthoptist is sensible for any child in whom there are any concerns about squinting. Their assessment will include:

1. Detection of a manifest squint

    The *cover test* detects manifest squints.

    The right eye is covered while the child's attention is fixed on a near object. The left eye is watched. If the left eye moves out to fix on the object then there is a convergent squint. If the eye moves in, there is a divergent squint.

    The cover is removed from the right eye and placed over the left. If the right eye moves outwards then there is a convergent squint, if it moves inwards a divergent squint is diagnosed.

2. Detection of a latent squint

    The *alternate cover test* detects latent squints.

    The cover is moved rapidly from one eye to the other while observing which eye fixes. The cover is then placed over the right eye and then removed. The movements in this eye are watched. If the eye moves inwards a latent divergent squint is present and if the eye moves outwards a latent convergent squint is diagnosed.

3. Other

    Visual acuity, eye movements and ophthalmoscopy. It is important to remember that epicanthic folds and facial asymmetry can mimic a squint.

Managing non-paralytic squints

Any refractive error should be corrected. Patching of the good eye helps stimulate the squinting eye and prevents amblyopia, with resultant improvement in visual acuity. Surgical realignment may be required, principally for cosmetic purposes.

Visual impairment affects many aspects of development (as shown in case 14.17). The motor skills may be delayed as children are unaware of their surroundings and have no desire to explore. Language development suffers because there is limited association between what the child hears and the object the child perceives. Parents find it difficult to know how best to interact and play with their child and this may further slow developmental progress. Subsequently the assessment and management of children with a severe visual impairment requires a specialist service. Developmental assessments are difficult. Accurate diagnosis is vital. It is unlikely that the impairment can be treated, but other health or developmental problems may be identified as a result.

See Box 14.2 for causes of severe visual impairment.

Box 14.2 Causes of severe visual impairment

- Retinoblastoma
- Retinopathy or prematurity
- Neonatal encephalopathy (cortical blindness)
- Trauma
- Congenital infection

Progressive loss of vision

Some children are born with normal visual acuity and lose it over time. The most devastating loss is a sudden one. Causes include trauma and retinoblastoma. Gradual losses can be accommodated gradually. The impact depends on the nature of loss – whether it is central or peripheral. Causes include the retinal dystrophies and Batten's disease, which is also associated with progressive intellectual and neurological deterioration and fatal outcome.

Case 14.17 A blind child

Alicia was born prematurely at 25 weeks' gestation. Routine screening of her fundi revealed retinopathy of prematurity. Despite aggressive management with laser therapy, she developed bilateral retinal detachment. It was clear by 6 months of age that she was blind. Much of Alicia's development had been delayed, although it was difficult to establish what aspects of her development were delayed by her visual impairment alone. Aged 18 months, her parents felt she was 'slow and unresponsive' and that 'We spend ages playing with her but she doesn't seem that bothered'.

The white eye

Retinoblastoma

Retinoblastoma is a tumour of photoreceptor cells with an incidence of 5 per million, almost all cases developing before the age of 4 years. The majority occur as sporadic cases but an autosomal-dominant inherited form exists due to deletion of the Rb gene on chromosome 13. Bilateral disease is uncommon in the sporadic form but occurs in up to 70% of genetic cases. Diagnosis is suggested by the finding of a white pupil ('leukocoria') and confirmed by detailed ophthalmoscopy under general anaesthetic (as in Case 14.18). Treatment involves localized cryotherapy with or without lens-sparing radiotherapy for small lesions and enucleation of the orbit for more extensive disease. Adjunctive chemotherapy is required for advanced disease.

Cataracts

A cataract may be detected at birth, or may develop subsequently. The parents notice a 'white eye'. The absence of the red reflex is a key indicator. Cataracts are one of the causes of visual impairment amenable to treatment. Removal of the lens and insertion of prostheses or the use of contact lenses is required. The causes of cataract include congenital infections and inborn errors of metabolism.

Case 14.18 A girl with a 'white eye'

Amie, aged 3 years, was seen after her mother noticed that her right eye sometimes appeared to have a white pupil. The eye did not react to light, and appeared blind. Retinoblastoma was diagnosed after examination under anaesthesia, and Amie underwent enucleation of the eye, with insertion of a prosthesis.

The red eye

Conjunctivitis

A diffuse redness of the conjunctiva is seen. This may or may not be associated with discharge.

There are viral, bacterial and allergic causes. Viral conjunctivitis is common in childhood. It is associated with a clear discharge and it resolves spontaneously. Bacterial conjunctivitis presents with purulent discharge. Allergic conjunctivitis presents with an itchy eye. Identifying the allergen and antihistamines are helpful.

Neonatal eye infection

In the neonatal period, consideration needs to be given to the possibility of herpes simplex, *Gonococcus* and *Chlamydia* as causative agents. *Gonococcus* in particular may cause rapid destruction of the eye and requires combined topical and parenteral antibiotics. It is a notifiable condition (ophthalmia neonatorum). 'Sticky eyes' are common in the neonatal period. If sticky eye persists for 3–4 days after birth, empirical treatment with topical antibiotics such as chloramphenicol may be indicated. *Chlamydia* swabs should be taken in an appropriate transport medium. Persistent sticky eyes may be due to inadequately treated infection, or more commonly, occlusion of the nasolacrimal duct. Treatment involves nasolacrimal massage and wiping away any debris. If necessary, the duct may be probed surgically under anaesthesia.

Glaucoma

Glaucoma in children is most commonly congenital. It typically presents in early childhood with the classic triad of lacrimation, photophobia and blepharospasm, all secondary to corneal irritation. The eye may enlarge – buphthalmos (bull's eye). Treatment is surgical.

Orbital cellulitis

In periorbital cellulitis, there is erythema and tenderness around the eye, face and eyelid. It is imperative to exclude orbital cellulitis with an appropriate examination of the eye and eye movements. This may require ophthalmological advice. The cause is bacterial and antibiotics are necessary.

Orbital cellulitis presents with a painful eye, sometimes proptosis, and decreased eye movements. These children are systemically unwell. They may experience a visual loss. Assessment with a CT scan of the orbit and prompt intravenous antibiotics are essential.

Iritis

Inflammation of the anterior eye may accompany a range of connective tissue diseases, most commonly juvenile idiopathic arthritis (see Chapter 6, p. 55). Presentation may be acute with a painful red eye, photophobia and lacrimation, or chronic with insidious loss of vision. The pupil may appear irregular, and the anterior chamber may appear cloudy or contain debris on slit-lamp examination. Complications include cataract and glaucoma. Treatment is with steroid eye drops with or without antiviral or antibiotic treatment.

The mind 15

(Nishi Puri, Nandu Thalange)

CHAPTER CONTENTS

INTRODUCTION

All children are different. Part of this difference is seen in how they behave.

Health professionals are asked to judge behaviour and decide if it is normal. This may be difficult. At all times our thoughts must be based on the wider view of that child and who they are.

HISTORY

Taking a behaviour history gives a doctor insight into functional as well as neuropsychiatric disorders. The information largely needs to be gathered from the parents, but this gives only one perspective. The family has already made a judgement about the behaviour – that is why they have come to the clinic. It is important to seek the opinions of others who know the child well, e.g. siblings, grandparents, teachers and other professionals; the mother may see the child's behaviour as irritating, while the friend sees it as good fun, the teacher sees it as enthusiastic and the grandparent sees it as lacking discipline. Do opinions tally? Is the concerning behaviour limited to one setting?

Ask the parents what they have done to try and resolve the problems; what has worked, and what has not. Talk to the child. Even very young children should be engaged. They may tell you things that others might not know. Bear in mind that you are unlikely to discover all that is important at the first meeting. Consider children as 'barometers' of the social context in which they live. Talking to siblings is invaluable and frequently sheds light on family dynamics. The family's focus on one child's behaviour may signal unacknowledged problems in other family members, including marital problems, or indeed the child may be made a scapegoat for these problems.

Transient behaviour problems occur in most children, and most resolve. Some children get stuck. Try to establish what it is about the child and their family that prevents them moving on.

EXAMINATION

Organic disease from constipation to brain tumours may present with problematic behaviour. On occasion, the abnormal behaviour leads to physical ill health, e.g. anorexia nervosa. A child's physical features may give clues about their behaviour. For example, a number of chromosomal disorders, such as fragile X, Prader–Willi and Klinefelter syndromes (see Chapter 18, Table 18.2) have particular behavioural characteristics. If necessary, any investigations should ideally be done at the beginning to identify physical health problems.

TANTRUMS

What are tantrums?

Toddlers like being 'in charge' (as can be seen in Case 15.1). This desire is often thwarted by their abilities and the limits set by their parents. For example, 2-year-olds may want to eat their meal with their parents' cutlery although they do not have the fine motor skills to do so, or their parents may prevent them from adding tomato sauce to their ice cream, for example.

Case 15.1 A 'naughty' girl

Daisy is 3 years old and her parents were anxious about her 'extreme mood swings'. Daisy would not follow her parents' instruction: 'We ask her nicely but she just ignores us and if we try and make her, she goes rigid and falls to the floor'. Daisy had started to vomit during these episodes.

Her father thought that these episodes might be fits, and when they happened he gave Daisy a cuddle and comforted her. Her mother tried to ignore her but felt she had to intervene when she vomited: 'I can't ignore her if she's sick'.

This lack of control causes frustration, and tantrums may follow. This is normal behaviour between the ages of 1 and 4 years.

Tantrums are usually dramatic. Crying, screaming, dropping to the floor and thrashing of limbs are common. Some children are able to induce vomiting. Occasionally these episodes may be mistaken for seizures. The key distinction is a history of provocation and the complex pattern of behaviours seen in tantrums.

Tantrums may be seen in children who receive inconsistent messages from different parents, and may in a sense mimic their parents' behaviour. Note that children, despite appearances, never really want to 'win the war' – to do so would be very frightening as it would affirm their own power and destructiveness.

Management

Is advice necessary?
Before giving parents advice on how to manage tantrums, stop and think. More advice has been given and received about tantrums than most other topics in paediatrics. Is advice what the family want? If you have not established what the family's expectations are, then now is a good time to do so. For some, all they want is an opinion as to whether or not these episodes are tantrums. It may be a way of alerting the doctor to other emotional problems in the family. Be prepared to listen

Are you the best person to advise?
Most people who seek advice about the management of tantrums do not see a doctor. There is a good reason for this: there are many other sources of knowledge and information on this subject, e.g. health visitors who may be able to offer greater support to the family

What advice has been given before?
If particular strategies did not work, establish why. A detailed minute-by-minute account of what happens before, during and after each tantrum will help determine this.

Specific strategies

Reasonable expectations
Have a reasonable expectation of what the child is able to comply with. Excessive expectations of a child may occur with parents who themselves have unmet needs.

Ignore bad, praise good
Children want responses to their tantrums. If no reaction is gained they get bored and eventually the behaviour stops. If good behaviour is greeted with cuddles and praise, the child will seek this sort of response again. Sanctions should quickly follow bad behaviour as delayed punishment is confusing to the child and ineffective.

Time out
Place the child alone in a safe environment to calm down. This works well if used for short periods. Usually only a few minutes is required.

Consistency
Consistency of approach is crucial. Children like certainty and respond badly to the parent reacting differently on different days. They find it confusing and their poor behaviour is perpetuated. Worse, they may simply learn to read (and manipulate) their parent's mood state, rather like a traffic light signal, instead of learning to understand the world around them.

Win sometimes

Allowing a toddler to be successful in their unreasonable demand is sometimes OK. There are some battles not worth having. Parents should only insist on compliance if able to carry out behaviour management to a successful conclusion. Anyway, only an angel or a behaviour therapist can be consistent all the time! It may be sensible to start with one specific behaviour. Do not choose the supermarket as the first arena. If the child behaves in one setting, generalization to other settings will usually follow.

Support

With the changing structure of society and families, many parents feel unsupported in managing behaviour problems. Other primary care professionals and voluntary agencies may be able to help. Befriending with emotional and material support may make the difference for vulnerable families between viability or not of the family unit.

HYPERACTIVITY

What is attention deficit hyperactivity disorder?

The girl's condition in Case 15.2 is an example of attention deficit hyperactivity disorder (ADHD) which is a triad of *inattention, impulsivity* and *hyperactivity*, with *impairment* of social or educational functioning as a consequence. In order to make the diagnosis, these difficulties should be seen before the age of 7 years and usually much younger. The patterns of behaviour need to be chronic (of at least 6 months' duration), pervasive – i.e. they affect the child in two or more situations, such as at home, at school, or with grandparents and friends – and cause functional impairment.

> ### Case 15.2 A girl who is always on the go
>
> Lauren is 7 years old and had always been 'hyperactive'. She found it difficult to concentrate on much, other than her computer. Her parents were worried about her schoolwork and her schoolteachers felt she was not fulfilling her potential. She was easily distracted in the classroom and found it difficult to sit at her table. Lauren liked school but got bored easily. She acted without thinking. She had recently been excluded from school for thumping a boy who had teased her.

The triad of impairments

- **Inattention.** The child:
  - Has difficulty concentrating
  - Moves quickly from task to task
  - May appear disorganized and forgetful.
- **Impulsivity.** The child:
  - Interrupts conversations
  - Has a 'short fuse' and there are regular outbursts of temper
  - Finds taking turns difficult.

- **Hyperactivity.** The child:
  - Is restless and fidgety
  - Struggles to sit still
  - Is always fiddling with things.

What is not ADHD?

The history should not only focus on identifying the key behaviours but should highlight other biological or psychiatric explanations that might mimic these behaviours (see Box 15.1).

In children, levels of activity and attention vary. This is related to age (lower in younger children), gender (worse in boys), environment and intelligence. These factors need careful consideration before labelling behaviour as ADHD. For example, in preschool children it is difficult to be certain that any pattern of behaviour represents ADHD. Many children who appear to be significantly hyperactive or inattentive at 3 or 4 years of age settle dramatically after starting school. Parental tolerance also varies. Factors such as the availability of additional welfare benefits or support may influence parental expectations. Do the parents show ADHD symptoms? Is there a dispute with the school over responsibility for conduct problems?

Family history

Family, twin and adoption studies show that ADHD has a strong genetic component. Also, later children in large families are at higher risk. One of the parents may report a similar pattern of behaviour as a child. Understanding that a parent has ADHD will help them and the child.

Making a diagnosis

ADHD, as yet, has no biological marker. No neuroimaging, genetic or metabolic studies make the diagnosis. The diagnosis is made on history and observation alone.

Information must be sought from a number of sources. This is important to establish the pervasiveness of the problem. Direct contact with the school is necessary. This information gathered may include the use of *Connors' rating scales*. These are standardized questionnaires that help identify significant patterns of behaviour.

Management

Understanding ADHD

Educating the child, the family and the school about what ADHD is a crucial first step. Increasingly, schools will be familiar with the issues. Indicating to the child's school what their ADHD-related strengths and weaknesses are is helpful.

Box 15.1 Mimics of ADHD behaviours	
Biological	**Psychiatric**
Hearing impairment	Autistic spectrum disorders
Visual impairment	Parenting problems leading to insecurity
Epilepsy	Post-traumatic stress disorder

'Medicalizing' patterns of behaviour, such as with ADHD, can send the wrong message to the child and family about how those difficulties have arisen and what should be done to help. It also places the doctor in the position of being the one to produce change. A wealth of written and electronic material is available to assist in communication.

An important aim is to assist the child in gaining benefits from education, the maintenance of a circle of friends, avoidance of being seen as simply 'naughty', and protection of family relationships.

Behavioural therapies

This attempts to modify the unhelpful behaviours. Praising good behaviour works and it needs to be immediate. Children with ADHD are unable to wait long for their reward.

Medication

Stimulant medication such as methylphenidate has had wide coverage in the worldwide press. Rightly, many groups are uncomfortable with young children being given amphetamine-based drugs. However, the 2009 NICE guidelines have recommended the use of these drugs as first-line treatment for severe ADHD. Non-stimulant drugs like atomoxetine are reserved for second-line treatment. Atomoxetine has been associated with suicidal ideation.

The mechanism of action of these drugs is via effects on dopamine neurotransmission.

For moderate ADHD, psychosocial/social intervention in the form of parent training/educational programmes should be used. If there is no response to the behavioural intervention then medication will be indicated. The ideal management course is often a combined approach of medication and behavioural therapy. The latter may be more easily utilized if children are more focused after medication.

Other

- **Diet.** It is reasonable to suppose that what children eat affects their behaviour. Epidemiological research indicates a link between additives and preservatives in the diet and levels of hyperactivity (e.g. McCann et al. 2007). A small proportion of children may be helped by a carefully applied exclusion diet. Many parents are keen to attempt dietary manipulation. A registered dietician can support this. It is important that dietetic support is provided by an appropriately trained dietitian, as there are a variety of 'nutritionists' offering services privately, often with little scientific foundation.
- **Long chain fatty acids.** Long chain fatty acids are suggested as being helpful in a number of behavioural and developmental disorders. There is some evidence that they improve ADHD behaviours.

AUTISTIC SPECTRUM DISORDERS

In recent years the diagnosis of autistic spectrum disorders has become more common. Parental anxiety about autism has been further raised by controversial reports allegedly linking the measles, mumps and rubella (MMR) vaccine with autism and inflammatory bowel disease. Despite the overwhelming evidence of MMR's safety, vaccination rates have fallen.

Case 15.3 describes a boy with autism and demonstrates some of the key features of the autistic spectrum.

Case 15.3 A boy who likes to be by himself

Jack is a 3-year-old boy. His parents were worried about his behaviour and speech. Jack only used one word 'Thomas', and showed no response when spoken to. He enjoyed playing with his Thomas the Tank Engine train set and liked grouping together the track and engines into separate piles. Jack preferred to play alone. He spent ages opening and closing the kitchen cupboard doors. He repeatedly rocked his body and flapped his arms. He was sensitive to loud noises and screamed and cried until they stopped.

Key features of autistic spectrum disorders

The key features begin before 3 years. They are *impaired social functioning*, *impaired communication*, *repetitive behaviours* and *stereotyped movements*. Diagnosis before 18 months may be difficult, but, in retrospect, parents may well recall very early concerns. Boys are more commonly affected.

Impaired social functioning

Children with autistic spectrum disorders struggle to interact meaningfully with the world around them and may appear aloof and indifferent. Interaction with peers and adults is on their own terms and initiated by themselves.

Impaired communication

Both expressive and receptive elements of language are impaired. Some children may never develop language and their language skills may be abnormal. Echolalia, the parrot-like repetition of words or phrases or even whole chunks out of story books, is classic, although rare. The normal intonation of speech may be absent. In severe cases, non-verbal communication with gesticulation or pointing may also be absent.

Repetitive and restricted behaviours

Children with autistic spectrum disorders do not like change. They develop routines and rituals for their day. They may be thrown by any unexpected change such as a new route to the shops. Their interests are restricted, e.g. the colour of cars or types of door handle. An 'obsession' with tractors for months may be followed by an equally intense interest in road traffic signals.

Normal children frequently develop special interests, but do not become obsessional to the exclusion of all else and their imaginative play is unaffected.

Stereotyped behaviours

Flapping, rocking and clapping movements are sometimes seen, especially if distressed. Tiptoe walking may be a feature.

The autistic spectrum

The patterns of behaviour characteristic of autism are the extreme end of the autistic spectrum. Less severely affected children show clear overlap with normal behaviour, and it may be more appropriate to describe these children as having *autistic traits*. Making a clear diagnosis in this area of overlap is difficult.

Asperger's syndrome

Autistic spectrum disorders without significantly impaired language skills, but with social impairment, may be described as *Asperger's syndrome*. Some sufferers even show gifted intelligence in particular areas, such as music, art or arithmetic.

Assessment and diagnosis

A detailed history from the parents usually highlights areas of concern. It is important to seek information from other professionals who know the child. These might include the health visitor, GP or a carer at the nursery.

Formal diagnostic tools are available to assist with diagnosis. Appropriately trained clinical psychologists, paediatricians or child psychiatrists usually conduct these.

Causes of autism

These patterns of behaviour are increasingly being recognized as attributable to a medical cause. Genetic markers for autism have been identified but are not yet useful as a diagnostic tool.

One widely regarded theory is that part of the problem can be explained by the child's lacking a sense of others having a separate point of view (theory of mind). Without that understanding, interpersonal relationships are impossibly confusing and the child withdraws.

Being a 'bad parent' is never a cause of autism. Acquisition of good expressive language by the age of 5 years indicates a reasonable prognosis.

Intervention

Intervention begins with early diagnosis. Interagency agreement about diagnosis and joint planning of intervention is essential (see also Chapter 3, p. 20). Key individuals include speech and language therapists, educational and clinical psychologists, specialist nurses and ideally an identified key worker to help the family negotiate the bureaucratic maze. Special schooling may be necessary. Transition to adult services is often fraught, as support is much less readily available.

DEPRESSION

> ### Case 15.4 A sad teenager
>
> Laura, aged 14 years, presented to her GP with somatic complaints. The GP perceptively noted that these followed the death of her grandmother. Chronicity of the symptoms and school absence prompted the doctor to suggest depression as the cause, but the family was reluctant to accept a psychiatric referral so she was referred to the paediatric clinic.

What is depression?

The resilience of children to cope with stress, including bereavement (as in Case 15.4), is dependent on the child's previous experiences coupled with the number and severity of other problems they have to face. A seemingly minor event may be more significant for a child than the parents realize (e.g. the death of a pet, loss of a friend) and normal sadness gives way to depression. There may be a family history of depression. Symptoms include diurnal variation in mood, being worse in the morning, irritability, low energy, poor self-esteem and thoughts of suicide. Interviewing the child may well elicit symptoms otherwise unknown to the parents. Poor appetite, sleep problems and other psychiatric conditions may be present.

Management

An experienced psychologist may be able to further clarify the diagnosis with the aid of appropriate rating scales. These can also be used to monitor progress. Psychological therapies are usually effective. Current NICE guidelines (October 2005) recommend cognitive behavioural therapy (CBT) for mild to moderate depression in adolescents (<18 years). Antidepressants should be used in conjunction with CBT in severe depression or if the patient is unwilling to try psychological intervention. CBT is used to explore the child's recurrent negative thoughts about self-worth and possibilities for change. Behavioural management includes maintaining activity and social contacts. Antidepressants should only be used under the direction of a child and adolescent psychiatrist.

DELIBERATE SELF-HARM

Whereas only a minority will be seriously mentally ill, all children and adolescents who self-harm deserve careful professional assessment. Thoughts of suicide are relatively common but are less often acted upon. Self-harm increases in the adolescent years, especially in girls. Poisoning is the commonest method; however, self-harm resulting in death is very uncommon. Repeated self-harm attempts are not uncommon. Ten per cent will harm themselves again within a year.

Good liaison needs to be established between the acute paediatric unit and the local Child and Adolescent Mental Health Service (CAMHS) which are likely to be seeing several such cases each week. A member of the CAMHS team should assess all children with self-harm, whether admitted or not.

The CAMHS team will explore what background factors are relevant, including family or peer problems, other social and emotional stressors and child abuse. Family members will need to be seen. Gentle enquiries by paediatric staff can help, but intrusive questioning should be avoided, especially if sexual abuse is suspected. Early disclosures may be subsequently withdrawn if not carefully handled. However, most patients will volunteer recent social stressors, express embarrassment, and declare a wish to not repeat the behaviour. Most will describe an immediate precipitant – typically a row – indicating a lack of serious forward planning.

SCHOOL REFUSAL

Difficult transitions in childhood can precipitate the onset of behaviour which presents to the doctor as 'illness' (as in Case 15.5). Perhaps it is better to view the child as stuck in a 'predicament' that brings him to professional attention.

Boys and girls in equal measure may try to avoid going to school, sometimes by playing truant, sometimes through symptoms of illness ('somatization'). School refusal usually boils down to anxiety about change, separation from parents and family conflict, or fear as a result of bullying

> **Case 15.5** A boy who does not like school
>
> Edward had been at high school for one term. At the start of the spring term he had had a week off with tonsillitis and had been reluctant to go back to school since then. He perked up at the weekend, but by the Sunday evening complained of a sore throat and felt too unwell to go on the Monday morning. The more he was challenged, the more it seemed that his conduct was manipulative of his exhausted parents. His father thought he needed a firm hand but his mother disagreed.

and, perhaps, for the health or safety of a parent. The parents are often ambivalent about school, which may contribute to the child's sense of insecurity and anxiety. The child may be grieving or depressed. Bullying, or fear of a particular lesson, may play a part, but changing the school regime or even changing school often fails to solve the problem.

The term 'school phobia' has been used, despite the fact that the child is not usually phobic about school. Nevertheless, getting the child back into school as quickly as possible is often the best way to overcome the problem, demonstrating to the child and family that school is not as bad as anticipated. Good liaison with the local education welfare service is essential. The child and parents need reassurance that it is medically safe to go to school. Addressing underlying separation anxiety or family problems, or an entrenched pattern of non-attendance, may require the skills of a child psychiatrist. Return to school is the norm, but more anxiety or phobic problems may emerge in later life.

Truancy

School refusal is distinct (at least in theory) from truancy, which is a term referring to a child who, for example, leaves home in the morning *as if* to go to school, but decides to do something more interesting instead. Social truanting with others may lead to delinquency. Isolated truants are more likely to be emotionally disturbed or otherwise unhappy or distressed.

CHRONIC FATIGUE SYNDROME/MYALGIC ENCEPHALOMYELITIS

> **Case 15.6** A boy who is tired all the time
>
> Ben was 12 years old. He had not been to school for 4 months. His tiredness started 9 months before with a throat infection that his GP thought was glandular fever. His mother was concerned that his immune system was not working properly and that that was why he was so tired. She thought he needed investigating. Ben was worried about becoming more active as he had started to feel a little better recently and thought he might relapse. Ben's school had stopped sending work home for him since his parents had arranged a home tutor.

Definition

Chronic fatigue syndrome/myalgic encephalomyelitis (CFS/ME) is defined as medically unexplained fatigue of at least 3 months' duration (as in Case 15.6). Post-exertional malaise and unrefreshing sleep are characteristic.

Causes of CFS/ME

The process by which some children develop chronic fatigue is poorly understood. It probably arises through a combination of biological, psychological and social factors.

Diagnosis

The diagnosis of CFS/ME should be considered in any child with persistent or, less commonly, recurrent symptoms of fatigue, often with post-exertional malaise, and consequent reduction in activity levels. The majority of children fall into three distinct symptom complexes:

- **Musculoskeletal:** prominent symptoms of muscle/joint pain with hypersensitivity to touch. Fatigue symptoms are usually more severe in this group.
- **Headache:** headaches with hypersensitivity to noise and light are prominent, usually associated with nausea, abdominal pain and dizziness. Anxiety symptoms are common. This subtype is associated with lower school attendance.
- **Sore throat:** symptoms of sore throat and lymphadenopathy, with lesser degrees of fatigue and malaise.

Investigation

It is important to investigate cases of fatigue carefully. Exclusion of medical causes for the symptoms must occur before embarking on managing the problem as CFS/ME. This certainly includes a detailed history and examination. It usually involves investigations such as full blood count and iron stores, electrolytes, kidney, liver and thyroid function.

It is important to ask the child and the family what their ideas are about this illness. Addressing these ideas and beliefs is a crucial step in the management. Explore the child's social anxieties as there may be hidden problems impeding recovery.

Management

General principles

It is important to formulate an individualized management plan, in conjunction with the child/family. In addition to the mainstays of treatment, graded exercise therapy and/or CBT, the plan should address the patient's specific symptoms. Pain symptoms are often prominent, but commonly poorly responsive to analgesia, and referral to a specialist pain team may be needed. Disordered sleep with poor sleep hygiene, may aggravate daytime fatigue and should be addressed within the management plan. The plan should set out specific care and treatment for symptom relapse, and support the child's educational and psychological needs. The plan should be reviewed regularly. Failure to respond adequately should prompt referral to a specialist CFS/ME service.

Graded exercise therapy

A structured increase in physical activity helps to alleviate the symptoms of fatigue. This should include a planned increase in school attendance.

This programme needs to be agreed by the child, the family and the school. The rate of increase in activity is not important. However, every step up should be maintained. Some aspects of this programme, particularly any exercise elements, may benefit from the supervision of a physiotherapist and/or occupational therapist.

Cognitive behavioural therapy
This aims to change a child's thought processes, behaviours, physiological responses and environment. It requires a skilled therapist to use this to target the thoughts and overt behaviours that might be perpetuating the symptoms of fatigue.

Outcome

The great majority of children recover, but this may take time. Many miss significant amounts of school and take years to regain full levels of activity. Co-morbid features such as school refusal and depression worsen the prognosis if not adequately addressed.

SUBSTANCE ABUSE

> #### Case 15.7 A boy smoking dope
>
> Tom was 15 years old and had been excluded from school. He was caught smoking cannabis at the bottom of the school playing field. His parents were concerned that his habit would lead to a wider drug problem and wanted to find Tom some help with giving up. Tom did not see what the problem was: 'Dad smokes and they both drink – that's more harmful than what I do'.

Children and adolescents are exposed to a variety of legal and illegal substances and the health effects vary. Rarely, acute intoxications of drugs or alcohol lead to hospital admission. Usually these behaviours do not precipitate immediate health problems, but can be the start of dependency or addiction that persists into adult life. The commonest substances used are tobacco and alcohol. Other than marijuana, illicit drug use under 16 years is relatively uncommon. As Case 15.7 illustrates the issues around these behaviours are complex both for families and society.

Smoking

In 2009 the proportion of English children who reported smoking at least one cigarette a week was 6% in those aged 11–15. Almost one-third of the children had tried smoking at least once. Girls were more likely to be regular smokers, and the prevalence increased with age. The health risks of smoking are well established but the incidence of smoking has remained static. Children start smoking for a number of reasons. The attitudes of their peers and siblings strongly influence children. The smoking habits of their parents similarly contribute to how socially acceptable it is for the child to smoke. Children whose parents smoke are more likely to start smoking. Children themselves report that tobacco advertising influences their decision to start smoking and which brands they smoke.

Alcohol

Regular alcohol consumption is common in older children. In 2009, 18% of boys and girls in England, aged 13–15 years, reported drinking alcohol in the past week. This proportion has decreased from 26% in 2001. Among those who drank, mean consumption in the past week was estimated as 11.6 units per week, with no significant difference between boys and girls. Drunk children are at risk of accidental injury and alcohol poisoning. Unplanned and unprotected sex may occur.

Cannabis

Cannabis is by far the most common illegal substance used by children. Since 2001 there has been a decline in cannabis use from 13.4% to 8.9% in 2009. In England and Wales, approximately 9.8% of boys and 8.1% of girls have tried the drug. The risks of cannabis are increased by regular and heavy use. This appears uncommon in children. Cannabis may cause a range of mental health problems, including acute anxiety and psychotic states.

Advice and support

National initiatives such as 'Connexions' and 'Talk to Frank' provide useful information to young people and families about these issues. Local support varies. For more significant drug use either in terms of frequency or substance, support from adult-orientated drug and alcohol services may be of help. Child and adolescent mental healthcare services may be similarly helpful.

Always consider the reasons why a child has become involved in these behaviours. To many children, drinking, smoking and cannabis use is part of 'growing up'. To others it may represent an escape from a difficult family or social circumstance. These children may at least need advice and support, and some will need protecting.

EATING DISORDERS

Food refusal

Some infants and young children persistently fail to consume adequate food, which affects their growth and development. It is usually helpful to view this as the outcome of subtle interactive difficulties between parent and child. Careful observation of feeding times, coupled with a detailed family history, will help discover the broader issues. Help for the parents, as well as the child, will need to be organized if problems persist.

Anorexia nervosa

Anorexia nervosa usually presents with insidious weight loss, often with excessive exercise and always with deception around food intake (as in Case 15.8). The child may like cooking and food, but denies having an appetite. Anorexia nervosa is much commoner in girls (the male to female ratio is 1:10), with as many as 1% of adolescent girls being affected. The characteristics are *inappropriately low body weight* (<15% under expected weight-for-height), *intense fear of fatness*, even when weight loss is achieved, and *disordered body image*, usually with accompanying physical sequelae such as amenorrhoea.

Pocket Essentials of Paediatrics

> ### Case 15.8 A girl who thinks she is fat
>
> Lucy is 14 years old. Her mother had taken her to see the doctor
> because she was uncertain about her daughter's weight loss.
> Lucy had been a little chubby 6 months previously, but had lost
> significant weight since then. The mother was initially rather
> pleased, as she herself had never been comfortable with people
> who over-eat. Lucy had started to refuse to sit down for any family
> meals. She exercised whenever she could, and had become very
> prudish about being seen undressed. The doctor discovered that
> she had been taking laxatives without her mother's knowledge.
> Lucy insisted all was well but half admitted to relationship problems
> with her friends at school.

Self-esteem is low, but the child usually denies emotional difficulties. The widening social life and sexual challenges of adolescence may well present the child with overwhelming anxiety, and a need to regain a sense of control over her life and her body. Denial of food stands symbolically for mastery over emotional turmoil.

Examination should include repeated weight measurements (at least weekly) in underwear and on the same scales. Where possible, female staff should weigh and measure. Lanugo hair may be seen. Blood pressure and the body mass index should be recorded.

Management involves stabilization of weight and exploration of the control issues beyond the food obsession. Confident handling reduces anxiety in both child and parents. Beware of the parents who are excessively enmeshed in the child's problems and who subtly undermine and frustrate the therapeutic regime.

The management of anorexia should be supervised by a child psychiatrist. Early referral and treatment is important. Partnership between paediatric services, child psychiatry/psychology and primary care is needed.

Cognitive therapy can be useful in challenging the child's mistaken negative thoughts about herself. Inpatient care should be avoided unless essential. It may be needed to stabilize weight. Wherever treated, advise on realistic weight for age, and target rates of gain (not to be exceeded or under-achieved) should be set for gradual improvement over a period of weeks. It is vital to address the child's underlying feelings. Low mood is common but usually resolves with weight gain.

Bulimia and binge eating disorder

This involves the eating of large amounts of food, followed by a sense of guilt, lack of control, and sometimes induced vomiting. The psychological dynamics may be similar to those for anorexia. Treatment for bulimia requires more intensive input, and is essentially similar in outline to the management of anorexia. Binge eating – i.e. uncontrolled eating, not characterized by induced vomiting – usually responds well to cognitive behavioural therapy.

TICS

Tics are repetitive, sudden motor movements. They may mimic expressive movements and frequently involve the face. Tics are common during childhood and may be prominent at times of stress or anxiety. About 10% of children develop tics. Usually nothing more than explanation and reassurance are required.

Tourette's syndrome is a state of chronic motor and vocal tics that begins in childhood. It has high co-morbidity with obsessive–compulsive symptoms. ADHD is similarly frequent. A child psychiatrist usually supervises management. Medication may be helpful.

Useful resources

Connexions http://www.connexions-direct.com.

Frank http://www.talktofrank.com.

McCann, D., Barrett, A., Cooper, A., et al., 2007. Food additives and hyperactive behaviour in 3-year-old and 8/9-year-old children in the community: a randomised, double-blinded, placebo-controlled trial. Lancet 370 (9598), 1560–1567.

Royal College of Psychiatrists. Mental health information and growing up. http://www.rcpsych.ac.uk.

Infectious disease and immunity 16

(Richard Beach, Nandu Thalange)

CHAPTER CONTENTS

INTRODUCTION

The newborn infant is immunologically naive, protected only by its inheritance of maternal antibodies and its inexperienced immune system. Babies and toddlers have to acquire immunity to a whole range of infections which they do by catching one illness after another.

Immunization protects children from a range of deadly infections (see Chapter 1, p. 3 for UK immunization schedule), but a 4-year-old can still expect 6 to 10 illnesses per year – usually viral. Thus, infectious disease is ubiquitous in children. In many countries, diseases such as measles and gastroenteritis remain major causes of death, especially when combined with malnutrition.

The challenge for the doctor is to sort the benign and self-limiting viral infections from those few deadly infections, such as meningitis, septicaemia and pneumonia, which are rightly feared by parents and doctors alike.

HISTORY

Symptoms of infection are often non-specific, especially in the early stages. Parents may describe children as not like their normal selves, listless, lethargic or not feeding well. Use direct questions to tease out the timings of fever, rash and other symptoms. Where did the rash start? Has it changed? How did it spread? Reluctance to eat or drink may indicate a sore mouth or throat, and children may rub miserably at a sore ear. Do not forget that these diseases may be infectious so ask about family contacts and friends with similar symptoms.

EXAMINATION

Examining the febrile child with an acute illness is always a challenge but with patience and gentleness a full examination is possible. Examining the ears and mouth and throat is essential but best left until last as it often upsets the fractious toddler. Look carefully for a rash and check if it is purpuric.

Rashes are often the reason for seeking medical advice. Most are non-specific, blanching, maculopapular rashes of viral origin, typically varying over time. Rarely, such rashes are the first signs of serious illness, such as meningococcal septicaemia, so always recommend that parents return if they are concerned their child is deteriorating, and show them how to check for non-blanching spots with a glass tumbler.

Non-blanching rashes are highly concerning. Petechiae are less than 1 mm in diameter and may signify bacterial infection but are common in viral illnesses where observation for a minimum of 4 hours is recommended. When present in the distribution of the area drained by the superior vena cava, look for causes of raised intrathoracic pressure – principally prolonged coughing or vomiting. Purpura (spots greater than 1 mm) in a child who is unwell and who has a temperature should be taken as evidence of meningococcal septicaemia and treated as an emergency (see Appendix I, p. 288).

Palpate the lymph nodes and spleen. Check carefully for a stiff neck but do not forget that this sign may not be present in children less than 1 year old. Check vital signs carefully – capillary refill, pulse, blood pressure, temperature and respiratory rate. Septicaemia and shock may complicate acute infections. Remember that falling blood pressure is a late sign. A tachycardia should be a cause for concern – there must always be an explanation.

INVESTIGATIONS

A urine sample is always important but not always easy to collect (see Chapter 11, p. 118). Take swabs from vesicles, purulent lesions and weeping skin. There are different swabs and transport media for bacteria, viruses and *Chlamydia* – make sure that the right one is used.

A throat swab is sometimes useful in sore throats but always important in meningitis where growth correlates with cerebrospinal fluid (CSF) findings. Lumbar puncture is the gold standard test for diagnosing meningitis and should be considered whenever meningitis remains a possible diagnosis. There is a small but significant risk of coning (see Chapter 14, p. 188) if lumbar puncture is performed in acutely ill infants. In these circumstances, delayed lumbar puncture is safer (see Box 16.1).

For lumbar puncture results and interpretation see meningitis, below.

Box 16.1 Contraindications to lumbar puncture

- Signs of raised intracranial pressure or depressed or abnormal conscious level
- Abnormal coagulation (platelets below 50 x 10^9/L)
- Respiratory distress
- Shock or signs of poor perfusion
- Recent seizure (within 30 minutes) or prolonged seizure (over 30 minutes)
- Focal seizures or focal neurological signs

ACUTE FEVER

It is often hard to be certain of the cause of infection in children who are acutely unwell. Are there signs of a serious infection? Check carefully for pneumonia and meningitis, or other features of sepsis such as impaired capillary refill, tachypnoea or tachycardia. In hospital practice it is usual to screen for any major infection. This septic screen usually includes blood culture, full blood count, ESR (erythrocyte sedimentation rate) or C-reactive protein (CRP), urine culture and a lumbar puncture. Collecting these samples before antibiotic administration improves the chances of growing an organism and clinching the diagnosis. Children screened for serious bacterial sepsis are usually, although not invariably, treated with antibiotics pending CSF and blood cultures.

Is there an upper respiratory tract infection? Otitis media and tonsillitis are very common, and it is crucial to look at the throat and ears carefully. Children with tonsillitis might appear surprisingly unwell. Think of urinary tract infection – collect a clean catch specimen for local and laboratory testing.

Is there a history of foreign travel? Infections such as malaria or viral haemorrhagic fevers may only become manifest after return to the UK.

If the child is not very ill, a wait-and-see approach is an acceptable policy. The rash in many viral infections may follow hours or days of fever.

POSSIBLE MENINGITIS

Unconscious or drowsy children should be assumed to have meningitis or encephalitis. Irritability implies cerebral irritation and may be hard to distinguish from children who are simply feverish, frightened and miserable. A smile, some desultory play or even well-organized objection to examination is reassuring. Children with a high-pitched cry or who cannot be comforted are of concern. Seizures with a fever are usually febrile seizures in children aged 6 months to 5 years (see Chapter 14, p. 190) but meningitis, encephalitis and brain abscess may also cause seizures – especially in infants.

Investigation

In Case 16.1, the clinical diagnosis is meningitis. The likely causes are listed in Table 16.1. Early treatment may be life-saving, and antibiotics should be given as soon as possible. Intramuscular or intravenous penicillin can be given by GPs or paramedics. In hospital, intravenous cannulation will allow blood for blood culture, blood count and clotting studies to be drawn before the first antibiotic dose is given. Lumbar puncture – provided there

---

Case 16.1 A boy with meningitis

Faisal, a 15-year-old boy, presented with a 2-day history of sore throat, fever and headache. He was brought in by ambulance having suffered a generalized seizure at home. On examination he was drowsy and combative. His temperature was 38.5°C. He was well perfused with normal blood pressure and a pulse of 130 beats per minute. He had marked neck stiffness.

Table 16.1 Organisms causing meningitis

Age	Pathogens	Treatment
Neonatal period (birth-28 days)	*Streptococcus* group B *Escherichia coli* Other coliforms *Listeria monocytogenes*	Amoxicillin and gentamicin or cefotaxime
28 days and older	*Meningococcus Haemophilus influenzae Pneumococcus*	Ceftriaxone
Any age	Viruses: enterovirus, mumps, influenza	Supportive
Any age	Tuberculosis	Seek specialist advice

is no contraindication – can be performed *once treatment is underway*. **Do not wait to give antibiotics in a child who is obviously unwell.**

Lumbar puncture will confirm the diagnosis of meningitis and help determine the cause (Table 16.2). Even if antibiotics prevent growth from CSF culture, polymerase chain reaction (PCR) will detect bacterial DNA in blood or CSF and enable a diagnosis.

Be sensitive when talking to the family: the word 'meningitis' is very powerful and surrounded by much myth in the media. It is important to be honest about the possible diagnosis whether it is a certainty or a suspicion. Most parents worry that an ill child has meningitis whether they say so or not – voice your thoughts and demonstrate that you are serious in investigating and treating this possibility.

Bacterial meningitis still has a mortality of around 5%; meningococcal septicaemia is even more dangerous, with reported mortality very high if the initial presentation is with shock. Of the survivors, 10% have sequelae – most commonly deafness, especially after pneumococcal meningitis. Hearing screening should be performed on all children after meningitis (see also Chapter 14, p. 206).

Do not forget that meningitis is an infectious and notifiable disease. Meningococcal infection, in particular, is recorded as occurring in household contacts of the index case. In the UK, cases should be reported to local public health authorities. Household and other close contacts should be treated with prophylactic antibiotics.

Table 16.2 Cerebrospinal fluid findings in infection

	Appearance	White cells	Protein	Glucose
Normal	Clear and colourless	0–5/mm³	0.15–0.45 g/L	2.2–4.7 mmol/L, and should be greater than two thirds of plasma glucose
Bacterial	Turbid	Polymorphs	High	Low
Viral	Clear	Lymphocytes	Normal/raised	Normal/low
TB	Variable	Lymphocytes	Very high	Very low

Encephalitis

> **Case 16.2** A boy with *Herpes simplex* encephalitis
>
> James, a 4-year-old boy, presented with a 3-day history of fever and lethargy. He had been rather irritable, off his food, and had had some diarrhoea. He then had a flurry of brief tonic-clonic seizures and was admitted unconscious – responding only to painful stimuli. He had no neck stiffness, was not shocked but had a fever of 38.9°C. His mother was noted to have a large cold sore. He was promptly treated with high-dose intravenous antibiotics and aciclovir. An EEG showed diffuse slowing, compatible with encephalitis. PCR testing of CSF later confirmed herpes simplex virus infection.

Diagnosis of encephalitis is a clinical dilemma, as shown in Case 16.2. Why is the boy so drowsy? He could have post-ictal drowsiness following febrile seizures, but the history suggests encephalitis. Lumbar puncture will normally show a CSF lymphocytosis suggesting brain inflammation secondary to encephalitis, tuberculous meningitis, or partially treated bacterial meningitis where there is a history of antibiotic use. Send CSF and stool for virology and seek specialist microbiological advice. Diarrhoea may indicate an enterovirus infection. Most viral encephalitis is self-limiting, but herpes simplex encephalitis is often aggressive and damaging. Children with encephalitis are therefore treated with aciclovir until the diagnosis is clear. Children may also get encephalitis after viral infections as part of the immune response to the original infection. Measles, mumps, varicella and rubella can all do this.

FEVER AND A RASH

This is a common presentation. It may help to sort these cases out using the following scheme:

1. *Could the child be seriously ill?* Many viral infections produce a non-specific rash and fever. It is often not possible to make an accurate diagnosis, in which case the trick is to sort out those who are worryingly ill from those who are not.
2. *Has the child been given antibiotics?* You could be observing a sensitivity reaction or a modified presentation of a bacterial infection.
3. *What is the appearance and distribution of the rash?*

Non-blanching rash

If the rash does not blanch on pressure, it could be meningococcal infection. A purpuric rash may also occur with Henoch–Schönlein purpura (see Chapter 6, p. 55), but the child does not appear markedly unwell, and the distribution of the rash over the buttocks, extensor forearms and lower limbs is characteristic (so-called 'gravitational' distribution of rash).

Meningococcal septicaemia

The cause of meningococcal infection – *Neisseria meningitidis* (meningococcus) – may present with meningitis, or, as is the case in Case 16.3, an overwhelming septicaemic illness. This occurs at any age and may progress with frightening speed.

> ### Case 16.3 A baby with meningococcal septicaemia
>
> Jasper, a 3-month-old baby, presented with a 6-hour history of being unsettled, off feeds and with a fever. On assessment he looked pale and unwell. The fontanelle was tense and he had persistent, high-pitched crying. His pulse was 160 beats per minute, capillary refill 5 seconds, and respiratory rate 40 breaths per minute. On examination he had a rapidly spreading purple rash that did not blanch on pressure, which is characteristic of meningococcal septicaemia.

He was immediately given a bolus of 20 mL/kg of normal saline, and high-dose intravenous antibiotics.

Antibiotic therapy is imperative, and shock and multiorgan failure are likely with such a presentation (for management, see Appendix I, p. 288). High dependency or intensive care is imperative. Lumbar puncture to confirm meningitis is deferred until the child is stable. The initial rash in meningococcal septicaemia may be a blanching, maculopapular rash, but it quickly changes character to become petechial or purpuric.

Generalized maculopapular rash

The principal differential diagnosis lies between measles, rubella, roseola infantum, slapped-cheek disease and drug/allergic reactions, particularly following aminopenicillin use in glandular fever (see below). Kawasaki's disease (see below) is distinguished by the presence of other features.

Measles

> ### Case 16.4 A boy with measles
>
> Sammy, a 2-year-old, presented with a rash which followed 48 hours of fever and coryza. The rash started behind the ears and spread rapidly to involve the whole body. He had a widespread maculopapular rash and was miserable and very unwell with a high fever and conjunctivitis. He had not received any immunizations.

Measles is uncommon where immunization rates are high. A decline in measles immunization rates in the UK lead to the reappearance of this previously rare, but highly infectious disease (as in Case 16.4). As public confidence in the MMR immunization has increased, so immunization rates nationally have risen (in April 2011, the Department of Health reported that 88.9% of children under 2 years had received at least one MMR immunization) but they remain too low to prevent measles outbreaks, particularly in urban areas. At the time of writing, a large measles outbreak was underway in France, (under 2 year immunization rate 87.0%), with nearly 5000 cases reported in the first quarter of 2011.

Measles is always a nasty illness and may be complicated by pneumonia, encephalitis and otitis media, leaving a significant morbidity and mortality, especially in the very young, and in adults. Koplik spots, which can make the diagnosis (described as like grains of white salt on a red background inside the mouth), are seen only in the first couple of days – usually before the rash. The period of infectivity ranges from about 4 days before the onset of the rash, to about 4 days after its appearance.

Rubella

Rubella is a relatively trivial illness. The rash typically lasts about 3 days, and comprises fine 1–4 mm pink maculopapules (as in Case 16.5). Particularly in adolescents, it may be preceded by an upper respiratory tract prodrome – painful eye movements are characteristic. A troublesome post-viral arthropathy may follow. Rubella is important because it causes significant damage to the fetus if acquired by a pregnant mother. Rubella embryopathy comprises the triad of deafness, cataracts and retinopathy, and congenital heart disease, coupled with other features. It is entirely preventable. Women found not to be rubella-immune in pregnancy are offered immunization after pregnancy.

> ### Case 16.5 A girl with rubella
>
> Julie, a 5-year-old girl, was under the weather one day with a slight fever. She developed a fine pinkish maculopapular rash over her body. Examination revealed tender, enlarged, occipital lymph nodes.

Roseola infantum

> ### Case 16.6 A toddler with roseola infantum
>
> Ryan, a 1-year-old, presented with a febrile convulsion, associated with a 2-day history of very high fever (>40°C), and malaise. There were no specific findings on examination. He had a neutropenia on his blood count. He was treated with intravenous antibiotics, pending blood cultures, but as the fever subsided on day 3 a rose-pink maculopapular rash appeared.

Roseola infantum is a harmless infection caused by human herpes virus 6B (HHV6B). Febrile seizures occur with it quite commonly, as in Case 16.6. The characteristic feature is the appearance of the rash, concurrent with remission of fever. The rash is a diffuse maculopapular, rose-pink rash, readily distinguished from measles by the remission of fever. Neutropenia, as in Case 16.6, is characteristically found.

Slapped-cheek disease

Case 16.7 gives an example of a condition that is caused by parvovirus B19. Children with sickle-cell anaemia or other haemolytic anaemias may develop a severe aplastic crisis (see Chapter 7, p. 61). The fetus may develop hydrops fetalis if a mother catches this infection while pregnant.

> ### Case 16.7 An outbreak of parvovirus
>
> There was an outbreak of illness in a local primary school one December. Several children developed a bright red rash over their cheeks with pallor around the mouth. The fever and the facial rash settled in a few days, although some children had a more generalized rash which might have fluctuated for a week or more. A few children developed arthritis in the following days.

Urticaria

Some of the most dramatic rashes you will ever see are urticarial. Large red wheals usually with an irregular, raised edge are found on the trunk. The rash may come and go within a few hours, sometimes leaving a slightly bruised appearance. Symptomatic treatment with antihistamines and prednisolone is effective. (see Chapter 8, p. 83).

Generalized vesicular rash

Chicken pox

> ### Case 16.8 A boy with chicken pox
>
> Thomas, a 5-year-old boy, had come into contact with chicken pox in his cousin 3 weeks previously. After a short prodrome with fever he developed scattered discrete spots. These were initially red papules but rapidly developed into small vesicles. These spots were very itchy and healed within a few days by crusting over only to be replaced by a fresh crop.

Case 16.8 is an example of chicken pox (varicella) which is caused by varicella zoster, a herpes group virus. In most children the systemic upset and the rash are mild but a few children are covered with spots and are thoroughly miserable. Following exposure, viraemia develops about 6 days after infection, with fever. Subsequently, fever, malaise and abdominal pain develop, before the onset of the rash about 10–14 days after initial contact (though it may be as late as 21 days).

Secondary infection is the commonest complication. Around 5–10% of children get secondary bacterial infection – usually from scratching. A small number get super-infection with group A *Streptococcus*, which may produce toxic shock, necrotizing fasciitis, or septicaemia, with a very high mortality rate. Viral pneumonia, typically about 3–4 days after onset of rash, is a serious complication in the immunocompromised, in older children and adults, with progressive respiratory failure necessitating intensive care. Chest pain, wheezing and tachypnoea, with diffuse lung involvement on X-ray, are characteristic. Acute encephalitis, with depressed conscious level, affects 1.7/100 000 cases, and has a mortality rate of 5–10%. Post-infectious cerebellar ataxia, typically occurring 2–4 weeks after initial infection, is much more commonly seen and is benign. Cerebral vasculitis resulting in stroke may occur months after initial infection.

Although chicken pox is relatively harmless in most children, it represents a major threat to those with reduced immunity. Children on steroids, those being treated for leukaemia and other malignancies, and the newborn, are at high risk and may develop lethal systemic or encephalitic infection. The parents and children in these cases should be warned of the risk and report any possible contact with chicken pox (or shingles). Oral or systemic aciclovir taken as soon as possible after exposure will attenuate disease severity. In very high risk patients, zoster immune globulin may be required. Specialist advice is required in all cases. The herpes zoster virus may lie dormant for years but re-emerge as shingles. This acutely painful vesicular eruption along one dermatome is rare in childhood.

Rash restricted to one site

Impetigo, erysipelas and cellulitis are cutaneous infections caused by staphylococci or streptococci (see Chapter 8, p. 84). Impetigo and erysipelas usually affect the face. There are obvious local inflammatory changes, sometimes with regional lymphadenopathy. Cellulitis may overlie osteomyelitis (see Chapter 6, p. 51). Treatment is with oral or intravenous antibiotics. Red, painful raised lesions over the shins, erythema nodosum, may occur with drug reactions and a variety of infections or inflammatory disorders (see Chapter 8, p. 84).

Fever and rash associated with sore throat or oral lesions

Pharyngitis or tonsillitis with rash occurs in scarlet fever, glandular fever and Kawasaki's disease. Cervical lymphadenopathy is often marked, especially in Kawasaki's disease. Mumps is characteristically associated with parotid enlargement, which is often unilateral at first.

Sore throat

Glandular fever

> **Case 16.9** A teenager with glandular fever
>
> Alan, a 15-year-old boy, presented with a 4-day history of fever and a terrible sore throat. On examination he had enlarged tonsils covered with a white exudate and petechiae on his palate. His breathing was partially obstructed and sounded noisy. He had enlarged tonsils and cervical and axillary lymphadenopathy. His spleen tip was palpable. He had a fine maculopapular rash. Alan was advised to avoid contact sports until the splenomegaly had resolved, due to increased risk of splenic rupture.

Case 16.9 is an example of glandular fever, a condition that has an ominous reputation among adolescents for causing prolonged illness. This reputation is offset to some extent by the kudos of catching a disease thought to be spread by kissing! The incubation period is about 6 weeks. Glandular fever can be very unpleasant in the acute stage but most children make a prompt recovery. Typical symptoms include sore throat, flu-like symptoms, malaise, swelling around the eyes (20%) and a diffuse maculopapular rash (10%). Subclinical hepatitis is usual, with derangement of liver function tests, but overt jaundice is uncommon. The causative agent – Epstein–Barr virus – may be detected on paired antibody titres. Cytomegalovirus and toxoplasmosis may cause a similar illness. A glandular fever-like illness accompanies seroconversion in some HIV-infected patients. The monospot and Paul Bunnell screening tests are useful for Epstein–Barr virus, but false positives and false negatives occur. Ampicillin or amoxicillin must be avoided in the empirical treatment of sore throat – as a florid maculopapular rash occurs, typically 10–14 days later – and may be complicated by Stevens–Johnson syndrome (Chapter 8, p. 84). Treatment is usually supportive. Steroids may be used to reduce airway obstruction or swallowing difficulty secondary to severe tonsillar enlargement.

Scarlet fever

> ### Case 16.10 A girl with scarlet fever
>
> Gemma, aged 6 years, became febrile with a sore throat. After 48 hours a bright red rash appeared initially in the axillae and groins, and spread rapidly. Her face was red but the area around the mouth remained pale (circumoral pallor). The tongue was white and furred (strawberry tongue). As the rash faded the surface layer of skin peeled away – desquamation.

The girl in Case 16.10 has scarlet fever. The primary cause is usually a toxin-producing beta-haemolytic group A *Streptococcus*, although staphylococcal scarlet fever may also occur. The toxin produces generalized erythema. Treatment is with a 10-day course of penicillin or a macrolide antibiotic such as azithromycin. Late complications include pneumonia, rheumatic fever (see Chapter 6, p. 57) and acute nephritis (see Chapter 11, p. 129). Kawasaki's disease may present similarly (see below).

Kawasaki's disease

Kawasaki's disease is a vasculitic disorder of unknown aetiology. The key feature is an unremitting high fever lasting for 5 days or more in a child who is irritable and unwell. It is rare but is serious and treatable. The principal differential diagnosis is scarlet fever (see above) (see Figure 16.1).

The rash can take many forms but typically it is a maculopapular rash that begins in the groin or perineum. Other features include conjunctivitis, a sore mouth (stomatitis) with strawberry tongue and lymph node enlargement. There may be swelling of the hands and feet and later in the illness the peripheral skin may peel, particularly around the nails. A chronic symmetrical arthritis affecting knees, hips and ankles may occur.

About 5% of children, especially young boys, develop coronary artery aneurysms. Follow-up echocardiography is necessary to monitor for this complication. Sudden cardiac death (see also Chapter 9, p. 98) is a rare complication of coronary artery aneurysms, or other cardiac complications.

Treatment with high-dose aspirin and immunoglobulins produces symptomatic relief and reduces the risk of coronary aneurysms. Recent evidence suggests that the addition of pulsed methylprednisolone may improve outcome.

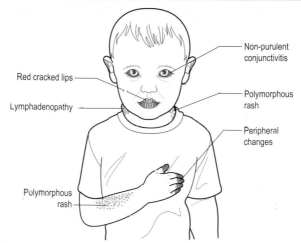

Non-purulent conjunctivitis

Red cracked lips

Polymorphous rash

Lymphadenopathy

Peripheral changes

Polymorphous rash

Figure 16.1 Features of Kawasaki's disease.

Fever and rash associated with mouth ulcers and lesions on the lips

Herpes simplex

Herpes simplex virus may cause cold sores in older children and adults. These are acutely painful red swollen lesions of the lips with a pus-filled centre. Younger children who acquire herpes for the first time may get herpetic gingivostomatitis. This produces an acutely painful ulcerated mouth, tongue and lips. Children may be unable to swallow and need intravenous fluids. Oral aciclovir treatment speeds recovery. Mouth ulcers also occur with enteroviral infections, particularly coxsackie virus (see also Chapter 8, p. 85).

Fever and rash affecting the palms or soles

The commonest infectious cause is hand, foot and mouth disease, caused by coxsackie viruses, which also produces vesicles on the skin and mouth ulcers. Erythema multiforme with its characteristic target lesions may also affect the hands and feet. Mucosal involvement may signify Stevens–Johnson syndrome (see Chapter 8, p. 84).

FEVER AND SPECIFIC SYMPTOMS

Specific symptoms accompany many infections:
- Dyspnoea and respiratory distress in pneumonia and bronchiolitis
- Intractable cough in pertussis
- Diarrhoea and vomiting in gastroenteritis
- Loin pain or dysuria in urinary tract infection
- Limp and pain in septic arthritis or osteomyelitis
- Jaundice in hepatitis
- Ear ache in middle-ear infection.
  These conditions are discussed in the relevant chapters.

Parotid swelling

Parotitis may occur with mumps (see below), HIV, parainfluenza and enteroviruses, or bacterial infections, and may be recurrent or chronic. Parotid swelling causes the pinna to be angled outwards, which is readily visualized from behind.

Mumps

Mumps is uncommon in the UK, thanks to immunization. The parotid swelling is usually unilateral at onset, but in 70–80% of cases both glands are affected. A truncal maculopapular rash occurs infrequently. Meningo-encephalitis occurs in 10%, but is usually benign. Deafness – usually unilateral – may ensue. Orchitis affects 35–40% of adolescents and adult males.

FEVER OF UNKNOWN ORIGIN

A persistent, unexplained high fever (fever of unknown origin, FUO) is rare and is a difficult diagnostic challenge. A logical approach is helpful, with severe symptoms prompting more invasive investigations. Clinical evaluation must be regularly repeated to detect new signs, such as heart murmurs.

Infection must be sought assiduously with repeated blood, urine and stool cultures. Viral studies should include glandular fever organisms. A chest X-ray, abdominal and pelvic ultrasound, and bone scan may be indicated if the fever is persistent and associated with significant symptoms. A tuberculin skin test may indicate underlying tuberculosis. Bone marrow aspirate for culture and to exclude leukaemia should be considered in protracted FUO. Neuroblastoma or lymphoma may also underlie FUO.

Inflammatory disorders such as Kawasaki's disease, systemic onset juvenile idiopathic arthritis (Still's disease), inflammatory bowel disease and polyarteritis nodosa may be responsible.

A history of foreign travel or insect bites should prompt appropriate investigations for malaria, Lyme disease, leptospirosis and rickettsial diseases.

Malaria

Worldwide, malaria is a very common cause of high fever and is seen from time to time in the UK. Think of it in children who have travelled recently to malarial zones. Thick and thin blood films will confirm the diagnosis, and indicate the parasite count. The most serious malarial infection is due to *Plasmodium falciparum*, which accounts for nearly all malarial deaths.

Classic symptoms are swinging fever, headaches, chills, rigors and night-sweats. Cerebral malaria results from occlusion of the cerebral microvasculature by infected red cells. Severe haemolysis may complicate *P. falciparum* infection, potentially leading to blackwater fever with acute renal failure. Artenusate is now recommended as optimum treatment for acute malaria. Quinine is no longer advised.

Lyme disease

Lyme disease is uncommon in the UK – there are about 2000 cases each year in the UK. It is caused by the spirochaete *Borrelia burgdorferi*, transmitted by the bite of the deer tick. A red macule or papule forms and progressively enlarges up to 30 cm in diameter, with partial central clearing. This rash – *erythema chronicum migrans* – is pathognomonic. This initial infection is followed months later by a mono- or pauciarticular arthritis of the knees and other large joints. Uncommonly, neurological and cardiac complications occur. Diagnosis is made on serological testing. Treatment is with tetracyclines or penicillins.

IMMUNE DEFICIENCY

The immune system comprises physical barriers to infection – skin and epithelial surfaces, and humoral and cell-mediated immunity. In practice, impaired immunity is most commonly seen with steroid therapy (supraphysiological) or other immunosuppressant or cytotoxic drugs. It is imperative that these patients and their physicians are aware of the risk and have a management plan for possible infection. In particular, they must be warned of the risk posed by chicken pox and measles infection.

Patients without a functioning spleen (e.g. following splenectomy, or in sickle-cell anaemia, where progressive splenic infarction occurs) are at increased risk of infection with polysaccharide encapsulated organisms – notably pneumococcus, *Haemophilus influenzae* B and meningococcus. Prophylactic penicillin V and targeted immunization based on antibody levels is recommended post-splenectomy.

Diseases causing immunodeficiency – congenital or acquired – most often present with frequent and/or unusually severe infections, failure-to-thrive and chronic diarrhoea. In older children, malignant disease, particularly non-Hodgkin's lymphoma, may supervene.

See Box 16.2 for investigation of suspected immunodeficiency.

Disorders impairing antibody-producing B-lymphocytes or granulocytes result in impaired bacterial killing with recurrent upper and lower respiratory tract, skin and bone infections. Complete antibody deficiency is usually an X-linked disorder – *Bruton's agammaglobulinaemia*. The commonest disorder of bacterial killing, *chronic granulomatous disease*, is additionally complicated by development of multiple granulomas leading to lymphadenopathy and hepatosplenomegaly. Partial antibody deficiencies are less severe. In *common variable immunodeficiency*, there is deficiency of IgG, and to a lesser extent IgA and IgM. IgG_2, IgG_4 and IgA deficiencies predispose to chest infections, particularly with *Pneumococcus*. Secondary antibody deficiency occurs in nephrotic syndrome.

Antibody deficiency may be treated with regular infusions of immunoglobulin.

Some immune deficiency disorders are associated with elevated immunoglobulins – notably *Job's syndrome* (elevated IgE with red hair, severe eczema and frequent bacterial skin and sinopulmonary infections).

Box 16.2 Investigation of suspected immunodeficiency

- Full blood count and blood film
- Lymphocyte subsets
- HIV test
- Immunoglobulins (including IgE) and IgG subclasses
- Specific antibodies to tetanus, *Haemophilus influenzae*, *Pneumococcus* (if immunized)
- Complement CH50, C2–C6 levels
- Alpha-fetoprotein, calcium, skin-prick tests

> **Box 16.3** Management of immunodeficiency
>
> - Prophylaxis
> - Antibiotics/antifungals, e.g. penicillin after splenectomy
> - Immunization, e.g. *Pneumococcus*, influenza
> - Specific immunoglobulin (chicken pox, measles)
> - Aciclovir
> - Avoidance of live vaccines
> - Gamma-globulin replacement
> - Thymus/bone marrow transplant

Complement deficiencies are rare, but lead to increased bacterial infections, especially with *Meningococcus* if the terminal complement pathway is affected (C5–C9).

Defective cell-mediated immunity is seen with *Di George syndrome* (see Chapter 18, p. 272) due to thymic hypoplasia, but normally a degree of recovery takes place. Thymus transplantation may be performed if necessary. More severe disorders of cell-mediated immunity include severe combined immunodeficiency (SCID) and HIV/AIDS.

SCID presents with severe and protracted infections with failure-to-thrive. Treatment is with bone marrow transplantation, although experimental gene therapy has been used for one variety – adenosine deaminase deficiency.

See Box 16.3 for the management of immune deficiency.

Human immunodeficiency virus

As of December 2008, there were 2080 children under 15 years living with HIV/AIDS in the UK. The great majority of these children were infected by mother-to-child transmission. Between 1986 and June 2009, 12 263 children were born to HIV-infected mothers, of whom 15% developed HIV infection. However, with improved anti-retroviral therapy transmission rates in pregnancy and breastfeeding have fallen dramatically. In the UK and Ireland, between 2000 and 2006, the National Study of HIV in Pregnancy and Childhood found 61 cases of vertical transmission of HIV from 5151 mothers (1.2%). This rate fell to 0.8% in those who received at least 2 weeks of anti-retroviral therapy.

Infection by other means (blood products, sexual contact) has a minimum incubation period of 6 months before a rapid increase in viral load occurs. Seroconversion may be associated with a glandular, fever-like illness. The viral load then drops to a static level, the virus may become dormant, and the child is asymptomatic. The lower the viral load, the longer the latent period before progression occurs. In time, the viral load increases and the CD4 (T helper cell) lymphocyte count drops, leading to 'full-blown' acquired immune deficiency syndrome (AIDS). CD4 counts are usually measured every 3 months to monitor progression. Lymphadenopathy, hepatosplenomegaly, dermatitis, parotitis and recurrent upper respiratory infections are early manifestations of HIV infection. In the UK, nearly all infected children have HIV1 infection. HIV2 is most likely to be observed in those of West African origin. Those infected with HIV2 progress to full-blown AIDS less quickly. Treatment of HIV2-infected patients is more problematic as HIV2 is inherently resistant to non-nucleoside reverse transcriptase inhibitors (first-line treatment in HIV1), and fusion inhibitors.

Diagnosis

Any HIV test should be discussed fully with the parents. Suggested tests:

- **Infants.** Maternal antibodies confound conventional serological testing, and may persist up to 18 months of age. HIV blood culture and PCR for HIV DNA are both highly reliable tests in infancy
- **Children >18 months.** ELISA antibody screen.

Treatment

- **Anti-retroviral therapy.** There are two classes of reverse transcriptase inhibitors, dideoxynucleosides and non-nucleoside reverse transcriptase inhibitors, which act to inhibit viral reverse transcriptase, thus suppressing HIV replication. Protease inhibitors inhibit formation of vital structural proteins. Combination anti-retroviral therapy (ART), with three drugs, delays progression of the disease. In the initial phase, highly active ART (HAART) is used to quickly reduce the viral load and prevent emergence of resistance, but treatment regimes are difficult and complex, and non-compliance with therapy is common.
- **Immunizations.** HIV-infected children receive the normal immunization schedule. As for all patients at increased risk of chest infection, pneumococcal and influenza vaccines are recommended.
- **Infection prophylaxis.** Routine antibiotic prophylaxis is not recommended because of problems with resistant organisms. Monthly immunoglobulin therapy may be given, but is of uncertain value. Prophylaxis with co-trimoxazole is used in infants to prevent *Pneumocystis carinii* pneumonia (PCP) until 1 year of age, or after PCP infection, or in children with low CD4 counts. Clarithromycin is used to prevent *Mycobacterium avium-intracellulare* complex (MAC) infection in children with very low CD4 counts. Children exposed to virus infections, such as measles, chicken pox or herpes, receive immunoglobulin and, if appropriate, aciclovir.

Complications

- **Serious bacterial sepsis.** There is a high risk of serious sepsis in HIV-infected children, including septicaemia (10% per year), particularly with *Pneumococcus*.
- **PCP.** This is common in infancy, when it is often the first presentation. PCP is often fatal (30–50%) and has a poor prognosis, with post-infection 2-year survival less than 50%.
- **Progressive multifocal leucoencephalopathy.** The peak incidence is between 9 and 18 months of age with progressive loss of intellectual and neurological impairment. Gross cerebral atrophy is seen on CT scan.
- **Lymphocytic interstitial pneumonitis.** This is common in preschool children, and may be asymptomatic, otherwise it presents with chronic cough and dyspnoea, and reticulonodular shadowing on chest X-ray. Prednisolone is effective.
- **Disseminated infection:**
  - Disseminated *Mycobacterium avium-intracellulare* complex (DMAC). DMAC affects school-age children with severe immune deficiency (CD4 <100). Symptoms include high fevers, night sweats, weight loss and abdominal pain.
  - Disseminated cytomegalovirus (CMV) infection may cause retinitis, pneumonitis, hepatitis and colitis.

- Disseminated candidiasis: oral and oesophageal candidiasis is common in older children and presents with retrosternal pain and dysphagia.
- **Non-Hodgkin's lymphoma,** particularly of the central nervous system, is the most common HIV-related malignancy in childhood.

Prognosis

Modern management of HIV infection has transformed the prognosis for infected children, and most will live to adulthood.

Further reading

For the most current information on management of HIV, visit aidsinfo. nih.gov.

Pregnancy, birth and the newborn 17

(David Booth)

CHAPTER CONTENTS

INTRODUCTION

The newborn period is a time to celebrate and to support and advise families about the health of their new baby. However, illness may present during this time, and this poses a particular challenge to the family and doctors involved.

The foundations of a child's health are laid in pregnancy. Many diseases in childhood are linked to the antenatal health of the mother and the wider family. Birth may similarly affect a child's long-term health, particularly:

- Infants with congenital anomalies (see Chapter 18)
- Premature infants (less than 37 completed weeks of gestation)
- Infants born small for gestational age (see Chapter 12, p. 147).

Infants in these categories have greatly increased neonatal infant mortality and morbidity in childhood. Additionally, there is a relationship between low birth weight and increased risk of premature cardiovascular disease, diabetes and mortality in adult life – *the Barker hypothesis.*

THE HEALTHY PREGNANCY

Antenatal care is important. It provides support and reassurance to the mother and her partner, and may detect early signs of ill health in either mother or child. Attendance for antenatal care is associated with improved pregnancy outcomes, whereas late presentation ('unbooked pregnancy') is associated with

Table 17.1 Health advice for women planning pregnancy

Advice	Reasoning
Folic acid prior to conception	Prevention of neural tube defects
Avoid excess alcohol	Prevention of fetal alcohol syndrome Improves maternal health
Stop or decrease smoking	Reduces the risk of premature birth, intrauterine growth retardation (see Chapter 12, p. 147) and respiratory disease in childhood
Avoid unpasteurized dairy products	Reduce risk of congenital *Listeria*
Avoid handling cat litter	Reduces risk of toxoplasmosis
Rubella immunization if not immune	Avoidance of congenital rubella (see Chapter 16, p. 235)

higher rates of maternal morbidity (e.g. anaemia, hypertension) and fetal morbidity (low birth weight) and mortality (stillbirth and early neonatal death).

See Table 17.1 for advice that can be given to women planning pregnancy.

ANTENATAL SCREENING

Pregnant women are screened for a range of maternal and fetal problems:

- Dating scan at 'booking' to confirm gestation
- Blood group and antibody screen for potential haemolytic disorders, e.g. rhesus incompatibility (see Chapter 7, p. 60)
- Rubella antibodies
- Hepatitis B, syphilis and HIV serology
- Alpha-fetoprotein for neural tube defects
- Triple test for Down syndrome (alpha-fetoprotein, human chorionic gonadotrophin, unconjugated oestriol) at 16 weeks' gestation. Ultrasound scanning to detect increased nuchal translucency (11–14 weeks' gestation) is being progressively introduced throughout the UK as a more sensitive test for detection of increased risk of Down syndrome and other congenital disorders
- Fetal anomaly scan at 18–20 weeks' gestation (see Box 17.1).

Box 17.1 Range of abnormalities detectable on fetal anomaly scan

- Neural tube defects (spina bifida, anencephaly, hydrocephalus)
- Cardiovascular (approximately 60%)
- Chest (diaphragmatic hernia)
- Gastrointestinal (cleft lip/palate, see below), duodenal/ileal atresia, exomphalos/gastroschisis, see pp. 259–260)
- Genitourinary (hydronephrosis, renal dysplasia, see Chapter 11, p. 120)
- Skeletal (achondroplasia and other skeletal dysplasias)
- Hydrops fetalis (skin oedema, pleural effusions, ascites)
- Chromosomal (suspicions may be raised by the pattern of anomaly seen)

Table 17.2 Medication with recognized teratogenic effects on the fetus

Maternal medication	Teratogenic effect on fetus
Carbamazepine	Neural tube defects
Lithium	Congenital heart disease
Phenytoin	Fetal hydantoin syndrome
Propylthiouracil	Hypothyroidism
Tetracycline	Enamel hypoplasia of the teeth
Valproate	Neural tube defects valproate embryopathy
Warfarin	Microcephaly, nasal hypoplasia

Ultrasound is also useful for monitoring fetal health and growth, potential abnormalities and amniotic fluid volumes in later pregnancy.

Some women are at higher risk of having problems in pregnancy and may be offered additional tests, e.g. amniocentesis for women over 35 years. Pregnancies at increased risk of abnormality include:

- Maternal age over 35 years
- Maternal diabetes and other disorders
- Previous child with a genetic abnormality
- Family history of an inherited disorder
- Parents who are known carriers of genetic disorders
- Consanguineous parents
- Maternal disease
  - Diabetes, maternal heart disease
  - Autoimmune disease, e.g. hyperthyroidism, systemic lupus erythematosus, autoimmune thrombocytopenia
- Maternal medication (see Table 17.2).

BIRTH

Neonatal resuscitation

Most infants do not require resuscitation. Some may not establish effective respiration and require help. Infant resuscitation is covered in Appendix I. The resuscitation routine is altered if the baby is premature or if the amniotic fluid is stained with meconium.

The Apgar score

The Apgar score (named after Virginia Apgar) is calculated at 1 and 5 minutes of life. It gives an indication of the condition of the baby at this time and provides a standard way of documenting the health of the baby in the first few minutes of life. Many parents know about this score. It is sometimes necessary to reassure worried parents that a score of less than 10 at 1 or 5 minutes is not an indicator for a lifetime of under-achievement! (see Table 17.3).

Table 17.3 Calculating the Apgar score

	0	1	2
Heart rate	Absent	<100	>100
Respiratory effort	Absent	Gasping	Regular
Muscle tone	Flaccid	Some flexion	Well flexed
Reflex irritability	None	Grimace	Cry
Colour	White/blue	Blue extremities	Pink

Adaptation to extra-uterine life

The process of delivery, temperature change and the clamping of the umbilical cord results in gasping and the removal of the remaining lung fluid. The pulmonary vascular resistance falls and pulmonary blood flow increases. The increased left atrial filling closes the foramen ovale and oxygenated blood flowing through the ductus arteriosus causes its eventual closure (see also Chapter 9, pp. 91–93).

THE NEWBORN

Examination of the newborn

Every newborn baby is examined soon after birth – usually within the first 24 hours of life. This examination is in part a screening tool but is also an opportunity for parents to raise concerns they might have about their child.

The objectives of the examination are to identify any congenital anomaly not identified by antenatal screening. The most important of these are structural heart lesions (see Chapter 9, pp. 91–95), congenital cataracts and other eye disease detectable through absence of the 'red reflex' (see Chapter 14, p. 210), and developmental dysplasia of the hip (see Chapter 6, p. 49) (see Figure 17.1).

Birth injuries

Deliveries following an obstructed labour or malpresentation and instrumental deliveries can cause injury. These include nerve palsies, soft-tissue injuries and fractures. The newborn examination will identify these.

Feeding

Breast-feeding

Breast milk is the best food for babies, irrespective of gestation. Exclusive breast-feeding is recommended for the first 4 to 6 months of life. Breast milk is nutritionally complete and ideal for feeding on demand. The benefits of breast milk include anti-infective properties, low allergenicity, improved digestion, fewer episodes of gastroenteritis and a reduced incidence of necrotizing enterocolitis in premature infants. There is some epidemiological evidence for improved cognitive function. Supplements may need to be added to breast milk to optimize growth in preterm infants.

The benefits for mothers who breast-feed are the promotion of attachment with their child, a reduced risk of breast cancer, and possibly a decreased risk of osteoporosis. Mothers who breast-feed show a quicker return to their pre-pregnancy weight.

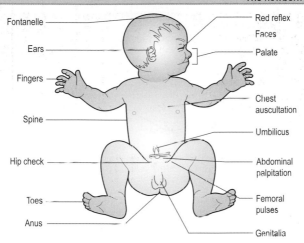

Areas of examination

Head – shape, fontanelle and suture separation, cephalohaematomas

Face – dysmorphism and nerve palsies

Eyes – red reflex for cataracts

Mouth – presence of natal teeth, cysts and cleft palate

Jaw – small mandible leading to airway obstruction

Chest – symmetrical movements

Heart – position of apex beat, heart rate and presence of murmur

Abdomen – liver edge palpable

Genitalia – clearly male or female, testes in scrotum in males

Groin – presence of femoral pulses and evidence of hernias

Anus – present, position and meconium passed

Hips – examination for developmental dysplasia

Spine – shape, naevi and sinuses

Neurology – assess feeding, behaviour and primitive reflexes

Skin lesions – stork marks

             capillary haemangioma

             milia

             mongolian blue spots

             urticaria neonatorum

Figure 17.1 The post-natal examination.

Whey and casein are the main proteins in breast milk. Whey forms a soft yoghurt-like curd in the stomach which produces a fine texture for digestion by enzymes. Gastric emptying is rapid. Breast milk comprises 60% whey.

Casein forms a firmer curd in the stomach, similar to cottage cheese. This is digested more slowly and gastric emptying is slower. Breast milk comprises 40% casein.

There are very few reasons not to breast-feed a baby. These may include:

- Maternal illness
- Infant illness
- Maternal medications.

Formula milks

Infant formulas have been developed to be either whey dominant or casein dominant. Standard formula comprises 60% whey and 40% casein (whey dominant).

These formulas are recommended for demand-feeding patterns similar to breast-fed infants. They are formulated for bottle-feeding from birth or when moving from breast-feeding, due to the similarity with breast milk composition. Standard formulas are suitable up to 12 months of age. It is important to remember that formula feed needs to be made up in a sterile fashion. The teat needs to suit the baby, and the temperature needs to be correct.

For more information on infant feeding and weaning, see Chapter 13, p. 160)

PREVENTING ILLNESS

Vitamin K

Babies have a limited ability to synthesize vitamin K. This persists for the first 3 months of life. In addition, during early infancy when fed entirely on milk, babies have very little supply of vitamin K, especially if exclusively breast-fed. A very small number of babies suffer bleeding due to vitamin K deficiency. This is called 'haemorrhagic disease of the newborn'.

Haemorrhagic disease of the newborn is prevented when a supplement of vitamin K is given to babies soon after birth. In the 1990s one study suggested a link between vitamin K administration to babies and the future risk of leukaemia.

In 1997 a panel of experts considered all the studies and concluded that, overall, the data do *not* support an increased risk of cancer caused by vitamin K. The Department of Health recommends that vitamin K supplements should be offered to all newborn babies. Intramuscular injections of vitamin K (phytomenadione, Konakion) prevent haemolytic disease of the newborn in virtually all babies. A single dose is recommended at birth.

Newborn screening

All babies in the UK are offered screening for phenylketonuria (PKU), congenital hypothyroidism, sickle-cell disease, cystic fibrosis (CF) and the rare but treatable fatty acid metabolism disorder medium-chain acyl-CoA dehydrogenase deficiency (MCADD). Blood for testing is taken via a heel prick sample at 5 days of age.

THE ILL NEONATE

Neonatal encephalopathy

Neonatal encephalopathy is most often caused by perinatal hypoxia ('birth asphyxia'). This situation arises as a result of a cerebral insult before or during labour or delivery. It occurs in 1–2/1000 deliveries. Prompt and effective resuscitation is an important start to the treatment of this serious condition.

Aetiology
● Before birth:
  • Inadequate oxygenation of maternal blood (anaesthesia, cyanotic heart disease, respiratory failure)
  • Low maternal blood pressure (spinal anaesthesia, inferior vena cava compression)
  • Inadequate contraction of the uterus (oxytocin)
  • Premature separation of the placenta
  • Impairment of cord blood flow (compression, drugs)
  • Placental insufficiency (toxaemia, post-maturity).
● After birth:
  • Severe anaemia (haemorrhage, haemolytic disease)
  • Severe shock (sepsis, blood loss)
  • Respiratory failure
  • Cyanotic heart disease
  • Inherited metabolic disease.
Neonatal encephalopathy is graded from I to III:
● **Type I** – this is usually benign and not associated with continuing brain damage
● **Type II** – eighty per cent of these babies have a good outcome. Only 20% will have a disability at follow-up
● **Type III** – most in this group die, and survivors usually have significant long-term neurodisability.

Hypothermia for hypoxic-ischaemic encephalopathy

Previously there was no specific treatment for asphyxia other than stabilization, intensive care and treatment to reduce seizures.

Since 2009, the use of whole-body cooling following perinatal asphyxia has become standard treatment for asphyxiated term infants. It is a safe treatment that improves survival and reduces neurological and neurodevelopmental impairments. Babies who have experienced moderate or severe asphyxia are cooled as soon as possible after birth (cooling should start before 6 hours of age). Cooled babies have their body temperature reduced to 33.5°C for 72 hours, followed by gradual re-warming.

Cooled babies have an increased rate of survival without neurological abnormality (cooling results in reduced risks of cerebral palsy and improved scores on neurodevlopmental assessments).

RESPIRATORY DISTRESS

The signs of respiratory distress include:
● Tachypnoea
● Chest wall recession
● Nasal flaring
● Expiratory grunting
● Cyanosis.

Pocket Essentials of Paediatrics

Table 17.4 Causes of respiratory distress in a term infant	
Pulmonary	Transient tachypnoea of the newborn Pneumothorax Pneumonia Meconium aspiration Persistent pulmonary hypertension
Non-pulmonary	Congenital heart disease Perinatal hypoxia Severe anaemia Metabolic acidosis
Rare	Diaphragmatic hernia Tracheo-oesophageal fistula Respiratory distress syndrome Pulmonary hypoplasia

Management is directed at identifying the cause and providing appropriate supportive and other treatment. Causes are detailed in Table 17.4.

Jaundice

Most newborn infants become jaundiced. Reasons for this include:
- Increased rate of turnover of red blood cells (red cell lifespan is 70 days in babies compared with 120 days older children and in adults)
- More bilirubin produced due to increased red cell turnover
- Immaturity of the liver, leading to reduced ability to excrete bilirubin in bile.

As increased red cell turnover and hepatic immaturity are normal physiological variants in newborn babies, the jaundice arising as a result is termed 'physiological jaundice'. This term separates it from jaundice that occurs secondary to disease – 'pathological jaundice'.

Jaundice appearing in the first day of life or persisting beyond 2 weeks of age is, until proven otherwise, assumed to be pathological – a proportion of babies with day 1 jaundice or persisting jaundice will have harmless physiological jaundice but this cannot be assumed until the jaundice is investigated for haemolysis or other causes. (For premature infants, in whom hepatic immaturity is more pronounced, jaundice is not considered abnormal until persisting beyond 3 weeks of age.)

Physiological jaundice starts after day 1 of life, peaks around day 4 or 5, and then gradually resolves over the next week.

Breast milk jaundice is physiological jaundice occurring in a breast-fed baby. Infants who are breast-fed are more likely than formula-fed infants to become jaundiced. Components of the breast milk act as inhibitors of hepatic bilirubin metabolism.

Investigation of neonatal jaundice

Day 1 jaundice or prolonged jaundice (as defined above) should be investigated. Judging bilirubin levels by examining the skin is unreliable; serum bilirubin levels should be measured to give a total value and individual levels for both unconjugated and conjugated bilirubin. A high level of conjugated bilirubin, sometimes in conjunction with pale stools and dark urine, suggests that the pathology lies in the liver and/or the biliary tree (failure to effectively handle and excrete the bilirubin following conjugation in the liver).

A high level of unconjugated bilirubin suggests that the mechanisms for bilirubin metabolism and excretion have been overwhelmed by an excess *production* of bilirubin or a failure to *metabolize* the bilirubin during the pre-conjugation steps of metabolism.

When the total bilirubin level and conjugated and unconjugated fractions are known, further investigations can be requested appropriately.

Neonatal jaundice may be a sign of excessive haemolysis (see Chapter 7, p. 60), infection or a metabolic disorder. Conjugated hyperbilirubinaemia suggests serious liver disease (see Chapter 13, p. 175) (see Table 17.5).

Harmful jaundice

A high level of conjugated bilirubin is in itself not usually harmful; however, it signifies potentially serious underlying pathology and a cause should be sought and treatment directed appropriately.

High levels of unconjugated bilirubin are potentially harmful as unconjugated bilirubin is neurotoxic at high concentrations as it can cross the blood–brain barrier. The cells of the basal ganglia are particularly sensitive. The neurotoxicity manifests as bilirubin encephalopathy or *kernicterus*, with initial lethargy and poor feeding progressing to irritability, increased muscle tone, rigidity and seizures. Kernicterus has a high fatality rate. Infants who survive often have permanent neurological damage in the form of choreoathetoid cerebral palsy and deafness (see Chapter 14, p. 200).

● **Treatment**. Poor feeding and secondary dehydration often exacerbate neonatal jaundice and establishing good feeding in conjunction with short-term rehydration therapy is all that is needed in most cases.

In some babies, the level of unconjugated jaundice becomes dangerously high and, in addition to rehydration, phototherapy is required to

Table 17.5 Causes of neonatal jaundice

Timing of onset	Cause
<24 hours of age	Rhesus incompatability ABO incompatability Glucose-6-phosphate dehydrogenase (G6PD) deficiency Spherocytosis Congenital infection
24 hours to 2 weeks	Physiological Breast milk jaundice Infection (e.g. urinary tract infection) Haemolysis (haemolysis/G6PD deficiency) Bruising Polycythaemia
>2 weeks	Physiological Breast milk jaundice Hypothyroidism Haemolysis Neonatal hepatitis Biliary atresia

reduce bilirubin levels. This utilizes light in the blue spectrum to pho-todegrade the bilirubin in the skin to a harmless isomer. The decision to start treatment with phototherapy is based on standardized charts, using the bilirubin level and the baby's age.

In some infants, phototherapy does not produce a sufficiently rapid decline in bilirubin levels and these infants need an exchange trans-fusion, in which blood containing high bilirubin levels is carefully exchanged for transfused blood.

HYPOGLYCAEMIA

The definition of hypoglycaemia in newborn babies is accepted as blood glucose <2.6 mmol/L, although this is a matter of ongoing controversy. Prolonged hypoglycaemia may be more damaging to preterm infants.

Symptomatic hypoglycaemia is rare in the well-grown term infant, although blood glucose falls after birth, even in normal healthy babies. At birth, the sudden discontinuation of nutrients from the mother's pla-centa causes a fall in plasma glucose. This then causes a counter-regulatory hormone response. There are rises in adrenaline (epinephrine), growth hormone, cortisol and glucagon. Infants can utilize ketone bodies and lac-tate as alternative cerebral fuels, contributing to their ability to tolerate hypoglycaemia.

In the term infant, the blood sugar level needs only to be checked if symptoms are present or if there is a risk of hypoglycaemia. Those 'at risk' include:

- Infants with intrauterine growth retardation
- Infants with hypothermia
- Infants with sepsis
- Infants of diabetic mothers.

Symptoms of hypoglycaemia include:

- Changes in conscious level; irritability, lethargy and coma
- Apnoea and cyanotic episodes
- Poor feeding
- Hypothermia
- Hypotonia (floppiness)
- Tremor, jitteriness and fits.

Blood sugars should be checked in *all* babies who exhibit these symptoms.

These symptoms are not specific for hypoglycaemia, and other causes, including sepsis as well as other neurological and metabolic abnormalities, need to be considered.

CONGENITAL INFECTION

Any mother can contract an infection during pregnancy. Some infections cause serious harm to the fetus. The most common bacterial infection to do so is Group B *Streptococcus*.

Important congenital infections include:

- Group B *Streptococcus* infection (see below) – pneumonia, meningitis, septicaemia
- Hepatitis B and C
- HIV
- **ToRCH** – Toxoplasmosis, Rubella, Cytomegalovirus (CMV) and Herpes simplex virus (HSV). Toxoplasmosis is associated with

macrocephaly/hydrocephalus and developmental delay, rubella infection in the first trimester with congenital rubella syndrome, CMV with microcephaly and developmental delay, and HSV with disseminated herpes infection in the newborn period

- Varicella zoster – varicella infection in late pregnancy exposes the newborn infant to a severe disseminated infection
- Parvovirus B19 (hydrops) – fetal anaemia results in high-output heart failure with *hydrops fetalis* – severe oedema of the fetus, which may be fatal
- Listeriosis – transplacentally acquired infection may present with preterm birth, commonly with meconium staining of the amniotic fluid, otherwise rare in preterm delivery, manifesting as meningitis and/or septicaemia
- Syphilis – although formerly rare in the UK, syphilis is increasing and results in stillbirth, premature delivery and congenital infection.

Group B *Streptococcus* infection

The incidence of Group B *Streptococcus* infection is estimated to be 0.7/1000 live births, although significant variation in incidence occurs around the world. Group B *Streptococcus* is a common inhabitant of the maternal genitourinary and gastrointestinal tract. It colonizes about 10–30% of pregnant women. Only 50% of carriers can be detected, and only 50% of these will have a positive culture at the time of labour. Rates of vertical *transmission and subsequent colonization* of the infant vary from 40% to 75%, but the *neonatal infection* rate is low. Screening for Group B *Streptococcus* is therefore too unreliable to be of use. Risk factors which substantially increase the risk of transmission include:

- Previous infant with Group B *Streptococcus* infection
- Prematurity
- Maternal intrapartum fever
- Prolonged membrane rupture (> 18 hours)
- Positive Group B *Streptococcus* culture on vaginal swab or in urine during pregnancy.

As 66% of Group B *Streptococcus*-infected infants will present within the first 7 days, any baby showing signs of illness needs to be investigated and treated promptly in order to exclude Group B *Streptococcus*. The overall mortality is 9.4% (6% for term infants and 18% for preterm infants). Suspected or confirmed Group B *Streptococcus* is treated with a penicillin or cephalosporin, coupled with an aminoglycoside, e.g. benzylpenicillin and gentamicin.

THE PRETERM INFANT

A significant number of infants are born prematurely. Spontaneous preterm labour is frequently associated with infection – notably Group B *Streptococcus*. The chances of survival and prognosis depend on gestational age. Infants born at less than 23 weeks and less than 500 g in weight currently have negligible chance of survival. These tiny babies look very different from a term infant. The skin is dark, transparent and very thin. Insensible water losses are high. The infants lie with arms and legs extended and muscle tone is poor .

The problems a preterm infant faces are considerable. Primarily these relate to the immaturity of the major organs, particularly the lungs. Adequate nutrition for these babies may be similarly difficult.

Principal causes of mortality are respiratory disease (acute or chronic), brain injury from intraventricular haemorrhage, and infection (as in Case 17.1).

Case 17.1 Extreme prematurity

Ella, an extremely preterm infant, was delivered vaginally after premature rupture of the chorioamniotic membranes and spontaneous labour at 24 weeks and 2 days of gestation, weighing 540 g. She was immediately placed in a plastic bag under a radiant heater. Her initial heart rate was under 60 beats per minute and she made little respiratory effort; her Apgar score was 2 at 1 minute. She was intubated, ventilated and received surfactant in the delivery room. She developed a patent ductus arteriosus (PDA), which exacerbated her chronic lung disease, and which failed to close with indometacin treatment, requiring surgical ligation at 34 days of age.

She required intravenous nutrition for 14 days until full milk feeds were established. Her bilirubin level peaked after a week of life, phototherapy being given from day 3 to 10. Infections were a persistent problem; she was initially treated with benzylpenicillin and gentamicin and then with a course of cefotaxime and vancomycin in the 2nd week of life for respiratory instability. Following this, she developed candidal nappy rash which spread across her abdomen and chest, necessitating oral and topical nystatin followed by fluconazole. In the 3rd week of life a blood culture grew coagulase-negative *Staphylococcus* which was treated with flucloxacillin and gentamicin. Cranial ultrasound on day 2 of life showed a moderate intraventricular haemorrhage on the right, and a larger haemorrhage on the left, with involvement of the surrounding brain. Ella had a further scan at 2 weeks of age showing that the area of haemorrhage had undergone necrosis, leaving a large periventricular cyst.

Despite the PDA ligation, on day 39, Ella developed abdominal distension and bilious vomiting with stress hyperglycaemia. Abdominal X-ray confirmed necrotizing enterocolitis, with gas within the biliary tree. She was treated with broad-spectrum antibiotics and abdominal drains were sited. Nevertheless, she developed Gram-negative shock with renal failure and a profound metabolic acidosis. Adequate ventilation eventually became impossible and she died in her parents' arms after intensive care was withdrawn on the 44th day of life.

See Table 17.6 for complications of prematurity.

Respiratory distress syndrome

Respiratory distress syndrome is caused by a deficiency in surfactant and is usually associated with prematurity. Surfactant is a mixture of lipo-proteins excreted by type II pneumocytes in the alveolar epithelium, lowering surface tension. Surfactant deficiency leads to a higher surface tension, alveolar collapse and inadequate gas exchange. Other causes of surfactant deficiency include sepsis, hypoxia, acidosis and hypothermia. Exogenous surfactant therapy is given to many premature infants but may also be used in term infants in certain conditions where surfactant

Table 17.6 Complications of prematurity	
General care	**Temperature instability**
Respiratory	Respiratory distress syndrome Chronic lung disease of prematurity
Cardiac	Hypotension Patent ductus arteriosus (see Chapter 9, p. 95)
Gastrointestinal	Feed intolerance Necrotizing enterocolitis Hypo- and hyperglycaemia
Liver	Jaundice Cholestatic obstructive jaundice (see Chapter 13, p. 175)
Renal	Electrolyte abnormalities Acute renal failure
Neurological	Periventricular haemorrhage Ischaemic brain injury
Vision	Retinopathy of prematurity, cortical blindness
Hearing	Sensorineural deafness
Haematological	Anaemia of prematurity Impaired leucocyte function
Infection	Septicaemia, meningitis Urinary tract infection Fungal and viral infections
Social	Parental anxiety and distress Family relationship disruption

deficiency is thought to be a contributing factor in a disease process. One major advance in the prevention of respiratory distress syndrome has been to give mothers antenatal steroids to stimulate fetal surfactant production (see Figure 17.2).

Management of respiratory distress is with respiratory support. The majority of babies below 28 weeks' gestation will require a period of mechanical ventilation. Ventilation is associated with lung injury which may manifest acutely as pneumothorax, and commonly leads to *chronic lung disease*, with prolonged oxygen dependence.

Chronic lung disease is defined as oxygen dependency (or other respiratory support) at the equivalent of 36 weeks of gestation. The likelihood of chronic lung disease is greatly increased in growth-retarded infants and those with patent ductus arteriosus (see Chapter 9, p. 95). Chronic lung disease renders the infant very susceptible to respiratory infection, particularly with respiratory syncytial virus and right heart failure (cor pulmonale). Steroids – usually dexamethasone – may improve lung function sufficiently to wean a child from respiratory support, but their use is associated with a high incidence of cerebral palsy (>30%) and does not improve long-term survival.

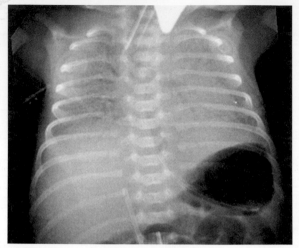

Figure 17.2 X-ray of infant with respiratory distress syndrome. Typical chest X-ray appearance of respiratory distress syndrome with 'ground glass' appearance of the lungs and air bronchograms.

Periventricular haemorrhage

The brain of the premature infant is highly susceptible to haemorrhage. Some degree of periventricular haemorrhage affects 50% of babies weighing less than 1500 g at birth. The floors of the lateral ventricles contain a rich network of vessels. These vessels involute in the 3rd trimester, making haemorrhage rare in infants above 32 weeks gestation. Infants who are unwell with infection, hypoxia, acidosis or hypotension are at particularly high risk.

Haemorrhages are graded according to severity:

- Grade I – haemorrhage within the germinal layer of the ventricle
- Grade II – haemorrhage confined to the ventricle
- Grade III – distension of the ventricle by haemorrhage
- Grade IV – extension of haemorrhage into the surrounding brain.

Grade I and II haemorrhages are not associated with adverse outcomes, but grade III or IV haemorrhages, particularly if bilateral, are associated with a high risk of cerebral palsy (see Chapter 14, p. 197).

Infection

Defence against infection relies on physical barriers to infection – the skin and respiratory and gut epithelium, as well as the immune system. The skin of the preterm baby is thin and porous and is frequently breached for venepunctures and cannulas.

The immune defences against infection in a term baby include an endowment of transplacentally acquired IgG antibodies received in the third trimester, and IgA antibodies in breast milk. Premature babies are deprived of their inheritance of antibodies and are often too unwell to feed, even if breast milk is available. The immunologically naive immune system is functional but demonstrates impaired responses to antigenic challenge.

Accordingly, premature infants are at extremely high risk of severe and invasive bacterial and fungal infections, and organisms such as coagulase-negative staphylococci, normally considered to be skin commensals, may become pathogenic.

Nutrition

Preterm infants have higher nutritional requirements by weight than term infants. Nutrient accretion occurs predominantly in the third trimester. Therefore, preterm infants have limited reserves of fat, glycogen and micronutrients. In addition, these infants have an accelerated growth phase and may be unable to tolerate large volumes of feed. Specialized breast milk fortifiers and preterm formulas are used for preterm infants to optimize growth and development.

CONGENITAL ANOMALIES

Cleft lip and palate

These embryological abnormalities may be diagnosed antenatally. They are common, affecting 1 in 700 infants. Careful examination is necessary to exclude other abnormalities that might suggest a syndrome such as D George syndrome (see Chapter 18, p. 272) or fetal alcohol syndrome. Most concerning is Pierre Robin syndrome, in which there is cleft palate and an underdeveloped jaw, causing the tongue to obstruct the airway.

Early feeding advice is necessary. Early repair of a cleft lip is possible. A cleft palate repair may be deferred until the baby is several months old. Alongside surgical intervention, speech and language therapy, ENT, audiology and orthodontic support are required.

Congenital gut abnormalities

Obstruction due to atresias and stenosis can occur at any level in the gastrointestinal tract, the more proximal the obstruction is the sooner the child presents.

Oesophageal atresia

Oesophageal atresia is usually associated with tracheo-oesphageal fistula and causes antenatal polyhydramnios, due to impaired fetal swallowing, and bubbly oral secretions are often seen at birth. A nasogastric tube should be passed in all babies if polyhydramnios was present in pregnancy. If oesophageal atresia is present, the tube coils in the proximal oesophagus at the point of obstruction (the 'upper pouch'). This is seen on X-ray. If air is visible in the stomach or gastrointestinal tract, this indicates a concomitant tracheo-oesophageal fistula (see below). Urgent surgery is required if oesophageal atresia is confirmed.

Tracheo-oesophageal fistula

The majority of these abnormal communications arise in association with oesophageal atresia. In 4% of cases an 'H' type fistula is seen. The oesophagus and trachea are continuous but the fistula allows communication between both. This may be a difficult diagnosis. It should be considered in babies who cough or choke during feeds, or in those who suffer recurrent aspiration.

Oesophageal atresia and tracheo-oesophageal fistula are commonly associated with other abnormalities, notably the VACTERL sequence (Vertebral anomalies, imperforate Anus, congenital Cardiac disease, Tracheo-oesophageal fistula, oEsophageal atresia, Renal anomalies and radial Limb defects).

Duodenal atresia

Duodenal atresia or stenosis present typically after the first feed. They may be associated with Down syndrome.

Meckel's diverticulum

Meckel's diverticulum is an embryological remnant of the vitelline duct, 40–60 cm from the ileocaecal valve. On average it is about 3 cm long. In about half, ectopic gastric mucosa is present, which may lead to copious rectal blood loss (haematochezia), which is the classic presentation. Other complications include chronic iron deficiency anaemia, intussusception and infection (manifesting similarly to acute appendicitis). It is found in 0.2–4.0% of children, but only rarely (<5%) causes symptoms.

Lower gastrointestinal obstruction

Lower obstructions, including imperforate anus and Hirschsprung's disease, may present with bile-stained vomiting, abdominal distension or failure to pass stool. Ninety-five per cent of normal infants pass stool within 24 hours of birth. Contrast studies may help determine the level of obstruction (see also Chapter 13, p. 165).

Diaphragmatic hernia

This is usually diagnosed antenatally. It is much commoner on the left. Confirmation of the diagnosis is with a chest X-ray. The presence of gut in the chest causes pulmonary hypoplasia and at birth these babies often require significant resuscitation, including ventilation. It is imperative to avoid bag-mask-valve ventilation until a nasogastric tube is sited to decompress the stomach (which is in the chest!). Repair of the defect proceeds when the baby's condition allows. Associated severe congenital abnormalities such as Edward's syndrome (see Chapter 18, p. 277) may make surgery inappropriate.

Gastroschisis and exomphalos

Diagnosis of both of these conditions is often with antenatal ultrasound. Gastroschisis occurs when bowel protrudes through a defect in the abdominal wall adjacent to the umbilicus. Surgical repair is possible. Large defects may require staged surgery, the herniated gut being contained within a

Table 17.7 Neural tube defects

Diagnosis	Pathology
Anencephaly	Absence of the cerebral cortex and much of the skull
Encephalocele	The brain protrudes through a midline skull defect
Meningocele	Dural and arachnoid tissue herniate through a defect created by an incomplete vertebral arch. The spinal cord remains normally sited
Myelomeningocele	Neural tissue from the spinal cord protrudes through the defect
Spina bifida occulta	Skin covers the defect. This skin may be abnormal – usually an incidental finding in an asymptomatic individual

silastic sack until the bowel can be accommodated in the abdominal cavity. Exomphalos is a similar protrusion of gut but it occurs through the umbilicus and the bowel is covered with amniotic membrane and peritoneum.

Neural tube defects

The incidence of neural tube defects has declined over the last 40 years. Antenatal screening (elevated alpha-fetoprotein and/or ultrasound) detects most cases during the early stages of pregnancy, allowing termination. Periconceptual folic acid reduces the risk of recurrence in subsequent pregnancies. The defects are described depending on the site in which the neural tube fails to close (see Table 17.7).

The neurological outcome for these children varies enormously. Early diagnosis, and neurological and neurosurgical assessment are necessary. Walking and continence are the major management issues in the defects compatible with life. Other congenital anomalies are discussed in relevant chapters.

Congenital and genetic disorders 18

(Nandu Thalange)

CHAPTER CONTENTS

INTRODUCTION

Congenital and genetic disorders are a major cause of morbidity and premature death in childhood. The presentation of these conditions may be at or before birth with congenital malformations, in early life with impaired development, or in the older child with learning difficulties or problems with growth or sexual development. Some disorders manifest as regressive conditions, with progressive loss of skills and functions, usually culminating in early death, such as Duchenne muscular dystrophy, or Rett's syndrome. Some genetic disorders do not become evident until adult life, such as Huntington's disease, or inherited forms of Parkinson's or Alzheimer's diseases.

The huge advances in genetics set in train by the Human Genome Project are now starting to feed into clinical practice, with better characterization of a range of disorders, and new diagnostic tools with ever more possibilities for diagnosis. Indeed, it is likely that, in the lifespan of this textbook, we will see a move towards whole-genome sequencing as a diagnostic aid.

Putting a label to a condition is very satisfying for a clinician. It may direct attention to key aspects of management (e.g. ultrasound surveillance for Wilms' tumour in Beckwith syndrome); it may enable a prognosis – developmental, intellectual, physical – to be pronounced on. However, for some parents or children, a label may be devastating – few parents will share the clinician's pleasure at an erudite diagnosis, particularly if there is the potential for future affected children (or grandchildren). Nevertheless, for many parents, a diagnosis is helpful in affirming the child's problems, charting the likely future course, and facilitating appropriate support for their child.

CONGENITAL ABNORMALITIES

Congenital abnormalities range from trivial morphological abnormalities, such as a rudimentary extra digit, to lethal conditions such as major brain malformations. At birth, 2–3% of infants are recognized to have a congenital malformation. By age 5, this rises to 4–6%, as abnormalities not initially evident become manifest. In 40–60%, the cause is unknown. A chromosomal/genetic cause is found in 10–15%. Environmental factors, such as congenital infections (see Chapter 17, p. 256), maternal disease (e.g. diabetes), nutritional deficiencies, hypoxia, drug and alcohol exposure contribute about 10%. The remainder arise from a combination of genetic and environmental factors.

Congenital abnormalities may be categorized as:

- **Malformations** – something occurs to disturb the normal development of an organ or structure. It may result in complete or partial absence, as occurs in most cases of congenital hypothyroidism, or alteration of structure, as occurs in congenital heart disease
- **Disruptions** – a disruption arises when the normal structure is affected by a process (usually destructive) after formation of the organ. For example, intestinal atresias are believed to result from a transient vascular insult during fetal life
- **Deformations** – the fetus is in a confined space. To develop normally, the fetus needs to move. Conditions which impair movement may lead to multiple postural deformities (arthrogryposis multiplex), as may occur in infants born to mothers with myasthenia gravis. Other 'packaging defects' are less severe, such as talipes (see Chapter 6, p. 44)
- **Syndromes** – a constellation of findings, which may themselves appear unrelated, may point to a syndromal diagnosis. Down syndrome (trisomy 21), is such an example. Other syndromes may not have a genetic origin, such as VACTERL (Vertebral anomalies, imperforate Anus, congenital Cardiac disease, Tracheo-oesophageal fistula, oEsophageal atresia, Renal anomalies and radial Limb defects). This arises from defective mesodermal development during embryogenesis.

Environmental factors

A number of environmental factors are implicated in the development of congenital abnormalities:

- **Congenital infection,** notably the ToRCH infections (Toxoplasma, Rubella, Cytomegalovirus and Herpes simplex), varicella and HIV (see Chapter 17, p. 256)
- **Hyperthermia** – fever secondary to infection, or use of hot tubs and sauna
- **Radiation** – studies of pregnant Japanese women exposed to radiation in Hiroshima and Nagasaki in World War 2 found that 28% miscarried, 25% of live born children died in infancy and 25% of survivors had CNS abnormalities – principally microcephaly and mental retardation
- **Environmental chemicals** – there is little definitive evidence about chemical exposure and congenital malformations, but growing circumstantial evidence implicates a number of chemicals as potential teratogens (e.g. arsenic, insecticides, lead, mercury, organic solvents, paint, polychlorinated biphenyls, toluene)
- **Alcohol** – fetal alcohol syndrome/fetal alcohol spectrum disorder may result from alcohol exposure (see below)
- **Prescribed drugs** – a number of drugs are known teratogens in pregnancy, but the severity of the underlying medical condition precludes their withdrawal. In general, drug use in pregnancy should be minimized, and known teratogens should be stopped prior to conception if at all possible (see Table 17.2, p. 249)
- **Recreational drugs** – drug use in pregnancy is often not disclosed, and often multiple drug exposures occur. Poor nutrition and concurrent alcohol use make attributing particular outcomes difficult. The best evidence is for cocaine use in pregnancy. Cocaine is a potent vasoconstrictor. Use is associated with miscarriage, intrauterine growth retardation, microcephaly, gastroschisis and genitourinary abnormalities.

Maternal disease

A number of maternal conditions have the potential to cause fetal malformations:

- **Maternal diabetes** – 2–5% of pregnancies are complicated by gestational diabetes mellitus (GDM), which accounts for 85–90% of diabetes in pregnancy. Often this is associated with maternal obesity. GDM arises during pregnancy, and is not associated with increased fetal malformations, but there is a high rate of miscarriage and fetal death, and neonatal morbidity and mortality from increased preterm birth, and complications of prematurity, coupled with macrosomia or growth retardation. Type 2 diabetes accounts for about 8–10%, with the remainder having type 1 diabetes. In contrast to GDM, hyperglycaemia during organogenesis may cause a range of fetal malformations, with an overall incidence of 5–15%:
  - Congenital heart disease – ventricular septal defect (VSD) transposition of the great vessels, hypoplastic left heart syndrome, complex congenital heart disease
  - Neural tube defects – anencephaly, holoprosencephaly, meningomyelocoele, spina bifida/caudal regression sequence (incomplete development of the sacrum and lumbar vertebrae, femoral hypoplasia, disruption of the spinal cord)
  - Renal agenesis and multicystic, dysplastic kidney
  - Pyloric stenosis, anorectal atresia, left micro-colon
  - Cleft palate
- **Congenital adrenal hyperplasia** – women affected by congenital adrenal hyperplasia need to take *suppressive* doses of hydrocortisone in pregnancy (or a suitable alternative steroid, e.g. prednisolone) to prevent virilization of a female fetus by the action of maternal androgens.
- **Phenylketonuria (PKU)** – phenylalanine is toxic to the fetus. Affected women must be scrupulous in their adherence to their diet and nutritional supplements to achieve near-normal phenylalanine concentrations. Spastic quadriplegia, microcephaly and mental retardation are the consequences of non-adherence. Use of supplemental tetrahydrobiopterin (a co-factor for phenylalanine hydroxylase, the deficient enzyme in PKU) may ease the dietary restriction, facilitating adherence.
- Maternal disease arising from the fetus – a fetus affected by long-chain 3-hydroxyacyl-CoA dehydrogenase deficiency produces toxic metabolites which cross the placenta and may result in severe maternal disease – severe pre-eclampsia, acute fatty liver of pregnancy, cholestasis of pregnancy and HELLP syndrome (Haemolysis, Elevated Liver enzymes and Low Platelets).

In an ideal world, women planning pregnancy would abstain from alcohol and recreational drugs, stop non-essential medication, be adequately nourished, including having folic acid supplements, and, if relevant, optimize care of pre-existing medical conditions, whether associated with fetal malformations or not. Unfortunately, 40–50% of pregnancies in the UK, especially in high-risk groups like teenagers, are unplanned. When pregnancy is confirmed, organogenesis is already substantially under way, meaning that harm may already have occurred. (See also Chapter 17, p. 247.)

Fetal alcohol syndrome

As shown in Case 18.1, the fetus is very vulnerable to the effects of maternal alcohol ingestion. There is strong evidence that binge drinking is more detrimental than regular alcohol intake. The effects of alcohol on the fetus are threefold:

- **Impaired growth** – resulting in reduced head size, intrauterine growth retardation (usually symmetrical), post-natal growth failure with poor catch-up growth (sometimes compounded by growth hormone deficiency)
- **Characteristic morphological abnormalities:**
  - Hypertelorism with epicanthic folds obscuring the inner canthi
  - Narrow palpebral fissures
  - Low nasal bridge and short nose
  - Thin upper lip with indistinct philtrum
  - Hockey-stick palmar creases
- **Cognitive impairment** with subsequent learning disability, behaviour problems (notably attention deficit disorder).

More severe fetal malformations may occur, such as VSD, cleft palate, hypoplasia or agenesis of the corpus callosum, joint dislocations, scoliosis, myopia, sensorineural hearing loss, etc.

Morphological abnormalities may not be evident if the mother did not drink heavily in early pregnancy, making the diagnosis more problematic, unless it is disclosed. Conversely, some women stop drinking heavily once they realize they are pregnant, and consequently the child has the characteristic appearance of fetal alcohol syndrome, but has relatively normal intellectual functioning.

The keys to optimizing success in education are structure and consistency. The child has a short attention span, so brief messages, repeated until embedded, are more successful.

Long-term prognosis is poor. Most go on to have long-term mental health problems, with few (<20%) living independently, and relatively few able to gain employment.

Case 18.1 A girl with fetal alcohol syndrome

Fiona, a 4 year-old-girl, was referred to the growth clinic with poor growth. The GP disclosed in the referral letter that her mother was receiving treatment for alcoholism. Aside from being small, her development was delayed – particularly her speech and language. On examination, she had microcephaly (head circumference below 2nd centile), and a heart murmur. She had typical features of fetal alcohol syndrome. Echocardiography showed a VSD, which was repaired, but there was no improvement in her growth She subsequently was found to have moderate learning difficulties with very poor concentration, and needed a high level of extra support at school. At age 7 years, she went to a special school, as she was unable to function adequately in a mainstream school. Her growth remained poor, with a projected final height of 140 cm.

INHERITANCE OF GENETIC DISEASE

It is important to understand the different patterns of inheritance of genetic disorders. There are four principle patterns of inheritance: autosomal recessive, autosomal dominant, sex-linked and mitochondrial. The inheritance pattern – and risk of recurrence – differs for each.

Autosomal inheritance

Autosomal recessive inheritance

Classic Mendelian inheritance describes traits as recessive or dominant. The human genome contains about 20 000–25 000 pairs of protein-encoding genes. Each individual carries a number of mutated genes, but as genes are inherited in pairs, the unaffected gene can compensate for the lost function. However, if an individual inherits a pair of defective genes, one from each parent, disease may result. The probability of such an event is 1:4 if both parents are carriers. Diseases inherited in an autosomal recessive pattern are typically severe. Examples include cystic fibrosis and phenylketonuria (PKU). Further children of the same relationship may be affected, but a family history would be very unusual, unless there is significant consanguinity in the family history.

Autosomal dominant inheritance

Some proteins have important functions, and require both genes to be functional. Loss of one gene results in haploinsufficiency, e.g. mutations affecting lipoprotein lipase, resulting in familial hypercholesterolaemia, or neurofibromin in neurofibromatosis type 1. Alternatively, the mutated gene may make a protein which has detrimental effects ('dominant negative') as in osteogenesis imperfecta, when defective collagen fibres affect the structure of collagen helices, thus weakening the structure of bone. In achondroplasia, the abnormal gene, a fibroblast growth factor receptor, gains function, and is 'switched on' even in the absence of the fibroblast growth factor ligand, resulting in skeletal dysplasia. Such conditions are referred to as autosomal dominant. The recurrence risk is 1:2, and there is usually a family history, unless the mutation has arisen de novo, which is not infrequent (as in Case 18.3).

Sex-linked inheritance

Sex-linked conditions arise from mutations on the X or, less commonly, Y chromosome. Females have two X chromosomes, and thus can compensate for the loss of a gene on one chromosome. Males, on the other hand, have only one X, and the loss of function is therefore manifest in males, but not usually in females. Examples include haemophilia A and B, fragile X (an important cause of learning disability in boys) and Duchenne muscular dystrophy. Occasionally females are affected, thus some female 'carriers' of fragile X have learning difficulties, but they are, nonetheless, much more mildly affected than males. Some sex-linked disorders are of such severity that male fetuses are not viable, thus only girls are known to have the condition. An example is Rett's syndrome, a neurodegenerative disorder almost exclusively affecting girls, due to mutations in the MECP2 gene at Xq28.

Certain dominant or X-linked conditions appear to worsen with successive generations – a phenomenon referred to as *anticipation*. Commonly such disorders have triplet repeat sequences which become expanded in oocyte formation. Thus, anticipation occurs only with mother to child transmission, as no expansion of the triplet repeat sequence occurs during spermatogenesis. An example is myotonic dystrophy, caused by mutations in myotonic dystrophy protein kinase on chromosome 19. In this condition, a mildly affected mother may give birth to a much more severely affected child, who may have a long period of ventilator dependence, with attendant morbidity and mortality.

Mitochondrial inheritance

Mitochondrial inheritance differs from the other forms of inherited disease, as it can only be passed down the female line. Inheritance may be traced in the family tree, and it will be evident that no children of affected fathers are themselves affected – only children of affected mothers. Certain forms of mitochondrial deafness are inherited in this way. There is great heterogeneity in the manifestations of mitochondrial disease. A number of well-recognized, but severe, mitochondrial disorders are recognized, e.g. MELAS (Myoclonic Epilepsy, Lactic Acidosis and Stroke-like episodes).

Imprinting disorders

The phenomenon of imprinting refers to the fact that certain genetic regions are only active on either the mother's or father's chromosomes. As a result, a deletion affecting the same region of a chromosome can have quite different effects depending on the parent of origin. Thus, deletion of the paternally derived chromosome 15q11 results in Prader–Willi syndrome, whereas maternal deletion results in Angelman's syndrome. The same result may arise if a child inherits two chromosomes from the same parent. For example, if a child inherits two copies of chromosome 7 from their mother, and thus the child lacks paternally expressed genes, Russell–Silver syndrome results. This phenomenon is referred to as *uniparental disomy*.

GENETIC INVESTIGATIONS

Chromosome analysis

For many years the first-line genetic investigation has been a *karyotype*. This has now been superseded by *low-resolution micro-array* which gives more detailed genetic information, more quickly, and at lower cost, than conventional high-resolution cytogenetic analysis.

Cytogenetic analysis is still required for analysis of chromosomal translocations, as balanced translocations will not be evident on micro-array analysis. In emergencies, e.g. where urgent fetal sexing or confirmation of aneuploidy (e.g. trisomy 21) is required, *fluorescence in situ hybridization (FISH)*, using appropriate probes, allows rapid diagnosis within 2–3 working days.

Antenatal testing

Sometimes, the need for genetic tests is evident before birth, due to a prior history of genetic disease, or the finding of morphological abnormalities on ultrasound, (see Chapter 17, p. 248). In early pregnancy, fetal sexing can be determined with high reliability on a maternal blood sample, between 7 and 9 weeks' gestation. This may indicate the need for further investigations. For example, with a family history of haemophilia, an X-linked disorder, if the fetus is found to be a male, then chorionic villous sampling (CVS) at 10–12 weeks will permit molecular genetic diagnosis. For disorders that are not sex-specific, CVS is the initial investigation of choice. Later in pregnancy, amniocentesis and subsequent culture of fetal amniocytes will allow a detailed karyotype to be done. This is, however, more time consuming, and pregnancy is more advanced, making decisions about possible termination of pregnancy more problematic.

Neonatal testing

The newborn infant may be recognized to have dysmorphic features or abnormalities which indicate a possible genetic diagnosis. In this circumstance genetic investigation is indicated without delay as it may aid in management and decision-making, as in Case 18.2.

Case 18.2 An infant with Edwards' syndrome

George was born at term, to a 41-year-old mother. She had declined antenatal screening for fetal abnormalities. At birth, George was growth retarded. He had a number of dysmorphic features, including microcephaly, 'rocker-bottom' feet and his thumbs were grasped in his hands. He had a loud heart murmur, and urgent echocardiography confirmed a diagnosis of tricuspid atresia (complex congenital heart disease). The clinical features led to a suspicion of trisomy 18 (Edwards' syndrome), which was confirmed by urgent genetic analysis, using FISH probes for chromosome 18. As Edwards' syndrome is uniformly fatal, cardiac surgery was felt inappropriate. An end-of-life care plan was put in place, and George died a few days later at a local children's hospice.

Table 18.1 Genetic tests in the newborn infant

Clinical problem	Test
Urgent confirmation of a suspected chromosomal aneuploidy (e.g. Down syndrome)	Fluorescence in situ hybridization (FISH) using appropriate probes
Urgent confirmation of genetic sex in an infant with ambiguous genitalia	FISH using appropriate probes
Confirmation of genetic status of a child born to a parent with a known balanced translocation	Karyotype (if not done antenatally)
Investigation of a child with multiple congenital anomalies	Low-resolution micro-array (or karyotype if array unavailable)*
Investigation of a specific genetic abnormality (e.g. cystic fibrosis)	Specific molecular genetic testing

*Note that low-resolution micro-array is replacing the karyotype as a standard first line investigation.

The finding of significant congenital abnormalities at birth should prompt genetic investigation. The nature of the problems will dictate the investigation performed (see Table 18.1).

Genetic investigation of older children

Indications for genetic investigation of the older child are primarily:

- Unexplained learning or developmental difficulties (see Chapter 4, p. 29, for a list of investigations to be considered in the child with developmental delay)
- Dysmorphic features
- Short stature and/or delayed puberty
- Confirmation of specific diagnoses (e.g. confirmation of a clinical diagnosis of cystic fibrosis).

As with any other part of medicine, genetic investigation begins with a careful history. This includes a careful family and pregnancy history, with careful inquiry into any illnesses and deaths. It is important to enquire specifically about miscarriages, as these may be an indication of a maternal balanced translocation.

The family tree should include both sets of grandparents, and any other first- or second-degree relatives. Exploring the family tree needs to done thoroughly and accurately, but with sensitivity. For an example of a complex family tree, see Figure 1.1, p. 4.

Careful physical examination may reveal clues as to the diagnosis, such as the typical hockey-stick palmar crease of fetal alcohol syndrome. It is very important to look closely at the face, hair line, ears and inside the mouth. Enquire about birth marks. Look at height, weight and body proportions – some conditions are characterized by asymmetry, e.g. Russell–Silver syndrome (see Table 18.2). Formal ophthalmological examination may be helpful for some conditions (see Case 18.3). For other cases, radiographic investigation may be decisive (see Case 18.4).

Case 18.3 A case of neurofibromatosis type 1

Ricky, aged 3 years, presented to hospital with gastroenteritis. He was noted to have multiple café-au-lait patches, although no other abnormalities were noted. His height was just above the 9th centile, whereas his head circumference was above the 75th centile. He was referred to the visiting genetics team with a possible diagnosis of neurofibromatosis type 1. The clinical geneticist was unable to confirm the diagnosis clinically, as the family history was negative, and asked for ophthalmological review. This confirmed the presence of characteristic Lisch nodules, which, in conjunction with the café-au-lait patches, was sufficient for a clinical diagnosis of neurofibromatosis, without the need for molecular genetic testing. Ricky was referred to the neurofibromatosis clinic for ongoing follow-up.

Case 18.4 A case of skeletal dysplasia

Iona, aged 4 years, was referred with short stature. She had normal development, but her head was relatively large. Her parents reported that they struggled to buy clothes that would fit, and measuring her sitting height confirmed that she had relatively short limbs, compared with her trunk. A skeletal dysplasia was suspected, and a skeletal survey suggested a diagnosis of achondroplasia or hypochondroplasia. Mutation analysis of the FGFR3 gene confirmed hypochondroplasia (a milder variant of achondroplasia). The diagnosis facilitated provision of appropriate help at school.

COMMON GENETIC SYNDROMES

The range of genetic diagnoses is large, and growing by the day! The assistance of a clinical geneticist in guiding appropriate investigations is invaluable. The commoner genetic conditions are shown in Table 18.2.

Table 18.2 Common genetic syndromes

Syndrome	Incidence	Genetics	Key features	Key problems	Outlook
Achondroplasia	1 in 20 000	Autosomal dominant Most spontaneous mutations in FGFR3 (chromosome 4)	Short stature Macrocephaly Limb shortening Frontal bossing Flat nasal bridge	Growth – the average final height is 126 cm for a woman and 131 cm for a man Movement – motor skills delayed. Walking and head control are a particular problem Hearing – conductive hearing loss secondary to glue ear is common Neurology – greater risk of hydrocephalus and spinal cord compression	Normal IQ – unless there are neurological complications Normal lifespan
Angelman	1 in 15 000	Deletion of maternal Chromosome 15q11.2-13 (70%), paternal uniparental disomy (2%), or imprinting defect (2–3%), mutation in ubiquitin-protein ligase EB3A (25%)	Puppet-like movements Inappropriate emotions/ bouts of laughter Microcephaly Tongue protrusion	Epilepsy – greater incidence of seizures with a characteristic EEG pattern Learning difficulties – a universal problem but there is some range of ability	Puberty is often delayed Seizures may continue into adulthood Scoliosis may develop in adolescence

Continued

Table 18.2 Common genetic syndromes—cont'd

Syndrome	Incidence	Genetics	Key features	Key problems	Outlook
Angelman - cont'd				Speech – limited speech development Movement – delayed motor skills. Walking with a characteristic ataxic gait	
Di George	1 in 3000	Deletion at chromosome 22q11.2	Hypertelorism Micrognathia Low-set ears with a notched pinna Short philtrum Fish-shaped mouth	This anomaly is caused by the defective embryological development of the 1st to 6th branchial pouches Hypocalcaemia – the parathyroid glands may be absent or hypoplastic, giving rise to low parathyroid hormone. This may present as tetany or as seizures Congenital heart disease – various abnormalities seen. Interrupted aortic arch, tetralogy of Fallot and VSD are common malformations	Heart disease – the nature and severity of the congenital heart disease will often determine the prognosis Immunodeficiency – requires careful investigation. Irradiated blood products should be used because of the potential for graft vs host disease

| Down | 1 in 800 | Trisomy of chromosome 21 | Up-slanting palpebral fissures
Brachycephaly
Single palmar crease
Hypotonia
Tongue protrusion | Immunodeficiency – thymic hypoplasia causes defective T-cell function | Congenital heart disease - over 50% of children. AVSD (atrioventricular septal defect), ASD, VSD, tetralogy of Fallot are all common
Bowel – greater incidence of duodenal atresia and imperforate anus
Learning difficulties – moderate to severe difficulties
Average IQ is 60
Airway – large tonsils, adenoids and glossoptosis may obstruct the airway
Glue ear and obstructive sleep apnoea are common | Life expectancy – average age at death is 49 years
Endocrine – routine screening for thyroid disease is required
Cancers – leukaemia is more common but other cancers are less common
Spine – atlantoaxial instability may give rise to neurological symptoms
Extension of the neck during intubation may be hazardous |

Continued

Table 18.2 Common genetic syndromes—cont'd

Syndrome	Incidence	Genetics	Key features	Key problems	Outlook
Edwards (trisomy 18)	1 in 7000	Trisomy of chromosome 18	Microcephaly Short palpebral fissures Low-set, malformed ears Small mouth Prominent occiput	Congenital heart disease – seen in 90% of cases. VSD, aortic and pulmonary valve defects, ASD, PDA, TGA (transposition of the great arteries) and tetralogy of Fallot are all common Bowel – structural gastrointestinal anomalies are seen Renal tract – congenital anomalies are common Endocrine – thymic, thyroid and adrenal hypoplasia may occur	60% of babies die before the age of 1 month Death arises from the associated congenital defects in the cardiovascular, gastrointestinal and renal tracts
Fragile X	1 in 2000 males 1 in 4000 females	X-linked inheritance of the FMR1 gene	Learning difficulties Prominent large ears Macro-orchidism Long thin face Prominent forehead	Learning difficulties - moderate to severe difficulties with an average IQ of 40 Behaviour – behaviours similar to children with ADHD may be seen	Normal life expectancy There may be significant psychological morbidity associated with the learning difficulty

| Fragile X – cont'd | | | | Autistic behaviours are also more prevalent
Mental illness – depression and obsessive compulsive disorder is more common
Neurodevelopment – global patterns of delay are seen | |
| Klinefelter | 1 in 500 males | Additional X chromosome producing an XXY genotype | Gynaecomastia
Tall adult stature
Small testes | Infertility – seminiferous tubule dysgenesis causes universal infertility
Learning difficulties – IQ generally normal. It may lower with each extra X chromosome, e.g. XXXY XXXXY
Mental illness – depression and anxiety disorders are seen more commonly
Gynaecomastia – caused by elevated oestrogen levels. There is a higher risk of breast cancer | Normal life expectancy
Many cases are not diagnosed until later life when adult males are investigated for infertility and hypogonadism |

Continued

Table 18.2 Common genetic syndromes—cont'd

Syndrome	Incidence	Genetics	Key features	Key problems	Outlook
Marfan	1 in 10 000	Autosomal dominant	Tall stature Arachnodactyly Pectus excavatum Scoliosis Hyperextensible joints	Cardiovascular–aortic root dilatation in up to 75%. Aortic dissection may follow Occular – lens dislocation occurs in 50% of cases Respiratory – spontaneous pneumothorax may arise Motor skills – the associated ligamentous laxity may delay fine and gross motor skills	The associated cardiovascular disease is the major cause of death Shortened life expectancy with an average of 45 years at death Normal IQ
Patau (trisomy 13)	1 in 10 000	Trisomy of chromosome 13	Microphthalmia Scalp defects (cutis aplasia) Cleft lip and palate Microcephaly Post-axial polydactyly Rocker-bottom feet	Congenital heart disease – seen in 80% of cases. PDA, VSD, ASD and dextrocardia are common Brain – holoprosencephaly is seen in 5–10%	Life expectancy is less than 3 days. Only 5% survive beyond 6 months of age Congenital heart disease is the major cause of death

Prader–Willi	1 in 10000	Defect on chromosome 15 inherited from the father	Almond-shaped eyes Short stature Small hands and feet Obesity Hypotonia	Feeding – early feeding problems secondary to poorly coordinated suck and swallow. Hyperphagia arises from the 2nd year of life. Neurodevelopment – global patterns of delay are seen Tone – hypotonia obvious in the neonatal period Behaviour – obsessive-compulsive and extreme food-seeking behaviours seen Learning difficulties – mild difficulties	Shortened life expectancy associated with obesity and its related cardiovascular and endocrine disease Behaviour problems may cause significant morbidity throughout childhood and into adult life
Russell–Silver	Unknown	Sporadic Loss of methylation at 11p15 due to mutations in telomere imprinting centre region 1 (ICR1) in paternal allele in about 30–40% Maternal uniparental disomy for chromosome 7 (mUPD7) in 10%	Short stature Small triangular face Blue sclera Micrognathia Hemihypertrophy	Growth – intrauterine growth retardation, followed by poor post-natal growth Development – patterns of global delay may be seen	Growth hormone may help final stature Some children may have a learning difficulty diagnosed in later life

Continued

Table 18.2 Common genetic syndromes—cont'd

Syndrome	Incidence	Genetics	Key features	Key problems	Outlook
Turner	1 in 2000 females	45XO (50%), 45XO/46XX Mosaicism 20%, abnormal X (30%)	Short stature Webbed neck Broad chest with widely spaced nipples Low posterior hairline Increased carrying angle of arms	Growth and puberty – short stature and primary ovarian failure is universal. Treatment involves growth hormone therapy and oestrogen replacement Congenital heart disease – this is more common than in unaffected females. Coarctation of the aorta is the most frequent lesion	Girls with Turner's syndrome have a normal intellect Life expectancy is slightly reduced. This is attributable to the associated cardiovascular disease
Williams	1 in 20000	Sporadic Deletion on chromosome 7q11.23	Prominent thick lips with open mouth Short upturned nose Stellate iris Periorbital fullness Long philtrum	Behaviour – friendly, outgoing nature with a 'cocktail party' personality Cardiovascular disease – congenital valvular stenosis is more frequent Learning difficulties – mild to moderate difficulties occur Hypercalcaemia – seen in the neonatal period. This is usually asymptomatic	The associated cardiovascular disease may cause death in infancy Most individuals remain healthy and have a normal life expectancy The level of learning difficulty will determine the adult's ability to live an independent life

Appendix I
Paediatric resuscitation

(Peter Bale, David Booth)

INTRODUCTION

Injuries are the largest single cause of death in children over 1 year of age. Road traffic accidents (mainly as pedestrians), drowning and fire account for a significant proportion. When faced with a casualty outside of hospital use the 'SAFE' approach (see Figure I.1):

- **S**hout for help: ask someone to get an ambulance and make sure they come back and help you
- **A**pproach with care: be vigilant for threats, e.g. broken glass, traffic, live electrical wires
- **F**ree from danger: prevent injury or risk to yourself
- **E**valuate the airway, breathing and circulation (ABC): perform basic life support (BLS).

BASIC LIFE SUPPORT

Check for responsiveness by asking 'Are you all right?' and gently stimulating the child. Do not shake a child with suspected cervical spine injuries.

A frightened child may not reply, so look for other signs of life. In all cases, immobilize the cervical spine first if trauma is suspected.

Airway

Open the airway using a chin lift or jaw thrust aiming for a neutral position in infants and a 'sniffing' position for older children.

Do the following, *each for 10 seconds*:

- Look for chest movement
- Listen for breath sounds
- Feel for breath against your cheek

Breathing

Give five rescue breaths if the child is not breathing. The usual mouth-to-mouth position works for larger children (pinch the nose); in infants you need to cover the nose with your mouth as well. Check that the chest rises as you give slow breaths (to avoid pressure trauma). Are you unable to get two good breaths in? Readjust the airway and try again. If this still does not work, suspect airway obstruction and follow the choking algorithm (see p. 282).

Circulation

Check for a pulse by palpation, for 10 seconds. Use the carotid except in infants, where the brachial artery is used (it is easier to find). If the pulse is absent or less than 60 beats per minute start cardiac compressions at a ratio of 15 compressions to 2 breaths (15:2). In 1 minute you should be delivering 4 cycles of 15:2 and the compression rate should be 100/minute.

Aim to depress the chest to a depth of one third. Hand position for compressions varies with age:

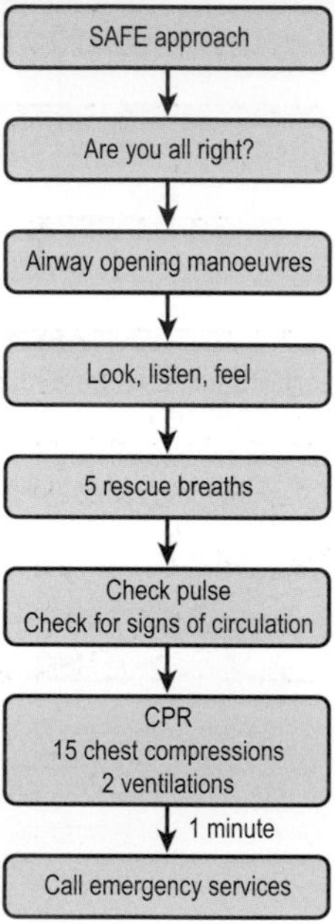

Figure I.1 The overall sequence of basic life support in cardiopulmonary arrest. CPR, cardiopulmonary resuscitation. (Reproduced with the kind permission of the Resuscitation Council (UK).)

- **Infants.** Encircle the chest with both hands, and press both thumbs together over the mid-point of the sternum. If alone, use the index and middle finger of one hand together, over the sternum, on a line that joins the nipples.
- **Child <8.** Use the heel of one hand, just above the level of the xiphisternum.
- **Child >8.** Use two hands to compress the chest, just above the xiphisternum. See Figure I.2 for the initial approach to cardiac arrest.

Key points

Most paediatric arrests are respiratory in origin. It is reasonable to deliver a minute of BLS as this may be enough to revive a collapsed child. After this time, if the emergency services have not yet been called, do this immediately. A smaller child may be carried with you to a phone. If the child recovers, place them on their side and continue to assess the ABC until help arrives.

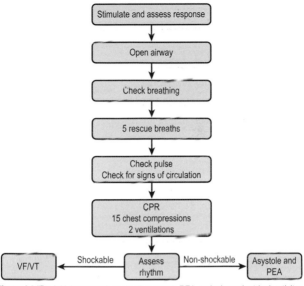

Figure I.2 The initial approach to cardiac arrest. PEA, pulseless electrical activity. (Reproduced from Advanced Life Support Group, 2010, Advanced Paediatric Life Support, BMJ Books.)

CHOKING

Coughing or gagging or a child who becomes suddenly quiet suggests airway obstruction. If the child is conscious, encourage coughing; other 'assistance' may cause total obstruction. If the child becomes quiet, or silent and cannot speak or cry, or if the cough becomes quiet and ineffective, or if they become cyanosed or lose consciousness, then you should call for help and start the interventions outlined in Figure I.3.

Obvious foreign bodies can be removed but do not perform a blind finger sweep. Obstruction due to infection, such as epiglottitis, should not be managed in this way.

ADVANCED LIFE SUPPORT

When help arrives with specialized equipment the ongoing management of the child depends on the cardiac rhythm. Remember to continue BLS while you assess this.

Weight

All drug doses in paediatrics vary with the size of the patient. Calculate an approximate weight using the formula:

Weight (kg) = (age + 4) × 2.

Thus an average 2-year-old will weigh: (2 + 4) × 2 = 12 kg.

Pocket Essentials of Paediatrics

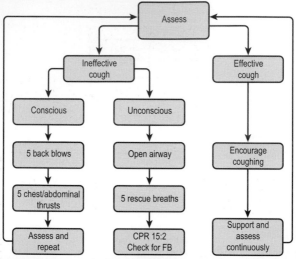

Figure I.3 The sequence of actions in a choking child. FB, foreign body. (Reproduced from Advanced Life Support Group, 2010, Advanced Paediatric Life Support, BMJ Books.)

Asystole

This is usually secondary to severe hypoxia and acidosis. Adrenaline (epinephrine) can be given via the endotracheal tube 100 μg/kg if there is no other access. Sodium bicarbonate is only used in refractory acidosis. Atropine is not routinely used in paediatrics.

Ventricular fibrillation and pulseless ventricular tachycardia

These rhythms are found in children with hypothermia, cardiac disease and tricyclic antidepressant overdose. The paddles are placed over the apex and the sternum in children. With infants, place one paddle on the front and one on the back (see Figure I.4).

Pulseless electrical activity

The most common cause for this is hypovolaemia (see Figure I.4).

Discontinuing resuscitation

A decision to stop may be taken by the team leader in agreement with the members of the team. This is usually after 30 minutes without any cardiac output. With cases of hypothermia or poisoning, expert advice is needed before such a decision is taken.

Paediatric Advanced Life Support

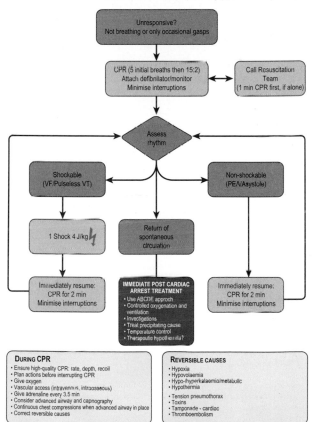

Figure I.4 4 J/kg on all shocks, not incremental. Adrenaline should be every 4 minutes, from before the 3rd shock and amiodarone before the 4th. Copyright European Resuscitation Council - www.erc.edu - 2012/037.

NEWBORN LIFE SUPPORT

The majority of babies require no help at birth. In those that do, most only require a little stimulation or a few inflation breaths to expand the lungs and displace the liquor. Cold, wet babies are harder to resuscitate so dry them and keep them warm.

PAEDIATRIC EMERGENCIES

Remember

In all emergency situations the first priority is to assess the airway, breathing and circulation (ABC) and provide appropriate life support. Reassess the situation frequently and respond quickly to the changing situation. Get help. Emergencies cannot be managed single-handed.

Shock

Shock results from failure of the circulation to perfuse the organs. Reduced oxygen delivery results in anaerobic respiration and acidosis, which is exacerbated by the accumulation of metabolic waste products in the tissues.

How to recognize shock

Children with shock are usually worryingly ill. Whatever their presentation, the onset of shock is heralded by deterioration with pallor, drowsiness and apathy. Examination can reveal sighing respirations, tachycardia, poor pulse volume, slow capillary refill and, in the later stages, hypotension. Poor brain perfusion results in agitation or depressed conscious level. Failure of peripheral perfusion causes cold peripheries, which can be measured using the difference between peripheral and core temperature (Box I.1). See Box I.2 for causes of shock.

Managing the shocked child

Airway and breathing come before supporting the circulation.

- **Airway.** Children unable to maintain their own airways may be managed with an oropharyngeal or nasopharyngeal airway.
- **Breathing.** Administer oxygen (15L/min via a face mask) to improve tissue oxygenation, even if the saturations are adequate. Support failing respirations with bag valve and mask ventilation. If the child becomes apnoeic, intubation and ventilation is needed; this should be attempted by a person proficient in intubation of children. In hospital, an anaesthetist should be called.

Box I.1 Capillary refill

This measure of skin perfusion measures how long the skin takes to go pink again after the examining finger squeezes the capillary blood out. It is assessed by pressing on the skin over the sternum or the pulp of a finger for 5 seconds. Return of capillary pinkness within less than 2 seconds is normal. Remember that other conditions can result in poor peripheral perfusion: fear or pain via adrenaline (epinephrine) release or a rapidly rising temperature.

Box I.2 Causes of shock

- Low circulating volume
- Dehydration (e.g. gastroenteritis)
- Haemorrhage
- Burns
- Intra-abdominal loss, e.g. peritonitis, volvulus
- Pooling of blood in dilated vessels
- Septicaemia
- Anaphylaxis
- Head or spinal cord injury
- Cardiac failure
- Arrhythmia
- Cardiomyopathy
- Heart failure
- Myocardial injury/infarct
- Obstruction to blood flow to or from the heart
- Tension pneumothorax/haemothorax/flail chest
- Pulmonary embolism
- Failed oxygen carriage by the blood
- Severe anaemia
- Carbon monoxide poisoning/methaemoglobinaemia

- **Circulation.** Assess the degree of shock and look for potential causes. Site two large-bore cannulas and take blood to look for a cause, e.g. infection, dehydration, hypoglycaemia. Repeated attempts at IV cannulation should be avoided, and the intraosseous (IO) route should be used instead. Do not forget to cross-match blood in trauma. Check for the signs of heart failure: raised jugular venous pressure, lung crepitations, gallop rhythm, enlarged liver.
- **Treatment.** Treat shock (except cardiogenic shock) with a fluid bolus of 20 mL/kg of 0.9% saline then assess the response. Some centres use colloid solutions such as 4.5% human albumin solution as primary replacement fluid in septicaemia. Haemorrhagic shock requires blood urgently. Blood group O negative blood may usually be obtained urgently. Continue to reassess as you treat the cause. The initial fluid bolus can be repeated as required, but bear in mind that two boluses are the equivalent of half the child's circulating volume. Ventilation is likely to be necessary, and appropriate arrangements should be made to transfer the child to a critical care environment.
- **Glucose.** Always check the blood glucose in any seriously unwell child. Treat hypoglycaemia with 5 mL/kg 10% glucose IV.

Anaphylaxis

Anaphylaxis results from massive histamine release following a type 1 allergic reaction. The allergen is often ingested – milk, peanut or egg are the commonest, but the reaction may follow insect stings or inhaled allergens.

How to recognize anaphylaxis

Signs of anaphylaxis include urticarial rash or flushing, facial swelling or itching, stridor, wheeze or difficulty breathing, abdominal pain and diarrhoea and circulatory collapse.

Managing anaphylaxis

1. **Remove the allergen** if still exposed
2. **Perform BLS** as required
3. **Airway:** anaesthetist should be called for airway management if stridor is present. Administer intramuscular (IM) adrenaline (epinephrine) 10 μg/kg of 1:1000
4. **Breathing:** wheeze as part of acute anaphylaxis should be treated with intramuscular adrenaline (epinephrine) as above. In milder cases, inhaled or nebulized salbutamol may suffice
5. **Circulation:** treat shock with a fluid bolus of IV 20 mL/kg 0.9% saline and give adrenaline (epinephrine) as above if this has not already been done
6. **Giving IV hydrocortisone 4 mg/kg and chlorphenamine** (an antihistamine) will also help. These drugs do not work quickly so maintain BLS and frequently reassess the child until stable
7. **Repeat fluid boluses** as required
8. **Explore the history** to identify the precipitant.

Cardiac arrhythmias

Primary cardiac emergencies are rare in childhood. When a child presents with a tachycardia do not forget to include cardiac disease in the differential diagnosis.

How to recognize a cardiac arrhythmia

There may be an abrupt onset of tachycardia and the child may be aware of palpitations. Tachycardias often present in infants. If they present in shock this must be distinguished from sepsis, dehydration and other causes of shock.

Managing a cardiac arrhythmia

Assess the child using the ABC sequence and commence ECG monitoring:
- Is the child shocked?
- What is the heart rate?
- Is the rhythm regular or irregular?
- Is the QRS complex on the monitor narrow or broad?

Supraventricular tachycardia

Suspect supraventricular tachycardia (SVT) with pulse rates over 220 beats per minute. The complexes are usually narrow – like a sinus tachycardia – but the heart rate does not vary from beat to beat and there is no preceding illness causing shock, although the patient may be shocked now (see Figure I.5).

Vagal manoeuvres:
- Stimulate the diving reflex by applying an ice-cold towel to the face, covering the face with a plastic bag containing iced water or immersing the baby's face in iced water. These sound and look frightening but are safe and effective

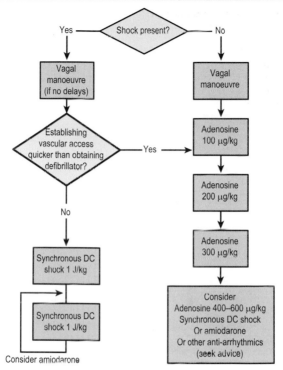

Figure I.5 Algorithm for the management of SVT (Reproduced from Advanced Life Support Group, 2010, Advanced Paediatric Life Support, BMJ Books.)

- Perform unilateral carotid massage
- Get an older child to perform the Valsalva manoeuvre – e.g., by blowing the wrong way into a syringe.

Ventricular tachycardia

In haemodynamically stable children with ventricular tachycardia (VT), ask about a history of cardiac surgery or poisoning. Discuss their management with a paediatric cardiologist urgently before the rhythm deteriorates. Shocked children require either IV amiodarone or asynchronous DC cardioversion. If there is no pulse, proceed with the pulseless VT algorithm (see Figures I.6 and I.7).

Bradycardia

In a sick child this is a preterminal sign. Maximize resuscitation efforts to treat the cause. Use adrenaline (epinephrine) (see Figure I.8).

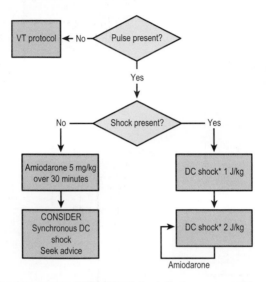

Figure I.6 Rhythm in ventricular tachycardia (a regular tachycardia with a heart rate of 240 beats per minute).

Figure I.7 Algorithm for the management of VT. (Reproduced from Advanced Life Support Group, 2010, Advanced Paediatric Life Support, BMJ Books.)

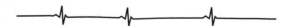

Figure I.8 Rhythm in preterminal bradycardia.

MENINGOCOCCAL SEPTICAEMIA

Meningococcal septicaemia causes shock as a result of a complex interaction of infection, toxin release and immune reaction. There may be rapid onset of vasculitis and deranged clotting with a purpuric rash, and shock from both poor cardiac function and pooling of blood within the circulation.

How to recognize meningococcal sepsis

Children with overt meningococcal sepsis deteriorate rapidly. This may be preceded by a prodrome of non-specific malaise, fever and lethargy. A rash

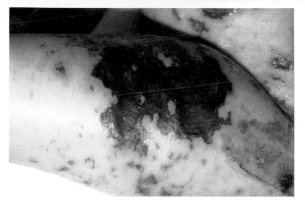

Figure I.9 Appearance of meningococcal purpura.

present at this stage is often maculopapular and blanching, making diagnosis difficult. Even blood tests may be normal (see Figure I.9).

The characteristic non-blanching, purpuric rash means shock and cardiovascular collapse are imminent, secondary to widespread endothelial injury, capillary leak and disseminated intravascular coagulation. Depression of consciousness may be secondary to concurrent meningitis or shock. Incipient cardiac failure and pulmonary oedema give rise to tachycardia and dyspnoea with elevated jugulovenous pressure or hepatic enlargement. Oliguria signals renal failure. Do not delay; give antibiotics (e.g., ceftriaxone 80 mg/kg OD) immediately!

Managing meningococcal sepsis

1. Approach and resuscitate using the ABC sequence.
2. Establish intravenous access and send blood for full blood count (FBC), urea and electrolytes (U&E), magnesium, phosphate, coagulation, glucose, cross-matching, and blood culture. Blood can be sent for a polymerase chain reaction (PCR) test for meningococcal antigens.
3. Give high-dose antibiotics as soon as possible (cefotaxime or ceftriaxone). Out of hospital, give parenteral benzylpenicillin. For children 3 months and older, if there are meningitic signs and no evidence of shock, give dexamethasone 0.15 mg/kg QDS (maximum dose 10 mg).
4. Treat shock with a fluid bolus of 20 mL/kg 4.5% human albumin solution or 0.9% saline. Monitor the response and repeat as required. Ask for an intensive care review after the second bolus as capillary leak is likely to make ventilation necessary along with further boluses and inotropic support.
5. Take a throat swab and send scrapings from a skin lesion on a slide for microscopy to look for Gram-negative diplococci.
6. Correct electrolyte and clotting abnormalities. Intensive or high-dependency care will be needed.
7. *Do not attempt lumbar puncture!*
8. Meningococcal disease is notifiable. As soon as practically possible, the local public health department should be notified. Contact tracing and antibiotic treatment will be required for all close contacts.

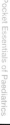

DIABETIC KETOACIDOSIS

Diabetic ketoacidosis (DKA) may be the first presentation of type 1 diabetes or it may occur in a known diabetic secondary to infection, trauma, or non-adherence to insulin therapy.

How to recognize diabetic ketoacidosis

The history usually comprises polydipsia, polyuria and weight loss followed by vomiting and abdominal pain. Look for dehydration, deep-sighing breathing ('Kussmaul breathing' – indicating severe acidosis). A fruity smell on the breath is acetone. Salicylate poisoning and uraemia may present in a similar manner. Confirm the diagnosis by finding hyperglycaemia (glucose >11.0 mmol/L), ketones in the urine (3+ or 4+) or blood (beta-hydroxybutyrate >3 mmol/L) and acidosis (pH <7.35, HCO_3 <15 mmol/L).

Managing diabetic ketoacidosis

1. Administer oxygen by face mask and monitor oxygen saturation and ECG.
2. Site two intravenous lines and take blood as above.
3. Treat shock with 20 mL/kg 0.9% saline, given over 30 minutes.
4. Calculate the maintenance fluid volume required and the volume required to correct the assessed dehydration over 48 hours. Use normal saline until the glucose is 12–14 mmol/L, then use 0.45% saline with 5% glucose.
5. Commence an IV insulin infusion at 0.1 u/kg/h, reduce to 0.05 u/kg/h if glucose falls rapidly, (more than 5 mmol/h), especially in young children, to reduce risk of cerebral oedema.
6. Add potassium when the child has passed urine as the child will have a total body potassium deficit, regardless of the presenting plasma sodium, and is at risk from hypokalaemic arrhythmias. Bicarbonate therapy is contraindicated, except for refractory shock with severe acidosis.
7. Observations should be frequent – quarter- to half-hourly – and include neurological observations. If consciousness is impaired, a nasogastric tube should be inserted to prevent aspiration.
8. Monitor the plasma glucose hourly, and check blood gas and electrolytes at least every 4 hours in the acute phase. Adjust the insulin rate to ensure a gradual reduction in blood glucose.
9. Identify and treat any precipitating cause.
10. Critically ill children need intensive care; these include those with severe shock, arrhythmias, aspiration, renal failure and cerebral oedema.
11. Once recovered, recommence their usual insulin and diet. Address any non-adherence to insulin therapy.

Key points

Overly aggressive fluid resuscitation may precipitate fatal cerebral oedema in children with DKA. Signs include headache, agitation, reduced conscious level, hypertension, bradycardia or abnormal pupil reactions. Treat promptly with mannitol 0.5 g/kg, intubate and commence ventilation.

STATUS EPILEPTICUS

Prolonged seizures put children at risk of brain injury, multi-organ failure and death.

How to recognize status epilepticus

Status epilepticus is easily diagnosed when a tonic-clonic seizure persists for more than 30 minutes or when there is no recovery between fits. More subtle seizure activity with stiffness or eye/head deviation may be the only sign in an unconscious child.

Causes of status epilepticus

- Epilepsy (either established or newly presenting)
- Meningitis or encephalitis
- Prolonged febrile convulsion
- Trauma (including non-accidental injury)
- Metabolic disturbance (e.g. hypoglycaemia)
- Poisoning.

Managing status epilepticus

1. Protect the airway, assess breathing and give oxygen. NB: steps 2–4 should be dealt with within 5 minutes to avoid delay in treatment.
2. Assess circulation and, if the child is shocked, treat with 20 mL/kg parenteral fluid bolus.
3. Consider antibiotics if there is any suspicion of sepsis.
4. Check glucose and treat if it is less than 5 mmol/L with 10% dextrose 5 mL/kg intravenously.
5. Control the seizure:
- If there is IV access, give lorazepam 0.1 mg/kg
- If there is no IV access, give buccal midazolam 0.5 mg/kg or rectal diazepam 0.5 mg/kg
- Repeat once after 10 minutes if the seizure is not controlled
- If there is no response, give rectal paraldehyde 0.4 mg/kg in saline
- If the seizure continues for more than a further 10 minutes, give:
  - Phenytoin 18 mg/kg IV over 30 minutes. If the seizure ceases during the infusion, complete the infusion.
  - In a known epileptic, already using phenytoin as maintenance medication, use phenobarbital 20 mg/kg, given as a 20-minute infusion, as an alternative.
- Monitor respiratory rate, ECG and blood pressure during administration.
- If the seizure is not controlled within 30 minutes of the phenytoin infusion being completed, reassess for possible causes. Rapid sequence induction by an anaesthetist may be required. Discuss with a paediatric neurologist for further advice.

Key points

Status epilepticus has a mortality of 5%, often from the underlying cause. Keep to time when administering the various medications. Avoid getting either too far behind or ahead of schedule.

COMA

In children a decreased conscious level is usually due to metabolic upset, poisoning or hypoxia, regardless of the underlying pathological process. Effective resuscitation will help to reverse hypoxia. Further treatment depends on the cause and an effective history, examination and appropriate investigation should elicit this.

Causes of coma

- Hypoxia (following respiratory or circulatory failure)
- Infection, e.g. meningitis or encephalitis
- Seizures
- Trauma – accidental and non-accidental
- Poisoning – accidental and intentional
- Raised intracranial pressure – shunt blockage, intracranial bleeding, brain tumours
- Metabolic, e.g. hypoglycaemia, diabetes, hepatic or renal failure
- Hypertension.

How to assess a child in coma

1. Assess the level of consciousness using either the AVPU or Glasgow Coma Scale (see below).
2. Check the eye movements, pupil size and reaction to light.
3. Look for decorticate (flexed arms, extended legs) or decerebrate (extended arms and legs) posturing.
4. Assess the fontanelle if present (is it bulging?) and determine whether neck stiffness is present or not.
5. Check the deep tendon and plantar reflexes.
6. A high blood pressure with a bradycardia and altered respiration is known as Cushing's triad. It is a late sign of raised intracranial pressure.

AVPU score

A   Alert
V   Res ponds to Voice
P   Responds to Pain
U   Unresponsive

The Glasgow Coma Scale

Originally designed to quantify altered consciousness with head injury, the GCS has now become a tool for all occasions. There is a modified version for young children. The maximum score is 15 and the minimum is 3. Eight or less is taken as coma (see Figure I.10).

Pupillary changes

Pin-point pupils	Narcotics ingestion or metabolic disorder
Fixed dilated pupils	Severe hypoxia, hypothermia or seizure
Unilateral dilated pupil	Expanding ipsilateral lesion/tentorial herniation

Managing the child in coma

1. Approach and resuscitate using the ABC method.
2. Assess the extent of the neurological abnormality as described above. (Sometimes included in the ABC sequence as D for disability.) Children with a GCS of less than 8 or responding only to painful stimuli should be considered for intubation to protect the airway.

GCS	Score	Modified GCS for young children
Eye opening		
Spontaneous	4	Spontaneous
To verbal stimuli	3	To verbal stimuli
To pain	2	To pain
No response	1	No response
Best verbal response		
Oriented and talking	5	Usual self
Disoriented	4	Spontaneous cry, less chatty
Inappropriate words	3	Cries to pain
Incoherent noises	2	Moans to pain
No noise	1	No noise
Best motor response		
Obeys command	6	Spontaneous movements
Localizes pain	5	Localizes pain or withdraws to touch
Withdraws from pain	4	Withdraws from pain
Flexion to pain	3	Flexion to pain
Extends to pain	2	Extends to pain
No response	1	No response

Figure I.10 The Glasgow Coma Scale (GCS).

3. Check the blood glucose and treat hypoglycaemia with 5 mL/kg of 10% glucose.
4. Once the airway is secure, and oxygenation and circulation are assured, the diagnosis can be sought via history, further examination and investigations. These will include a blood gas (preferably arterial), FBC, U&E, blood culture and blood group or save serum (in case blood product transfusion required). Obtain urine for toxicology.
5. Cranial imaging is likely to be needed in a comatose patient without an obvious cause. A CT scan is quickest and will show most major intracranial events, although the child will need to be stabilized and possibly ventilated beforehand.
6. Cover any suspected infection with a broad-spectrum antibiotic (e.g. cefotaxime).

Pocket Essentials of Paediatrics

7. Children with signs of raised intracranial pressure should be managed in the intensive care unit. Neurosurgical advice should be sought.
8. Mannitol 1 g/kg may temporarily relieve raised intracranial pressure.

> **Key points**
>
> Determine the child's health and activities over the last day or two. Was there an illness or infectious contact? Is there a history of trauma or a risk of non-accidental injury? Are there any chronic medical conditions? Did the child have access to alcohol, medication or drugs, including drugs of abuse?

EMERGENCY CHILD PROTECTION

Children who require safeguarding present to health professionals in a number of ways. Some will do so as an emergency, often out of hours. This section gives a broad outline of what to do. It should be read in conjunction with the chapter on child protection (Chapter 5). Preparation for these situations is vital. Know and read your local child protection procedures before the event (see Figure I.11).

Recognition

Recognizing harm is covered in detail in Chapter 5. Key considerations in the history and examination include:

- Inappropriate history or inconsistent history
- Delay in presentation
- Presence of exacerbating social factors such as:
  - Domestic violence
  - Social isolation
  - History of drug or alcohol problems
- Worrying injuries including fractures, burns, bites, unusual bruises or marks, or any injury to a non-mobile child.

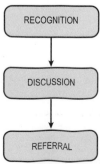

Figure I.11 Algorithm for the management of child protection concerns.

> ### *Personal safety*
>
> Investigating and managing protection issues can create strong emotions. Families, whether they are responsible for harm or not, can become confrontational. Careful and sensitive communication can almost always prevent this. However, it is necessary to be aware of your surroundings and risks. Let colleagues know what you are doing. Do not place yourself in a vulnerable setting. Secure your escape route before you need it. Let a security team and/or the police know if you predict or sense violence.

Discussion

Early discussion is vital. This must involve a conversation with your senior colleagues. It is not the responsibility of junior doctors to take these decisions alone. In all situations, other than when to do so might endanger the safety of the child or yourself, this discussion should include the parents and/or carers. It is not acceptable to make onward referral, admit or otherwise make decisions about children without letting the family know why. This may be a difficult conversation and senior support is needed. The first task is to offer appropriate medical care and the second is to keep the child safe. Remember that siblings must be kept safe. Urgency of onward referral depends in part on the severity of the injury. If a child is admitted dead or critically ill as a result of possible non-accidental injury it is essential to inform police and social services at once to ensure proper investigation of any crime and proper care for the family and any other children.

Referral

Social services

Onward referral to social services may be able to wait for working hours. However, useful information can be gathered from referral at any time. Access to the local child protection register is available at any time. This information is rarely vital in immediate decision-making, but it may give some detail about previous contact with the family. A telephone referral should be followed up by a written referral within 48 hours.

The police

It may be necessary to inform the police. Assistance with protecting a child in a family that refuses to cooperate with enquiry, e.g. attempting to remove the child from hospital, can be achieved with a police protection order (PPO). A crime against a child may have been committed. The police need to be given the opportunity to investigate. This might require forensic work and/or the arrest of possible perpetrators. Referral in this situation cannot wait.

Support and reflection

This out-of-hours emergency work involves some of the most upsetting and distressing aspects of child protection work and indeed paediatrics as a whole.

When it is over stop and reflect. All doctors should have an opportunity to do this regularly. In particularly harrowing cases, a formal 'de-brief' for all the professionals involved is extremely valuable.

ACUTE STRIDOR

Children often wake in the night with stridor – panic in both the child and parents can make the situation worse. Unless the child has ineffective respiratory effort or reduced consciousness, do not immediately confront them with face masks, drips and ECG leads as this may make panic worse. A calm approach, maintaining parental involvement is best.

How to recognize acute stridor

Severe stridor presents with supraclavicular in-drawing, subcostal and intercostal recession and reduced air entry. Stridor may not be loud if the airway is compromised. Hypoxia, if it is due to upper airway obstruction, is a sign of severe disease.

Managing acute stridor

Oxygen, if required, should be given in a non-threatening way. Nebulized adrenaline (epinephrine) may be useful as a holding measure, but its effects are short-lived. Intubation has become rarer, as the use of steroids for croup has increased. If necessary, intubation is ideally performed in theatre by an experienced ENT surgeon with a skilled paediatric anaesthetist.

If the airway is compromised, intubation may be essential to save life, in less than ideal circumstances. See Figure I.12 for a detailed management plan.

HEAD INJURY

Head injuries are common in children. Most are minor, require no treatment, and have no sequelae. Unfortunately, significant head injuries occur and survivors may be left impaired. Behaviour problems, intellectual impairment and post-traumatic epilepsy may arise.

Careful assessment and appropriate resuscitation at presentation will decrease secondary brain injury (caused by hypoxia, acidosis, hypo- or hyperglycaemia, or poor cerebral perfusion). 'Primary brain injury' refers to the neural damage sustained at the time of the accident and is currently beyond our skills to treat.

Assessment

Start with the ABC approach and consider cervical spine injury in all children with head trauma. Ascertain the mechanism of injury; ask about any loss of consciousness and symptoms since the injury, such as vomiting or seizures. In the initial assessment, include the level of consciousness (GCS), pupillary and deep tendon reflexes and plantar reflexes. Look for signs of focal neurological defect on your secondary survey.

Management

Children with minor head injuries are often fit to be discharged after initial assessment. Admit all children who are unconscious for over a minute, have a skull fracture or CSF leak, are still experiencing headache or vomiting after 4 hours or have had a seizure. When children present with head injury, consideration must be given to the possibility of non-accidental injury, particularly in non-mobile children.

Adequate fluid resuscitation helps maintain the cerebral perfusion pressure, but too much fluid risks cerebral oedema. Treat seizures and use antibiotics if

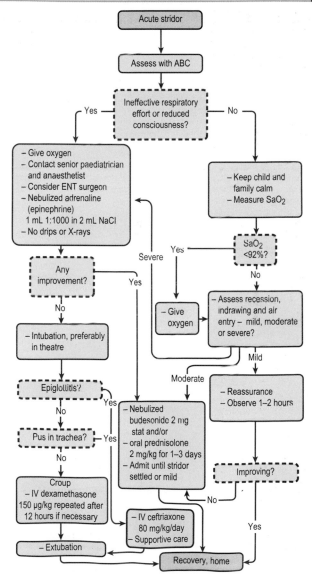

Figure I.12 Algorithm for the management of acute stridor.

there is an open injury. Children with severe head injuries require a CT scan; this is performed only when the child is stable and ventilated if necessary.

Neurosurgical referral will be required if there is a depressed or compound skull fracture, penetrating injury or intracranial bleeding. Focal neurological signs, coma or decreasing conscious level are also indications for referral.

Types of intracranial haemorrhage

- **Extradural haematoma.** This is typically found in teenagers, often as the result of a direct blow leading to a ruptured meningeal artery. Treatment involves urgent craniotomy and evacuation.
- **Subarachnoid haemorrhage.** This presents with headache, vomiting, fever, drowsiness and neck stiffness. It may follow a minor injury or be secondary to a ruptured berry aneurysm in an older child.
- **Subdural haematoma.** Blood leaks from venous tears caused by deceleration injuries (including shaking). It may present acutely and require surgical drainage or may follow a more chronic course, detected by an increasing head circumference.
- **Intracerebral haemorrhage.** An elastic skull makes these more common in children; especially in the posterior parietal region.

BURNS

Burns are a common injury in childhood. Toddlers exploring their environment may reach for the power cable of an iron or vessels containing scalding liquid. Serious burns occur with house fires, although it is usually the inhalation of smoke that kills, rather than the thermal injury.

Approach

Be wary of cervical spine and other injuries, as with serious fires there may be explosions or children may jump/fall to safety.

Use the ABC sequence

- **Airway.** The airway may be involved, with the inhalation of hot smoke leading to progressive laryngeal oedema which may then asphyxiate the child. Involve an anaesthetist early in this situation
- **Breathing.** The lungs may also be damaged by smoke or heat inhalation. Give oxygen; look for physical signs and monitor oxygen saturation
- **Circulation.** Obtain intravenous access as burns greater than 10% of the child's surface area draw fluid out of the circulation that will need replacing. Discuss the exact regime with a burns centre. Give a 0.9% saline 20 mL/kg if the child is shocked and repeat as necessary. If more than 40 mL/kg is required, seek advice from an intensive care unit and check for other causes of fluid loss.

> **Key points**
>
> **Signs suggestive of airway involvement are:**
> Fire with smoke in a closed space
> Soot around the mouth
> Carbonaceous sputum
> Singed nasal hairs

Make analgesia a priority once life-saving manoeuvres have been performed. Burns are extremely painful and children will cooperate with treatment and recover better if they are pain free. Care of the wounds varies with different centres. A sterile cover will keep it clean and stop air moving across it (which causes pain). Clingfilm allows subsequent assessments of the burn to be made without painful dressing changes and reduces insensible fluid losses from the burned area.

Further management

You need to assess the depth of the burn and the surface area it covers.

Depth

- **Superficial.** Erythematous, painful areas which are usually dry.
- **Partial thickness.** Painful pink skin with blisters; may be moist.
- **Full thickness.** The skin is white or charred and may be painless.

Measuring surface area is done by first carefully documenting the extent of the burn on a diagram. Use a chart to calculate this as a percentage. A rough rule of thumb is that the palm of the child's hand with the fingers closed is equivalent to 1% of their surface area. Refer burns covering 5% that are full thickness or 10% partial thickness (do not include erythema). Experts should also see burns to special sites such as the hands, feet, face or perineum.

ACUTE SEVERE ASTHMA

See Figures I.13 to I.15.

POISONING

Children eat most things – animal, vegetable or mineral. They are frequently 'rushed to hospital' as a result. In the majority of cases, they come to no harm. The commonest presentations are the inquisitive toddlers who discover and eat something while unsupervised, and the impulsive adolescents who ingest tablets after an upset and quickly regret their actions.

One of the important parts of management is to establish what and how much the child has taken. It is useful if the family brings with them an example of what the child has ingested. Excellent support and advice about management can be gained from the national network of Regional Poisons Information Centres in the UK, and on-line databases such as Toxbase.

After the child has recovered, consideration must be given to prevention of a repeat episode. Communication with the health visitor and GP is essential in all cases involving young children. An accurate assessment of the mental health of a child, who took a poison intentionally, is imperative.

Paracetamol

Paracetamol (acetaminophen) is the commonest analgesic used worldwide. It is available over-the-counter in most countries. An intended overdose is more likely to cause harm than accidental ingestion.

When large quantities of paracetamol are ingested the liver glutathione stores are depleted and paracetamol metabolites accumulate. This causes hepatic necrosis and acute renal failure. The liver function tests become

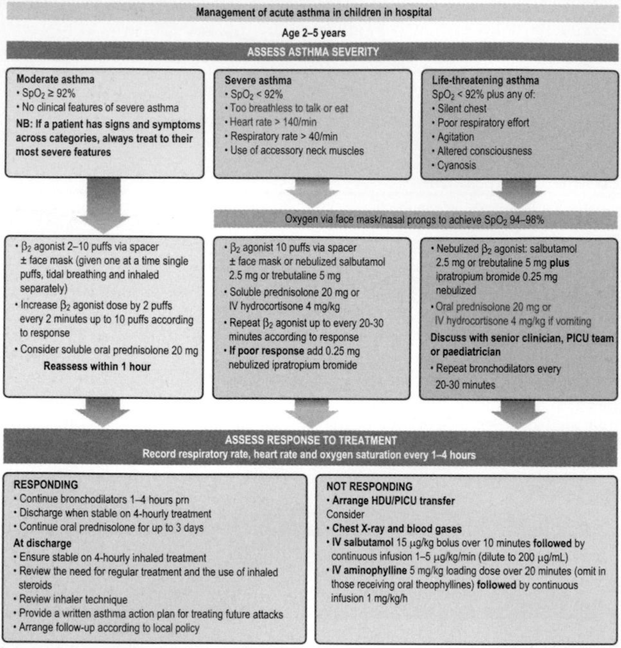

Management of acute asthma in children in hospital

Age 2–5 years

ASSESS ASTHMA SEVERITY

Moderate asthma
- SpO2 ≥ 92%
- No clinical features of severe asthma

NB: If a patient has signs and symptoms across categories, always treat them to their most severe features

Severe asthma
- SpO2 < 92%
- Too breathless to talk or eat
- Heart rate > 140/min
- Respiratory rate > 40/min
- Use of accessory neck muscles

Life-threatening asthma
SpO2 < 92% plus any of:
- Silent chest
- Poor respiratory effort
- Agitation
- Altered consciousness
- Cyanosis

Oxygen via face mask/nasal prongs to achieve SpO2 94–98%

- β2 agonist 2–10 puffs via spacer ± face mask (given one at a time single puffs, tidal breathing and inhaled separately)
- Increase β2 agonist dose by 2 puffs every 2 minutes up to 10 puffs according to response
- Consider soluble oral prednisolone 20 mg

Reassess within 1 hour

- β2 agonist 10 puffs via spacer ± face mask or nebulised salbutamol 2.5 mg or terbutaline 5 mg
- Soluble prednisolone 20 mg or IV hydrocortisone 4 mg/kg
- Repeat β2 agonist up to every 20-30 minutes according to response
- **If poor response** add 0.25 mg nebulized ipratropium bromide

- Nebulized β2 agonist: salbutamol 2.5 mg or terbutaline 5 mg **plus** ipratropium bromide 0.25 mg nebulized
- Oral prednisolone 20 mg or IV hydrocortisone 4 mg/kg if vomiting

Discuss with senior clinician, PICU team or paediatrician
- Repeat bronchodilators every 20-30 minutes

ASSESS RESPONSE TO TREATMENT
Record respiratory rate, heart rate and oxygen saturation every 1–4 hours

RESPONDING
- Continue bronchodilators 1–4 hours prn
- Discharge when stable on 4-hourly treatment
- Continue oral prednisolone for up to 3 days
At discharge
- Ensure stable on 4-hourly inhaled treatment
- Review the need for regular treatment and the use of inhaled steroids
- Review inhaler technique
- Provide a written asthma action plan for treating future attacks
- Arrange follow-up according to local policy

NOT RESPONDING
- Arrange HDU/PICU transfer
Consider
- Chest X-ray and blood gases
- IV salbutamol 15 μg/kg bolus over 10 minutes **followed by** continuous infusion 1–5 μg/kg/min (dilute to 200 μg/mL)
- IV aminophylline 5 mg/kg loading dose over 20 minutes (omit in those receiving oral theophyllines) **followed by** continuous infusion 1 mg/kg/h

Figure I.13 Management of acute asthma in children 2–5 years in hospital. (Reproduced from British Thoracic Society.)

abnormal 18 to 36 hours after ingestion. Peak disturbance in liver function occurs 4 to 6 days after ingestion.

Serum paracetamol levels should be measured 4 hours after ingestion. If the serum level is greater than 200 mg/L, N-acetylcysteine should be given intravenously. For paracetamol levels taken at other times, refer to an appropriate chart to guide treatment. Treatment may be required at a lower level if there is existing liver disease. Treatment may be started before a serum level is available if there is a history of ingestion of more than 150 mg/kg. Treating an ingestion of paracetamol over many hours or days requires expert advice.

Aspirin

Aspirin is contraindicated in childhood. Aspirin poisoning is uncommon. Poisoning occurs as a result of an accumulation of salicylic acid. Subsequent stimulation of the respiratory centres of the brain causes hyperventilation and alkalosis. The body compensates by excreting bicarbonate, sodium and potassium ions and water in the urine, resulting in electrolyte imbalances, dehydration and decreased buffering capacity. This leads to a later metabolic acidosis.

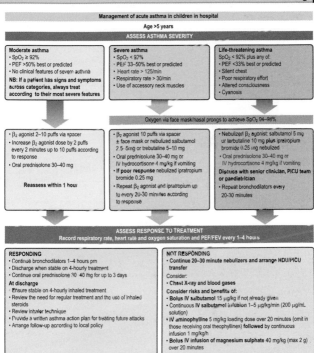

Figure I.14 Management of acute asthma in children >5 years in hospital. (Reproduced from British Thoracic Society.)

The symptoms of poisoning are nausea and vomiting followed by tachypnoea, tinnitus, sweating, epigastric pain and sometimes fever. Later, if poisoning is severe, the child can develop light-headedness, drowsiness, confusion, seizures and difficulty in breathing.

If the ingestion is recognized within 60 minutes, activated charcoal is advised. If the plasma salicylate level is greater than 350 mg/L, forced alkaline diuresis may be necessary. Dialysis and intensive care may be necessary in severe toxicity, indicated by a serum level of >700 mg/L.

Iron

Iron tablets are commonly prescribed to adults and may look invitingly like sweets. In overdose there is early gastrointestinal upset with vomiting, malaena and gastric irritation. Coma, liver failure and hypotension are late effects. Serum iron levels should be measured. Serious toxicity, as indicated by the serum iron level, may require chelation of the iron with desferrioxamine. This can be given earlier if the history suggests a significant ingestion of greater than 60 mg/kg. Radiography is sometimes helpful as iron tablets are radio-opaque and may be detected on an abdominal X-ray.

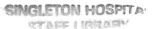

Management of acute asthma in infants aged < 2 years in hospital

ASSESS ASTHMA SEVERITY

NB: If a patient has signs and symptoms across categories, always treat according to their most severe features

Moderate
- $SpO_2 \geq 92\%$
- Audible wheezing
- Using accessory muscles
- Still feeding

Severe
- $SpO_2 \leq 92\%$
- Cyanosis
- Marked respiratory distress
- Too breathless to feed

Most infants are audibly wheezy with intercostal recession but not distressed

Life-threatening features include apnoea, brachycardia and poor respiratory effort

Immediate management

Oxygen via close fitting face mask or nasal prongs to achieve normal saturations

Give trial of β_2 agonist: salbutamol up to 10 puffs via spacer and face mask or nebulized salbutamol 2.5 mg or nebulized terbutaline 5 mg

Repeat β_2 agonist every 1–4 hours if responding

If poor response:
Add nebulized ipratropium bromide 0.25 mg

Consider: soluble prednisolone 10 mg daily for up to 3 days

Continuous close monitoring
- heart rate
- pulse rate
- pulse oximetry
- supportive nursing care with adequate hydration
- Consider the need for a chest X-ray

If not responding or any life-threatening features discuss with senior paediatrician or PICU team

Figure I.15 Management of acute asthma in infants <2 years in hospital. (Reproduced from British Thoracic Society.)

Tricyclic antidepressants

Toxicity arises from the anticholinergic effects. Dry mouth, blurred vision and agitation should be expected. Cardiac arrhythmias are the commonest cause of death. Convulsions and coma are common. Activated charcoal may be useful if given within 1 hour of ingestion; it adsorbs some of the drug. Treatment is supportive.

SUDDEN DEATH IN INFANCY AND CHILDHOOD

- Children are four times as likely to die in the first year of life from both natural and unnatural causes than at any other time.
- It is recommended that all children who die suddenly and unexpectedly in the community be transferred to the hospital A&E department, regardless of whether the chances of successful resuscitation are thought to be negligible, so that the death can be properly investigated.
- Post mortem examination of a dead body is not a sufficient investigation or explanation for the vast majority of sudden child deaths, and the chances of making a diagnosis are greatly improved by undertaking a thorough history, examination and appropriate investigations.
- The death of a child is a terrible tragedy for their family and they need support to help deal with their loss. Families want to know what happened, how the event could have occurred, what the cause of death was and whether it could have been prevented.
- A thorough and sensitively handled initial approach will help with grieving, and also with the family's anxiety about future pregnancies. It may identify some hidden underlying cause, such as a genetic problem.
- Social services and the police should be informed of the death at an early stage.

Informing the family of the death and subsequent events

An experienced paediatrician should inform the family that their child is dead. This should take place in a private and appropriate room. It is better not to speculate on the cause of death, unless this is obvious, and explain that the cause of death will be established after the post mortem examination. Tell the family that all unexplained deaths have to be reported to the coroner and he will require that a post mortem is carried out and that the police, who also have a duty to investigate unexplained deaths, will be directed by the coroner to carry out a visit to the family home. Explain to the family why a detailed history needs to be taken (this can be done later) and why the history, in conjunction with the investigations, are needed by the pathologist to inform the findings of the post mortem. Parents need to know what the post mortem examination involves and that consent from them is not required to perform a coroner's post mortem.

Examination of the child

This should be carried out as soon as possible after the end of resuscitation attempts, by an experienced paediatrician. A detailed, contemporaneous record should be made of the examination findings, remembering that this is a legal document. The following should be noted:

- General appearance and any dysmorphic features
- State of nutrition and cleanliness

- Growth parameters
- Skin and rectal temperature
- Skin marks secondary to resuscitation attempts and any other rashes, bruises or abrasions
- Signs of bony injuries
- Retinal appearance
- Lesions in the mouth, genitalia or anus
- Keep all of the child's clothing in labelled paper bags, closed with tape.

Specimen collection for investigations

Remember that a chain of responsibility has to be established for all samples, in case they form part of a forensic investigation. Samples must be handed to the laboratory staff and signed for.

- Blood
  - If there is insufficient blood collected during resuscitation attempts, samples should be collected by cardiac puncture. Blood glucose should be measured as part of resuscitation attempts.
  - Samples should be sent for microscopy and culture, toxicology, inherited metabolic diseases (Guthrie card sample), genetic testing.
- Cerebrospinal fluid (CSF)
  - Fluid obtained by lumbar puncture should be sent for inherited metabolic disease and microscopy and culture.
- Urine
  - Obtained by aseptic catheterization, urine for microscopy, culture, toxicology and inherited metabolic conditions.
- Swabs
  - Skin surface swabs for microbiology should be obtained from any visible lesions and nasopharyngeal aspirate, throat and nose swabs for microbiology.

History

Taking a history from the family needs to be done carefully and sensitively – it may need more than one interview and discretion should be used when dealing with the grieving family. Records should be detailed, legible and signed. Important components of the history include names and dates of birth of the infant, mother and father and other members of the household. A family medical history, paying particular attention to any deaths in infancy or childhood. A social and family history and medical history of the parents.

The history of the child who has died must be obtained in as much detail as possible, to include medical and developmental history. A detailed account of the 2 weeks prior to death should include feeding, sleeping and activity levels and an hour-by hour narrative of the 48 hours leading up to death should be sought.

Remember

It is every family's right to have their child's death properly investigated and that careful history, examination and specimen collection are vitally important components of this difficult and complex process.

Appendix II
Practical procedures

(Peter Bale, David Booth)

INTRODUCTION

Undertaking a painful practical procedure on a child is a big undertaking. There are no routine investigations in paediatrics. Children and babies experience pain. They react and respond to pain in ways that adults may not recognize. As a result their pain may be missed or ignored.

Before performing one of these procedures make sure you know why it is being carried out and how any results will affect management.

More complex procedures are unusual in children but are part of everyday neonatal practice. Where there are differences in technique for neonates these are indicated in the text.

COMPETENCE, CONFIDENCE AND SUCCESS

Practical procedures in sick children can be daunting. Powerful feelings of anxiety and fear are common in both the child and the operator. A successful procedure that causes the child minimal hurt or distress is a tremendous achievement. A theoretical understanding of the skills involved is helpful but competence is gained only through demonstration, observation and practice. Performance should be under supervision until competence is achieved. With competence comes confidence, and being aware of your own levels of competence and confidence is the key to success.

ANALGESIA FOR PROCEDURES

- **Neonatal.** There is now increased awareness that premature neonates can feel pain and that this can influence pain thresholds and behaviour in later life. Oral sucrose 24% is a useful analgesic in this patient group. It should be given 2 minutes before the painful procedure starts.
  Dosage:
  - 0.5 mL for 37 weeks' gestation and older
  - 0.25 mL for 32–36 weeks' gestation.
- **Children older than 1 year of age.** Various procedures are better tolerated if prophylactic analgesia is employed.
  - Venepuncture/cannulation/PICC lines:
    i. Topical anaesthetic cream – either amethocaine (Ametop) or lidocaine and prilocaine (EMLA). These require application over the site 30–45 minutes prior to the procedure.
    ii. Topical ethylchloride spray is a useful tool if delaying the procedure for topical anaesthetic to become effective is not possible, or if the child has a skin reaction to the cream.
  - Lumbar puncture
    i. Topical anaesthetic cream – lidocaine and prilocaine (EMLA).
    ii. Local anaesthetic 1% lignocaine can be infiltrated at the chosen site to minimize pain on passage of the needle through the skin and subcutaneous tissue.

Adequate preparation and consideration of non-pharmacological factors play an important role in the successful completion of potentially painful procedures in children. Some factors to consider include:

- Well lit and properly equipped room
- Use of a play specialist
- Use of an appropriate number of experienced assistants
- Correct holding and positioning of the child – this allows for a successful procedure attempt without restraining the child against their will
- Presence of parents – this is a matter for individual parent choice.

PREPARATION

Locate all the necessary equipment before starting. An experienced and able assistant is vital. Do not undertake any practical procedure on a child alone.

Preparation for the child is just as important. The play therapist, children's nurse and parents should play a role. An age-appropriate explanation to the child is needed. Do not try to deceive children. If it is going to hurt, tell them. Appropriate distraction therapy is valuable in children and young people of all ages. Sucrose solution on a dummy reduces symptoms of pain in neonates undergoing minor procedures.

BASIC PROCEDURES

Blood sampling and cannulation

Requirements
- Non-sterile gloves
- Distraction therapy
- Alcohol swabs
- Syringes
- Butterfly needles or cannulas
- 0.9% saline flush
- Assorted bungs and connectors
- Splints and dressings to secure
- Capillary tubes and/or blood bottles.

Venepuncture
Topical anaesthetic cream will reduce the discomfort. It takes time – about an hour for lidocaine (EMLA) or 15 minutes for amethocaine (Ametop) – to work. They may cause redness and swelling, particularly if left on for too long. Many children will get upset simply because their arm is restrained, so use distraction – ask a parent or the play specialist to oblige.

An assistant should hold the child and act as a tourniquet. Use a syringe with a butterfly needle (Figure II.1). Children's small veins may not tolerate using vacuum systems. Blood can also be collected from a cannula at the time of insertion, minimizing the number of needles the child has to endure. Neonatal blood sampling needles have no hub and minimal dead space – the blood can be allowed to drip into bottles.

Cannulation
- Find a vein. Commonly used sites: back of hand/foot, antecubital fossa. Less common: ventral wrist, forearm, and scalp
- The person acting as a tourniquet should apply gentle traction to the skin from above to keep the vein position constant

- Wiping with an alcohol swab may make the vein more visible through thin skin
- Introduce the cannula at an angle of 45° through the skin and into the vein (Figure II.2a). Flashback (blood visible in the hub of the needle) may not occur in small veins. If the vein was not entered, pull back (but not out), re-check the position and advance in a different line
- Once in the vein, reduce the angle and go a very small way along the vein
- While holding the needle still, advance the cannula over the needle and into the vein – usually carried out in one movement using the index finger of the same hand (Figure II.2b). Blood may flow up the cannula (secondary flashback)
- Remove the needle and dispose of it in a 'sharps' container
- Sample blood with a syringe, then attach a T-piece or other appropriate connector and flush with 0.9% sodium chloride. Never use water to flush (it hurts!)
- Seal the end with a bung or, if appropriate, connect an infusion
- Secure the cannula firmly. A splint may be required if it is near a joint.

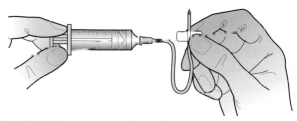

Figure II.1 Butterfly needle and syringe used for venepuncture.

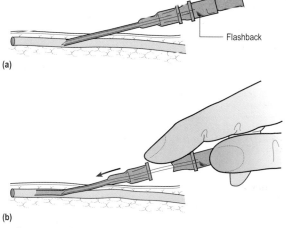

(a)

Flashback

(b)

Figure II.2 Insertion of venous cannula.

Long lines are thin catheters introduced into peripheral veins and advanced centrally. They may be inserted through a needle or over a guide wire. These lines are useful for certain drugs, such as inotropes, or for parenteral nutrition. These lines have a longer lifespan, which is useful for prolonged courses of therapy.

Capillary samples

Requirements

- Alcohol swabs
- Petroleum jelly
- Sterile lancet
- Spring-loaded lancing device
- Capillary tubes and blood collection bottles.

Procedure

- Make sure the extremity is warm
- In babies, use the sides of the heels (Figure II.3), never use the sole of the foot. In older children the side of the thumb or big toe can be used
- Clean the area with an alcohol swab. Application of a thin layer of petroleum jelly makes blood collection easier, but is not always used because of concerns about possible cross-infection – check your local policy
- Use a sterile lancet to make two punctures close together, approximately 2 mm deep. A spring-loaded automatic lancing device is convenient and probably less painful
- Collect the blood onto reagent strips or into capillary tubes. Blood can be allowed to drip into bottles but venepuncture samples are preferred.

MORE DIFFICULT PROCEDURES

Intraosseous access

Requirements

- Non-sterile gloves
- Alcohol swabs
- Intraosseous needle
- Saline flush
- Syringes, bungs and connectors.

Procedure

This is an emergency procedure, contraindicated in pelvic fracture or long-bone fracture in the same leg.

- Use an intraosseous needle or, if unavailable, a bone marrow needle
- The site used is the flat anterior surface of the tibia, a finger's breadth below and medial to the tibial tuberosity. Clean with an alcohol swab
- Consider local anaesthetic if the child is conscious and there is time
- Support the leg on a rolled up towel. Do not put fingers behind the limb in the path of the advancing needle
- Firmly insert the needle using a turning or boring motion. There is a sudden 'give' when the needle enters the bone marrow. The needle should then stay upright unsupported (Figure II.4)
- Remove the stylet. Try to aspirate marrow; send this for the usual samples but tell the lab that it is marrow and not venous blood

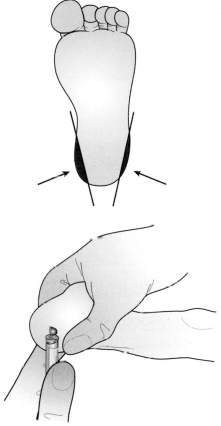

Figure II.3 Heel-prick sites and technique for capillary blood sampling.

- Some units stock a specially designed drill/gun to introduce the intra-osseous needle. A new needle should be used for each attempt. Drill until you feel a 'give' as the bone marrow is entered. Detach the gun and connect a syringe to sample the marrow
- Flush with saline. If there is swelling, the needle is not in the correct position and should be removed
- Secure the needle. Any drug or fluid may be given by this route. Resistance to flow is high, and a syringe may be necessary to push through fluids. Replace with more secure intravenous access when possible
- Complications include tibial fracture, osteomyelitis, compartment syndrome and skin necrosis.

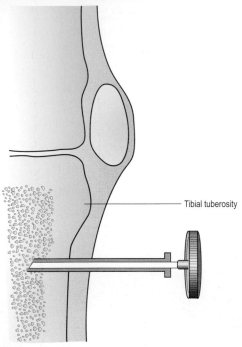

Tibial tuberosity

Figure II.4 Insertion of intraosseous needle for emergency vascular access.

Lumbar puncture

Requirements
- Full aseptic technique with gloves, gown and patient skin preparation and sterile drapes
- Local anaesthetic
- Lumbar puncture needle and manometer
- Bottles to collect spinal fluid – three plain and one fluoride tube for glucose
- Dressings
- Ability to resuscitate child if condition deteriorates.

Contraindications (see also Chapter 16, p. 230)
- The child's condition is unstable
- Abnormal clotting (known bleeding diathesis, or prothrombin ratio (INR) >2; platelet count less than $50 \times 10^9/L$
- Signs of raised intracranial pressure
- Reduced level of consciousness.

Procedure
A cerebrospinal fluid (CSF) sample is necessary to confirm meningitis. The key to success is correct positioning with an experienced helper.

- Use topical anaesthetic cream on the skin at the site of the lumbar puncture if time permits
- The child should be in the left lateral position for a right-handed operator. The lumbar spine should be as flexed as possible, with the plane of the back perpendicular to the bed. The assistant should hold the shoulders and behind the knees, rather than flex the neck
- Scrub up, then clean the skin with antiseptic
- The landmark is the top of the anterior superior iliac spine. A vertical line downwards leads to L3–4 or L4–5 spaces (Figure II.5). Both are suitable
- In older children, local anaesthetic can be instilled. This is painful, and the single pass of a spinal needle may be less so
- Hold the needle bevel upwards and pass it between the vertebral bodies, aiming towards the umbilicus. Keep the needle horizontal. There is moderate resistance through the ligaments and then a 'give' as it passes into the CSF space
- Remove the stylet – if pressure measurement is needed, connect the manometer and record the pressure
- Drip the CSF into sterile pots and a fluoride bottle (for glucose), with 6 drops in each. Remove the needle and dress the site
- The serum glucose should be measured at the time of the lumbar puncture to enable comparison between serum and CSF glucose.

Tips

No CSF?	Gently rotate the needle or withdraw/advance slightly
Bone hit?	Either adjust the angle or the point of insertion
Still not successful?	Make sure the needle is truly horizontal. Try another space
Bloodstained?	Wait a few drops: the CSF may start to clear

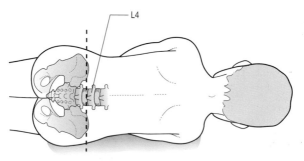

Figure II.5 Position and site for lumbar puncture.

Suprapubic aspiration of urine

Requirements

- Sterile gloves, aseptic technique
- Alcohol swabs
- 10 mL syringe (5 mL in neonates), 21 G needle.

Procedure

This is the 'gold standard' urine sample. Urine in the bladder should be sterile. Suprapubic catheterization should only be attempted after ultrasound confirmation that the bladder contains urine. A catheter specimen of urine may be obtained as an alternative if antibiotics are to be started pending the result.

- Clean the perineal area first. This may stimulate the baby to pass urine so have a sterile pot ready. Now clean the suprapubic area
- With an assistant holding the baby's legs, insert a 21 G (blue) needle on a 10 mL syringe a finger's breadth above the symphysis pubis. Angle towards the feet. Advance slowly, applying gentle suction with the syringe until urine appears (Figure II.6).

UMBILICAL CATHETERIZATION

Requirements

- Full aseptic technique with gloves, gown and patient skin preparation and sterile drapes
- Scalpel, two pairs of fine-toothed forceps, scissors, dilators, silk stitch, needle holders
- Umbilical lines
- Saline flush, syringes
- Bungs and connectors
- Sterile tape.

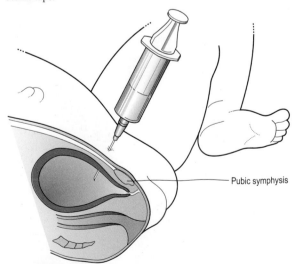

Pubic symphysis

Figure II.6 Suprapubic aspiration of urine.

Procedure

A newborn baby has easily accessible umbilical vessels. Usually two arteries and one vein are present in the umbilical cord (Figure II.7). The vein is large and may ooze blood. Muscular walls make the arteries stand proud but they are smaller.

Emergency umbilical venous catheter insertion

- Flush an umbilical venous catheter (UVC) or thin feeding tube with 0.9% saline. (An empty catheter and syringe may be used and will allow blood sampling as the line is inserted)
- Clean the cord and place a tie lightly around the base (to tighten if it bleeds)
- Cut the cord to about 4 cm long
- Identify the vein and insert the UVC only so far as to be able to withdraw blood – usually about 5 cm
- Administer resuscitation fluids and drugs according to protocol – then replace with definitive access.

Elective UVC insertion

- Calculate the distance to insert the line using a formula (see below) or chart
- Prepare and drape the patient
- Flush the line with 0.9% saline and leave the syringe on the end
- Wrap a tie loosely around the base then cut the cord down to 2–3 cm
- Holding the cord with the forceps, insert the UVC to the calculated length and check that it samples
- Secure the line by taping it to stitches through the cord. Do not apply tape directly onto the baby's fragile skin. Make sure it is secure
- Check the position with a chest and abdominal X-ray.

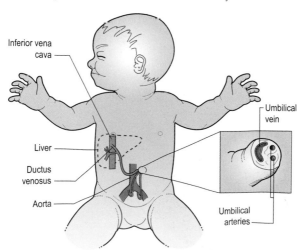

Figure II.7 Anatomy of the umbilical cord.

Umbilical arterial catheter insertion

An umbilical arterial catheter (UAC) is more difficult to insert than a UVC, so attempt it first if both are required.

- Decide the distance for insertion using a formula (see below) or chart
- Prepare and drape the patient
- Flush the line with 0.9% saline and leave the syringe on the end
- Wrap a tie loosely around the base then cut the cord down to 2–3 cm
- Stabilize the artery by holding the adjacent cord with forceps and gently locate the opening using fine-toothed forceps. Encourage it to open with a dilator. Rough handling of the artery will result in arterial spasm
- Gently ease the UAC tip into the artery. Some pressure is needed but too much and there is a risk of making a 'false passage' in the surrounding tissue. As the catheter enters the abdomen gently pull the cord superiorly to aid passage into the iliac artery
- Once in to the predetermined length, secure as above
- Always connect arterial lines to locking taps, bungs or connectors
- Check the position with a chest and abdominal X-ray.

Aim to site a line tip above T10 (high position) or below L4 (low position) to avoid interference with the mesenteric and renal vessels. Lines should not end in the heart or near the abdominal branches of the aorta. If there are signs of compromised circulation to the legs, a UAC must be removed.

Distance to insert umbilical lines

- Umbilical venous catheter: (weight (kg) × 1.5) + 5 cm
- Umbilical arterial catheter: (weight (kg) × 3) + 9 cm
  Do not forget to add on the length of cord to the umbilicus.

ADVANCED PROCEDURES

Radial arterial cannulation

Requirements

- Non-sterile gloves
- Distraction therapy
- Cannula
- Alcohol swabs
- Appropriate locking bungs and connectors.

Procedure

- Pick either a radial or posterior tibial artery
- When using the radial artery, first perform Allen's test, to ensure the patency of the ulnar artery. The hand is elevated and, if old enough, the child is asked to make a fist for about 30 seconds. Apply pressure over both the radial and ulnar arteries, so as to occlude them. Open the hand – it should appear blanched and pallid. Release pressure on the ulnar artery, and the hand should quickly suffuse with blood, becoming pink again. If colour does not return to the hand within 10 seconds, the ulnar artery is compromised, and it is unsafe to proceed with radial cannulation or catheterization
- Support the wrist slightly extended for the radial artery (Figure II.8)
- Find the pulse and insert the cannula towards it. The angle is shallower than for venous cannulation. Flashback will be pulsatile. Advance the cannula and remove the needle
- Connect to lockable bungs or connectors

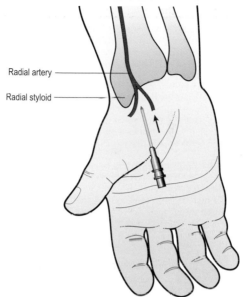

Radial artery

Radial styloid

Figure II.8 Radial artery cannulation.

- If the artery is punctured but the catheter will not advance, remove it and apply firm pressure for 5 minutes
- If there are any signs of ischaemia remove the cannula
- When sampling blood and flushing peripheral arterial lines, do so slowly to prolong their lifespan. Too much haste and the artery will go into spasm.

Endotracheal intubation

Requirements
- Non-sterile gloves
- Monitoring of oxygen saturation and heart rate
- Bag-valve-mask with oxygen supply
- Suction
- Laryngoscope (and spare) with a bright light and different-sized blades
- Suitably sized endotracheal (ET) tube plus one size above and one below
- A means of securing the tube
- A stethoscope.

ET tube sizing
Tube size in children can be calculated using the formula age/4 + 4, and tube length from age/2 + 12. Term newborn infants need a tube size of 3.5. Premature infants will need a 3.0 or even a 2.5 tube.

Procedure
Most children can be maintained using bag-valve-mask ventilation while awaiting an experienced operator to intubate. Learn intubation by being

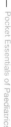

supervised performing elective tube changes. Monitor oxygen saturation and heart rate during the procedure. Stop if it is not tolerated. A struggling child will require sedation and/or paralysis before intubation – an anaesthetist should normally supervise this in an older infant or child

- Pre-oxygenate with bag-valve-mask ventilation
- A neonate needs a neutral head position; for older children extend the neck ('sniffing position')
- With the laryngoscope in the left hand, introduce the blade in the right side of the mouth and centralize, moving the tongue out of the way (see Figure II.9a)
- Insert the laryngoscope blade down to the vallecula before the epiglottis (Figure II.9a). In babies it is easier to go into the oesophagus and pull back until the cords appear (Figure II.9b). Be careful not to traumatize the larynx
- Pressure on the cricoid helps bring the cords into view – use the little finger of the left hand or ask a helper to do it
- Gently suction out secretions
- Insert the ET tube and stop once the black mark (near the tip) is past the cords. Note the length at the lips. Do not insert the ET tube if the cords cannot be seen. Do not push against closed cords

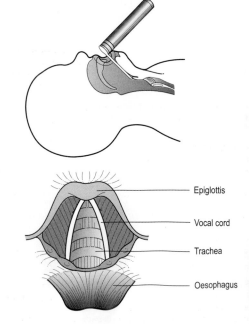

(a)

Epiglottis

Vocal cord

Trachea

Oesophagus

(b)

Figure II.9 Endotracheal intubation: (a) laryngoscope position; (b) view of vocal cords.

- Once the ET tube is in, listen to air entry (while bagging) in both axillae and over the stomach. Louder sounds on the right indicate the tube is in the right main bronchus; pull it back slightly and listen again. If the sounds are loudest over the stomach with little chest expansion then the tube is in the oesophagus: remove it
- Secure the ET tube and confirm position with a chest X-ray.

Chest drains

Requirements

- Full aseptic technique with gloves, gown and patient skin preparation and sterile drapes
- Monitoring of oxygen saturation and heart rate
- Chest drain
- Scalpel
- Forceps for blunt dissection
- Suture material and needle holder
- Dressings
- Underwater seal equipment.

Procedure

Chest drains are used to treat pneumothorax, pleural effusion, empyema and haemothorax. They are painful to insert and in children are often performed by surgeons under general anaesthetic. Insertion of chest drains in the newborn is easily performed under local anaesthesia.

Tension pneumothorax

- Do not delay for an X-ray unless you are uncertain as to the diagnosis
- Insert a cannula or green butterfly needle (in neonates) in the 2nd intercostal space, mid-clavicular line on the same side as the tension pneumothorax
- Connect to a valve or underwater seal
- When things are more stable, insert a chest drain and perform the chest radiograph.

Chest drain

- Support the child with the affected side up
- Aim for the 4th or 5th intercostal space in the mid-axillary line. The position should be guided by ultrasound in empyema
- Infiltrate local anaesthetic using an orange needle. In larger children use a blue needle to infiltrate deeper
- Make an incision just above and parallel with the rib, avoiding the intercostal vessels and nerve that lie inferior to each rib (Figure II.10). With fine forceps bluntly dissect down to the pleura
- Do not use the trocar in the chest drain – use the forceps to insert it. After initial resistance it will pop through the pleura. Advance it so all the holes are inside the chest
- Connect the drain to the seal/valve. Stitch the incision closed. Secure the tube with a stitch and use an occlusive dressing over the whole site
- Confirm drain position with a chest X-ray
- If the drain is not bubbling, applying a small amount of suction may help
- The drain can be removed once it has stopped bubbling for 24 hours. Remove it on expiration (crying). Close the incision and perform a chest X-ray after 2–4 hours.

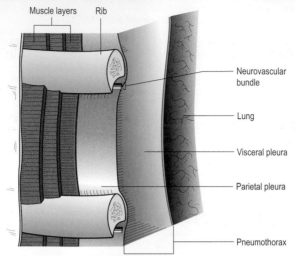

Fig. II.10 Anatomy of the chest wall for chest drain insertion.

Appendix III
Prescribing

(Rosalind Howe, Nandu Thalange)

The principles of good prescribing are relevant for all ages, but for children there are specific issues that include documentation, doses and preparations. Guidance is given here for these.

DOCUMENTATION

The name, date of birth and weight should be indicated on the front of the drug chart. It may be appropriate to record the surface area in children receiving drug doses based on this measurement. The first doctor or nurse to use the drug chart should fill in the drug sensitivities/allergies box and sign it. Prescriptions should be legible, and block capitals should be used. Each prescription should be signed and dated. The date should include the year.

DOSES

All paediatric and neonatal prescribing should be based on the Children's British National Formulary (BNF-C) or an suitable alternative formulary. This facilitates checking of doses. Expert advice from an appropriately skilled pharmacist may be required for drugs not included in this book or if you need to prescribe a drug at variance with the formulary. Drugs should be prescribed by weight rather than by volume. If a volume is prescribed, the strength of the solution should be stated. The term micrograms should be written in full and not abbreviated to 'mcg' to avoid confusion. The prescribed dose should not exceed the maximum dose for adults.

It is important to use the 'yellow card' system for suspected adverse drug reactions in order that vital safety data may be obtained. For example, the antibiotic ceftriaxone has been implicated in deaths of neonates receiving calcium-containing intravenous fluids.

Reporting using the yellow card system may be done on-line: yellowcard. mhra.gov.uk

PREPARATIONS

Young children struggle to take tablets. All children struggle with injections. Many drugs are available as suspensions or syrups. Individual pharmacy departments may be able to help create liquid preparations for drugs not usually available in this form. If intravenous injections are required on a regular basis then an intravenous catheter should be sited. Intramuscular injections are painful and, other than immunizations, there are very few drugs that need to be administered by this route.

PRESCRIBING ERRORS IN PAEDIATRICS

Paediatrics is an area particularly prone to errors. Prescribing errors may have a fatal outcome. Prescribing in young children frequently requires complex dose calculations, particularly for drugs given by infusion. It is vital to double-check dose calculations, independently, especially for potentially hazardous agents.

Prescribing errors occur much more frequently than is reported using standard incident reporting systems; one prospective study found 13.2% of prescriptions contained prescribing errors. Moreover, paediatric prescribing errors are estimated to be 3–4-fold more likely to result in harm, compared with adults. Neonatal prescribing is an area particularly fraught with risk.

The following drugs have been the subject of recent safety alerts in children:

- Opiates
- Gentamicin
- Insulin
- Intravenous paracetamol
- Ceftriaxone and calcium-containing infusions
- Intravenous fluids.

Appendix IV
Fluids and electrolytes

(Nandu Thalange)

VOLUME

Healthy children tolerate marked fluctuations in their daily fluid intake. If they drink lots, they pass lots of urine. If they drink little they become thirsty and seek fluid. However, during illness, and assuming a thermally neutral environment, requirements are calculated according to weight. Note that fluid requirements of a newborn baby change considerably during the first week of life, and vary according to gestation and birth weight (Table IV.1).

Insensible losses – there will usually be an increase of about 20% of normal requirements if there is fever or tachypnoea. Surgical drains and other fluid losses also need to be accounted for. Sometimes transfusions or drug infusions may constitute a significant fluid load and need to be taken into account also, especially in the intensive care setting.

ELECTROLYTES

The electrolyte requirements of a child vary. In good health without significant gastrointestinal, renal or skin loss, they can be approximated (Table IV.2).

DEHYDRATION

The most accurate method of judging an existing deficit is to compare a pre- and post-illness weight. In the absence of a recent weight, clinical judgement is important. The signs of dehydration vary according to severity; this is detailed in Chapter 13, p. 168–169. A summary of the clinical findings is detailed in Table IV.3. Note that, in hypernatraemic dehydration, the usual signs of dehydration are absent (see Chapter 13, p. 169).

FLUID AND ELECTROLYTE REPLACEMENT

Example

A child of 22 kg presents with gastroenteritis and is estimated to be 7% dehydrated.

The fluid requirement is:

$10 \times 100 = 1000$ mL

$+ 10 \times 50 = 500$ mL $+ 2 \times 20 = 40$ mL

Total $= 1540$ mL in 24 hours

To which must be added the allowance for dehydration:

10 mL/kg $\times 7$ (%) $= 1540$ mL

Total $= 3080$ mL over 24 hours $= 128$ mL/h

Table IV.1 Normal fluid requirements

Weight	Volume
1st 10 kg	100 mL/kg/day or 4 mL/kg/h
2nd 10 kg	50 mL/kg/day or 2 mL/kg/h
Subsequent kg	20 mL/kg/day or 1 mL/kg/h

Table IV.2 Electrolyte requirements

Weight	Sodium	Potassium
	(mmol/kg/24 h)	(mmol/kg/24 h)
1st 10 kg	2–4	1.5–2.5
2nd 10 kg	1–2	0.5–1.5
Subsequent kg	0.5–1	0.2–0.7

Table IV.3 Signs of dehydration

Severity	Signs
Mild (5%)	There may be few signs
Moderate (6–9%)	Dry mucous membranes, sunken fontanelle, decreased skin turgor, decreased urine ouput, poor peripheral perfusion, tachycardia
Severe (10%)	Shocked, lethargic, hypotensive with reduced conscious level

The fluid used is ideally normal saline (0.9%) with 5% glucose, if necessary. Potassium is added (up to a maximum of 40 mmol/L, or 20 mmol in a 500 mL infusion bag), depending on electrolyte results.

It is important to replace ongoing losses *in addition* to maintenance fluid requirements. The best way of replacing losses is enterally, ideally with a suitable oral rehydration solution. In situations in which this is not possible, e.g. vomiting or shock, parenteral fluids may be used. Intravenous fluids are not always necessary in children who refuse, or are unable, to drink as a nasogastic tube can be used. The rate of fluid replacement depends on the clinical situation and it needs to be determined after careful consideration of the severity and nature of the dehydration. In general, it is sensible to replace lost fluids slowly, over at least 24 hours.

ELECTROLYTE BALANCE

Disturbances of sodium and potassium are rare, except in acutely ill children, and an explanation should be sought. The most common reason for electrolyte imbalance is the administration of intravenous fluids.

Hyponatraemia is a consequence of excessive sodium losses or, more commonly, excessive water intake of hypotonic fluids, or retention (e.g. syndrome of inappropriate ADH secretion (SIADH); see Chapter 11, p. 134). Hyponatraemia treatment depends on the cause. If secondary to infusion or consumption of hypotonic fluids, fluid restriction (e.g. 2/3 normal maintenance requirements), with or without diuretics, is appropriate. This is also appropriate for patients with SIADH. If secondary to sodium depletion, as occurs in gastroenteritis, then treatment is with normal saline, as described in the example above.

Hyponatraemia, and misguided attempts to treat it, may have fatal results. In March 2007, the National Patient Safety Agency issued a Patient Safety Alert on hyponatraemia, following the deaths of 4 children, associated with infusion of hypotonic fluids, between 2000 and 2007.

Hypernatraemia results from excessive losses of free water or, rarely, excessive sodium intake. Treatment of hypernatraemia is with 0.9% saline, as this will still reduce the plasma sodium, whilst avoiding an overly rapid fall.

Hypokalaemia most often results from excessive urinary losses of potassium. *Hyperkalaemia* is most often a consequence of renal impairment, but also occurs in adrenal insufficiency (see Chapter 11, p. 138) and following widespread cellular injury such as crush injuries and burns.

In determining the cause of electrolyte imbalance it is helpful to measure urinary electrolytes, but this must be done in conjunction with total urinary output, e.g. a hyponatraemic child may be appropriately conserving sodium, but the urinary sodium concentration may still be high if the hyponatraemia is secondary to dehydration with reduced urine output.

Any child receiving parenteral fluids should have regular (daily or twice daily) measurement of electrolytes.

Multiple choice questions

MULTIPLE CHOICE QUESTIONS

1. **Good record keeping. Which of the following are true?**
   a) Keeping good medical records is essential to protect against future litigation
   b) It is a legal requirement to write in black ink
   c) Abbreviations may be used
   d) It is important not to record sensitive information, as the parents or child may subsequently view the notes
   e) Time must be recorded using the 24-hour clock

2. **Which of the following are true of health inequalities?**
   a) Child poverty is associated with obesity
   b) There is a strong relationship between child poverty and educational attainment
   c) Death from meningococcal disease is more common in deprived families
   d) Children from minority ethnic groups are more likely to live in poverty
   e) ADHD may be caused by child poverty

3. **Which of the following represent good practice when telling the parents of a 4-year-old that their son has Duchenne muscular dystrophy?**
   a) It is important for the doctor seeing them in clinic to share the news at once
   b) The news should be delayed until the parents can be seen together
   c) All other staff and relatives should be asked to leave
   d) To avoid causing distress to the parents, the doctor should be kind to them
   e) A written report to the parents is good practice

4. **Which of the following patterns of development give cause for concern?**
   a) A 16-month-old child who does not walk
   b) A child of 24 months who is only able to say 'Mum', 'Dad' and 'dog'
   c) A 2-year-old who has tantrums when she does not get her own way
   d) A 4-year-old with persistent faecal soiling of his underpants
   e) A 6-year-old who wets the bed 4 nights a week

5. **Which of the following are true statements of child protection practice?**
   a) Sexual abuse of children is most often caused by strangers
   b) It is good practice to inform a family of an intended referral to social services for child protection concerns
   c) Normal rules of patient confidentiality are waived in child protection cases
   d) In any confirmed case of child abuse, the child's name must be placed on the child protection register
   e) In cases of sudden unexpected death of children, the police must be informed immediately

6. **Which of the following should be considered as possible child abuse?**
   a) An infant being seen for their first immunization at 8 weeks is noted coincidentally to have a tiny bruise on the upper arm
   b) A child who is smacked for bedwetting
   c) A child of 8 years who is allowed to play truant from school by his parents
   d) A young teenager who is allowed to smoke by her parents
   e) A primary school child showing sexualised behaviour

7. **Which of the following scenarios should lead you to suspect child abuse?**
   a) A 4-week-old baby with a bruise on her cheek. Her mother explains that she banged it on a toy in her cot
   b) A 6-week-old baby who falls below the 10th centile for height and weight
   c) A 3-year-old with lots of bruises on his shins. His mother says he is always falling over
   d) A 5-month-old with a fractured skull. His mother says he rolled off the bed
   e) A 4-year-old with strap marks on his bottom where his father chastised him for not eating his dinner

8. **If you have concerns that a child may have been abused or neglected you should:**
   a) Take a detailed history and write careful notes
   b) Call the police to question the parents
   c) Avoid detailed questioning for fear of aggravating the parents
   d) Tell your senior colleagues of your concerns
   e) Refer to social services

9. In sickle-cell anaemia:
   a) Thrombocytopenia is common
   b) Growth is usually unaffected
   c) Infection with *Streptococcus pneumoniae* is more common
   d) Painful crises are rare
   e) Massive splenomegaly may occur

10. The management of childhood eczema includes:
   a) Topical tacrolimus
   b) Long-term antibiotics
   c) Emollients
   d) A cow's milk-free diet for all
   e) Corticosteroids

11. In the newborn period, the following are common skin conditions:
   a) Molluscum contagiosum
   b) Erysipelas
   c) Erythema toxicum
   d) Milia
   e) Psoriasis

12. Bronchiolitis:
   a) Is commonly caused by the respiratory syncytial virus
   b) May be treated acutely with monoclonal antibodies
   c) May necessitate nasogastric feeding
   d) Causes asthma
   e) Is treated with steroids

13. The following statements are true of pertussis (whooping cough):
   a) Pertussis immunization is more than 99% effective in preventing whooping cough
   b) Whooping cough may be associated with a severe encephalopathy
   c) The lymphocyte count is reliably raised
   d) Antibiotics do little to affect progression of the disease
   e) Cyanosis with coughing paroxysms augers a poor prognosis

14. The following are true of cystic fibrosis:
   a) Antibiotics to protect against staphylococcal infection are routinely used in young children
   b) *Pseudomonas aeruginosa* infection is difficult to eradicate
   c) Pancreatic enzyme therapy is needed in all patients
   d) Hepatitis may complicate cystic fibrosis
   e) Dietary therapy is a mainstay of management

15. The following statements are true of childhood diabetes:
a) Diabetes complications are rare in childhood
b) Insulin treatment must continue during illness, even if the child is not eating
c) Good control of diabetes is associated with a higher risk of severe hypoglycaemia
d) Insulin should be reduced before strenuous exercise
e) Children with diabetes should be screened annually for auto-immune thyroid disease

16. The following statements are true of congenital hypothyroidism:
a) The outlook for treated congenital hypothyroidism is excellent
b) Treatment is with recombinant human TSH
c) The thyroid gland is usually absent or ectopically placed
d) Screening for hypothyroidism and other disorders is normally done within the first 72 hours of life
e) Severe mental retardation results when the diagnosis is missed

17. The following statements are true of calcium metabolism:
a) The principal regulator of serum calcium is vitamin D
b) There is insufficient sunlight in the winter months in the UK for photochemical synthesis of vitamin D in the skin
c) Rickets will result from lack of activated vitamin D
d) Acute hypocalcaemia may be fatal
e) The principal dietary source of vitamin D is green vegetables

18. Which of the following statements about sexual development/intersex are true:
a) Without male hormonal influences, a fetus will develop a female phenotype
b) The sex of rearing is usually determined by the genetic sex
c) In a genetically female infant, the most likely cause of intersex is congenital adrenal hyperplasia
d) A child with intersex should be commenced on hydrocortisone until the diagnosis is made
e) The most useful investigation in the first few days is a pelvic and abdominal ultrasound scan

19. Causes of abdominal pain in childhood include:
a) Pneumonia
b) Abdominal migraine
c) Gastritis
d) Constipation
e) Henoch-Schönlein purpura

20. **Features of toddler diarrhoea include:**
    a) Offensive stools
    b) Unchanged food seen in the stool
    c) Poor weight gain
    d) Vomiting
    e) Urticaria

21. **In tension headache:**
    a) Symptoms have usually been present for more than 6 months
    b) There is associated vomiting
    c) Simple analgesia is often ineffective
    d) The headache is episodic with bouts of severe pain separated by days or weeks
    e) Symptoms are worse in the morning

22. **The following clinical cases should be diagnosed as cerebral palsy:**
    a) A 7-month-old child presents with a stiff, poorly functioning right arm. Reflexes are brisk down the right hand side. MRI scan shows left middle cerebral artery infarction which is thought to have occurred in early fetal life
    b) A 7-month-old child has a floppy poorly functioning right arm. The reflexes are absent in the arm but the legs seem normal. The cause was thought to be damage to the brachial plexus during a difficult delivery
    c) A 7-year-old child who develops a stiff poorly functioning right arm as a result of brain damage sustained after a fall from a horse when she was 6 years old
    d) A 7-month-old has a stiff poorly functioning right arm. The problem seems to be getting worse and an MRI reveals a tumour on the left side of the brain pressing on the motor area
    e) A 7-year-old child has pins and needles down the right arm. Careful testing shows a loss of sensation to touch

23. **The following statements are true of attention deficit hyperactivity disorder (ADHD):**
    a) MRI is a useful diagnostic tool
    b) The features of ADHD may be seen in children who are abused or neglected
    c) Sedatives may be useful
    d) Compulsive behaviours are a key feature
    e) Impulsivity is a key feature

24. **Which of the following food items should not be taken in pregnancy?**
    a) Liver
    b) Pasteurized dairy products
    c) Folic acid
    d) Opiate drugs
    e) Anticonvulsant

25. **The following are more common in breech delivery:**
    a) Developmental dysplasia of the hip
    b) Down syndrome
    c) Cord prolapse
    d) Neonatal encephalopathy ('birth asphyxia')
    e) Neonatal jaundice

26. **The following are true of cleft lip and/or palate:**
    a) Cleft lip is more commonly right-sided
    b) Cleft lip and palate are normally repaired in the first year of life
    c) Prolapse of the tongue into a cleft palate may produce airway obstruction
    d) Cleft palate may be associated with cardiac abnormalities
    e) Hearing problems commonly occur

Extended matching questions

27. **Match the following ages with the appropriate developmental milestone(s):**
    1) 6–9 months
    2) 1 year
    3) 2 years
    4) 3 years
    5) 4 years

    Responses
    a) Building a tower of 7 blocks
    b) Smiling
    c) Sitting
    d) Object permanence
    e) Walking
    f) Speaking simple sentences
    g) Dry by day and night
    h) Dressing, mostly unaided
    i) Counts to 10

28. **Read the following case histories and select the diagnosis that most closely matches the description:**

Cases

1) Finn, a 7-year-old boy, was dry by day and night from the age of 4 years, but following the break-up of his parents' marriage, he has begun bedwetting

2) Luke, aged 8 years, has soiling. Laxatives aggravated the soiling. Luke has a long-standing dislike of going to the toilet. On examination he has lower abdominal distension and tenderness with stool palpable per abdomen

3) James, aged 3 years, is a solitary child. His favourite activity is playing with his toy trains. He speaks a few single words. He dislikes change from his normal routines. His motor milestones were normal

4) Alice, aged 5 years, is a clumsy child. She has very poor handwriting and it takes her a long time to complete a task. When younger, Alice was diagnosed with benign congenital hypotonia after concerns about delayed motor skills. She also received speech therapy because of poor articulation of words

5) Danny, aged 6 years, had normal early milestones, except that his speech development was slow. His maternal uncle has seizures and went to a 'special school'. Danny is struggling at school, with very poor literacy and numeracy

Responses

a) Autistic spectrum disorder
b) Dyspraxia
c) Global developmental delay
d) Hemiplegic cerebral palsy
e) Encopresis
f) Constipation and soiling
g) Primary enuresis
h) Secondary enuresis
i) Learning difficulty

29. **For each of the following case scenarios select the most likely diagnosis from the list below:**

Cases

1) A previously well 2-year-old girl refuses to walk. She is generally unwell, has a temperature and is off her food. Examination reveals a miserable girl with a warm and swollen left knee, held still. She cries when you try to move it

Investigations show:
Hb 9.2 g/dl (10.5–12.5)
WCC 22 109/L (4.5–12.0)
Neutrophils 16×109/L (2–7.5)
Lymphocytes 6×109/L (2–4.5)
Platelets 350×109/L (150–400)
Autoimmune screen negative
Serum ferritin 32 ng/ml (10–140)
C reactive protein 83 mg/L
Erythrocyte sedimentation rate 22 mm/h (1–10)
X-ray of knee normal
Serum Ca 2.2 mmol/L (2.1–2.6)
Serum phosphate 0.9 mmol/L(0.8–1.8)
Alkaline phosphatase 320 U/L (145–420)

2) **A previously well 2-year-old girl refuses to walk. She has been unwell with temperatures, flitting rashes and has been off her food for a few weeks. Limping has got worse and now she will not stand. Examination reveals a miserable girl who is unwilling to move. Her left knee is warm and swollen and her ankles look puffy**

Investigations show:
Hb 9.2 g/dl (10.5–12.5)
WCC 13 109/L (4.5–12.0)
Neutrophils 8×109/L (2–7.5)
Lymphocytes 3×109/L (2–4.5)
Platelets 467×109/L (150–400)
Autoimmune screen negative
Serum ferritin 142 ng/ml (10–140)
C reactive protein 15 mg/L
Erythrocyte sedimentation rate 102 mm/h (1–10)
X-ray of knee normal
ASOT negative
Serum Ca 2.2 mmol/L (2.1–2.6)
Serum phosphate 0.9 mmol/L (0.8–1.8)
Alkaline phosphatase 320 U/L (145n420)
Hb 9.2 g/dl (10.5–12.5)

3) **A previously well 8-year-old boy is walking with a limp and complaining intermittently of pain in his right knee. He is unhappy at school and refusing to go. Examination reveals a healthy boy. His musculoskeletal examination is normal except that he winces on internal rotation of the right hip**

Investigations show:
Hb 11.2 g/dl (10.5–12.5)
Serum ferritin 27 ng/ml (10–140)
WCC 11

Neutrophils 7
Lymphocytes 3
Platelets 258
Autoimmune screen negative
C reactive protein 3 mg/L
Erythrocyte sedimentation rate 6
X-ray of right knee normal
ASOT negative

4) **A previously well 8-year-old boy is walking with a limp and complaining intermittently of pain in his right knee. He is unhappy at school and refusing to go. Examination reveals a healthy boy. His musculoskeletal examination is normal, but he holds his right knee in fixed flexion, winces when you touch the skin over it and shouts out in pain when asked to move it**

Investigations show:

Hb 11.2 g/dl (10.5–12.5)
Serum ferritin 27 ng/ml (10–140)
WCC 11
Neutrophils 7
Lymphocytes 3
Platelets 273
Autoimmune screen negative
C reactive protein 3 mgA
Erythrocyte sedimentation rate 6
X-ray of right knee normal
ASOT 200 (normal for age)

Responses

a) Perthes' disease
b) Generalized hypermobility
c) Idiopathic nocturnal leg pains
d) Juvenile idiopathic arthritis
e) Reactive arthritis
f) Rheumatic fever
g) Chronic fatigue syndrome
h) Localized pain amplification syndrome
i) Ulcerative colitis
j) Septic arthritis

30. **Choose the most likely diagnosis for the following cases from the list below:**

Cases

1) A 4-year-old boy from west Africa is admitted to hospital with *Plasmodium falciparum* malaria. After receiving chloroquine, he rapidly deteriorates with a sharp fall in haemoglobin and mild jaundice of his conjunctivae. His urine is dark and tests positive for haemoglobin, but no red cells are seen on microscopy

2) A 4-year-old girl is noted to be bruising easily. A blood count shows: Hb 10.1, WCC 5.2, platelets 12. On examination, she is mildly febrile and has hepatosplenomegaly

3) A 9-year-old girl is referred with pallor and bruising. Her blood count shows pancytopenia. An urgent bone marrow examination shows hypocellularity

4) A 3-year-old Turkish girl presents with pallor following a recent illness. She is otherwise well and eats a satisfactory diet. Her blood count shows a hypochromic, microcytic anaemia (haemoglobin 7.8 g/dl). Target cells are visible on the blood film. Serum ferritin is within the normal range

5) A 9-year-old girl is referred for investigation after severe post-operative bleeding following dental extractions. She has a history of easy bruising and epistaxis. Clotting studies show a prolonged aPTT (activated partial thromboplastin time)

Responses
a) Iron deficiency anaemia
b) Thalassaemia trait
c) Sickle-cell anaemia
d) Hereditary spherocytosis
e) G6PD deficiency
f) Idiopathic thrombocytopenic purpura
g) Haemophilia A
h) von Willebrand's disease
i) Aplastic anaemia
j) Acute leukaemia

31. **Choose the most likely diagnosis for the following scenarios from the list below:**
Cases
1) A 5-year-old boy presents with headache and unsteady gait. On examination he has mild neck stiffness and papilloedema

2) A 14-year-old girl presents with a painful lower femur with a palpable mass just above the knee. An X-ray showed elevation of the periosteum and calcification in the overlying soft tissue in a 'sunburst' pattern

3) A 4-year-old boy presents with haematuria. On examination, he has a massive right flank mass up to the midline of the abdomen. His blood pressure was normal, and urinary catecholamine metabolites were negative

4) A 7-year-old boy presents with severe short stature. He is found to be growth hormone, TSH and cortisol deficient, with an elevated prolactin. Visual examination reveals bitemporal hemianopia and mild optic atrophy

Responses
  a) Wilm's tumour
  b) Neuroblastoma
  c) Lymphoma
  d) Craniopharyngioma
  e) Prolactinoma
  f) Medulloblastoma
  g) Ewing's sarcoma
  h) Osteosarcoma

32. **Choose the most likely diagnosis for the following cases from the list below:**

Cases
  1) A 6-month-old infant has poor weight gain. He has had numerous chest infections since birth. Clinically he looked thin and had a 5 cm liver. There was a machinery murmur continuous throughout the cardiac cycle under the left clavicle. His chest X-ray revealed pulmonary plethora

  2) A 3-month-old infant is taking smaller and smaller volumes of feed. His weight gain is well below expected. There is no family history of note and his discharge examination at 2 days of age was normal. He is pink in air with a heart rate of 160 beats per minute and a respiratory rate of 75 breaths per minute. He demonstrates intercostal recession and his apex beat is displaced to the anterior axillary line. There is a pansystolic murmur which is loudest along the left sternal border. His liver is 4 cm below the costal margin, his ECG reveals biventricular hypertrophy and a chest X-ray shows a large heart with pulmonary plethora

  3) An 8-year-old child presents to the GP with a chest infection and a systolic murmur is detected. This murmur is heard in the second intercostal space just lateral to the sternal border. It is mid-systolic in timing, low intensity (2/6), and nearly disappears in the supine position. The heart sounds are normal, as is the rest of the examination

  4) A 4-year-old is at the GP's for a preschool check. A loud systolic murmur is heard in the pulmonary area. There is a parasternal heave and there is a thrill in the upper left sternal border. There is a delayed pulmonary second sound. The chest X-ray is normal and an ECG reveals right ventricular hypertrophy

Responses
  a) Fallot's tetralogy
  b) Coarctation of the aorta
  c) Transposition of the great vessels
  d) Ventriculoseptal defect

e) Atrioseptal defect

f) Pulmonary stenosis

g) Innocent murmur

h) Patent ductus arteriosus

33. **Choose the most likely diagnosis for the following cases from the list below:**

Cases

1) A 14-year-old girl presents acutely unwell with severe tonsillitis leading to a moderate degree of upper airway obstruction. She has cervical lymphadenopathy

2) A 4-year-old boy from a travelling family presents severely unwell with inspiratory stridor and high fever. He is sitting upright on his mother's lap and appears anxious. He has not had any routine immunizations

3) A 17-month-old child presents acutely unwell with stridor on inspiration and expiration. He is cyanosed and in extremis. The onset was sudden, and he had not appeared unwell prior to sudden onset of dyspnoea

4) A 2-year-old girl presents acutely with a dramatic 'barking' cough, having been unwell with cold symptoms for a few hours

5) A 2-month-old child is referred with inspiratory stridor, which was worse with a recent upper respiratory tract infection, although he is better now. He is thriving

Responses

a) Croup

b) Epiglottitis

c) Anaphylaxis

d) Inhaled foreign body

e) Glandular fever

f) Otitis media

g) Laryngomalacia

34. **Choose the appropriate organism for the following cases of respiratory disease, from the list below:**

Cases

1) A 10-month-old boy presents with severe respiratory distress and hypoxia. He is known to have HIV infection and has been having regular co-trimoxazole. His chest X-ray shows widespread pulmonary infiltrates

2) A 5-week-old baby presents with cold symptoms over the previous 48 hours and increasing respiratory distress, with intercostal and subcostal recession. He is dyspnoeic and unable to feed

3) A 4-year-old boy presents with a 7-day history of high fever, malaise and tachypnoea with cough. On examination he has a left pleural effusion, subsequently confirmed on chest X-ray

4) A 6-year-old boy, originally from Bangladesh, presents with a history of cough (initially diagnosed as asthma) and more recently, with drenching night sweats and weight loss

Responses

a) *Streptococcus pneumoniae* (pneumococcus)
b) *Mycoplasma pneumoniae*
c) *Mycobacterium tuberculosis*
d) Human immunodeficiency virus
e) Respiratory syncytial virus
f) *Pneumocystis carinii*

35. **For the following cases, match the most likely diagnosis:**

Cases

1) An infant has low birth weight (2.1 kg at 36 weeks gestation) and is noted to have microcephaly (head circumference <0.4th centile), length <2nd centile, hepatosplenomegaly and thrombocytopenia

2) An infant is born weighing 4.5 kg by emergency caesarean section after an otherwise uncomplicated pregnancy. The baby appears to have a large tongue, which impedes his initial resuscitation. Later he develops persistent severe hypoglycaemia requiring a glucose infusion

3) An infant is born markedly growth restricted, weighing 2.4 kg at 39 weeks gestation. She is symmetrical. She has a distinctive appearance with widely spaced eyes, is floppy, and slow to establish feeds

4) An infant of 4 weeks is referred with prolonged jaundice, found to be predominantly conjugated (i.e. of hepatic origin). Routine blood glucose testing shows asymptomatic premeal hypoglycaemia

Responses

a) Congenital infection
b) Down syndrome
c) Beckwith syndrome
d) Maternal diabetes mellitus
e) Hypopituitarism
f) Congenital hypothyroidism

36. **Select the single most appropriate investigation from the list below, for the following cases:**

Cases

1) A 15-year-old boy presents with delayed puberty and short stature. His father also had delayed puberty. He is otherwise healthy

2) A 6-year-old girl is referred with disproportionate short stature with relatively short limbs

3) An 8-year-old girl is referred with early menarche. On examination she is short and in early puberty

4) A 10-year-old boy is referred with short stature. His height is on the 2nd centile but his weight is well below the 0.4th centile. He has several mouth ulcers and is pale

5) A 17-year-old boy is referred with delayed puberty. He is tall (>91st centile), and is in early puberty, with testicular volumes of 2–3 mL (i.e. prepubertal in size)

6) A 3-year-old boy presents with poor weight gain. He is short and very miserable, with abdominal distension and obvious wasting of the buttocks

7) A 7-year-old girl is referred with short stature. She has always been one of the smaller children in her class, but is now the smallest. She has had hearing problems requiring insertion of grommets. On examination she has a broad chest, a low hair-line and a high-arched palate

8) A 5-year-old boy is referred with extreme short stature. His 2-year-old brother is the same height. He is otherwise healthy, but was born with cleft lip and palate, repaired in infancy

Responses

a) X-ray of left hand and wrist
b) Skull X-ray
c) Skeletal survey
d) Cranial MRI scan
e) Abdominal ultrasound scan
f) Growth hormone test
g) Karyotype
h) Thyroid function tests
i) Full blood count and ESR
j) Coeliac screen

37. For each of the clinical scenarios described below choose the investigation most likely to reveal the diagnosis:

Cases

1) An 8-year-old girl is admitted with a widespread purpuric rash over her legs and trunk. She requires two fluid boluses for hypotension and subsequent inotropic support. Her conscious level is fluctuating. She receives IV antibiotics and is transferred to a paediatric intensive-care unit (PICU)

2) A 5-year-old boy presents with a 2-week history of cough and pyrexia. He has had a 5-day course of antibiotics (amoxicillin) from the family doctor. In spite of this he continues to be unwell and now complains of headache and myalgia. He had some loose stools 2 days ago. On examination there is tachypnoea but only a few crepitations to be heard in the chest. A chest X-ray demonstrates bilateral infective changes

3) A 6-month-old boy is brought to the A&E department with a history of a generalized seizure lasting for 1 minute associated

with a high temperature. He was previously well, although he had been off colour for a few hours beforehand. He is observed on the ward where he remains pyrexial in spite of paracetamol. Examination reveals an irritable child with no rash and an otherwise normal examination (including ENT)

4) A 1-year-old boy is referred with a high temperature and a history of some vomiting. He looks otherwise well but with no clear focus for the temperature demonstrated on examination

5) A 4.5-year-old girl is admitted with a high temperature and abdominal pain. She initially started with a runny nose 5 days before and has developed a cough since then. Her respiratory rate is raised. Abdominal examination is entirely normal. A urine dipstick reveals a trace of protein and ketones

Responses

a) Abdominal X-ray
b) Erect PA chest X-ray
c) Sputum sample
d) Paul–Bunnell test
e) Mid-stream sample of urine
f) PCR for *Neisseria meningitidis*
g) PCR for herpes simplex
h) *Mycoplasma* serology
i) Lumbar puncture
j) Stool sample

38. Match the following cases with the diagnoses below:

Cases

1) A 5-week-old infant is referred with increasing jaundice and failure-to-thrive. On examination, he has an olive complexion, and is wasted with a distended abdomen, although he has been feeding well. His stools are putty-coloured, and urine analysis shows a large quantity of bilirubin, but no urobilinogen

2) A baby is noted to be jaundiced at 12 hours of age. A direct antiglobulin (Coombs) test is positive. His blood group is A positive, whereas his mother's blood group is O positive (see Chapter 7, p.60)

3) A 5-day-old infant is admitted with lethargy and poor tone. He has been breast-feeding but does not seem to be satisfied after feeds and is now not waking for feeds. He is deeply jaundiced but responds well to phototherapy and nasogastric feeding

4) A 4-week-old, thriving, breast-fed baby is noted to be mildly jaundiced. He has a blood test which shows: total bilirubin 196 μmol/L, conjugated bilirubin 0

Responses

a) Physiological jaundice
b) Breast-milk jaundice

c) Rhesus haemolytic disease of the newborn

d) ABO incompatibility

e) Galactosaemia

f) Biliary atresia

39. **Match the following case descriptions with the epileptic and non-epileptic events below:**

Cases

1) A 7-year-old is noted in school to have poor concentration and blank spells. Her parents notice her staring into space. They have to speak sharply to her to terminate the attack which may otherwise last for several minutes

2) A 7-year-old has been noted in school to have poor concentration and blank spells. Her family notice that she may stop abruptly in mid-activity for a few seconds before continuing

3) A 2-year-old collides with another child in nursery with a clash of heads. He starts to cry and moves towards a carer. He stops, goes pale and collapses. He remains stiff on the floor for 20 seconds and then there are a few coarse jerks of the whole body before he returns to consiousness. He is a bit subdued for 30 minutes in the aftermath

4) A tall, thin 7-year-old attends school even though she has a mild upper respiratory tract infection. She is queuing to get her lunch when she sways and falls against her friend. She is helped to the floor where she is found by a teacher to be pale and sweaty. There are some trembling movements of her limbs for a few seconds. She makes a rapid recovery

5) A 3-year-old child gets into a disagreement with his mother over a trip to the shops. He begins to cry but rapidly loses control of himself. He lashes out at his mother, throws his toys and lies on the floor where his arms and legs are threshing around violently. He is red or blue in the face. He recovers gradually. Twenty minutes later he is asleep

Responses

a) Vasovagal syncope

b) Epileptic seizure

c) Reflex anoxic attack

d) Daydreaming

e) Tantrums

f) Blue breath holding

g) Self gratification

h) Non-epileptic attack

i) Absence epilepsy

j) Post-traumatic epilepsy

Answers

1. **(a), (c)**

   The principle purpose of good note-keeping is to ensure effective care for the child and communication with colleagues, but good note-keeping is also important to protect against complaints and litigation. Many hospitals require notes to be written in black ink but this is not a legal requirement. Abbreviations in the notes are acceptable but should be unambiguous and never abusive. It is vitally important to record potentially sensitive information, e.g. child protection concerns, but note that this information may in the future be viewed by the child or parents. There is no legal requirement to record time using the 24-hour clock, although this is good practice.

2. **(a), (b), (c), (d)**

   Obesity is much more common in children living in poverty. Children from poor backgrounds are much less likely to remain in school after 16 years, and attain lower exam grades. Death from infectious disease is more common in poor children. Children in marginalized groups such as ethnic minorities, refugees and asylum seekers, travelling families, etc. are more likely to live in poverty. Poverty is associated with higher levels of mental health problems but is not a direct cause of ADHD.

3. **(b), (e)**

4. **(b), (d)**

5. **(b), (e)**

   Child abuse of all types is most commonly perpetrated by members of the immediate family or friends. Although sometimes difficult to do, it is best to inform the family of your proposed actions before making a referral to social services (or the police). Normal rules of confidentiality apply in child protection cases. The basis for disclosure of information is the over-riding need to protect the child. The appropriate course of action, e.g. placement on the child protection register, is decided at the case conference. This would be unnecessary for children removed into local authority care. As with any sudden unexpected death, the police should be informed without delay.

6. **(a), (e)**

   Any bruise, however insignificant in such a young child, should be regarded as suspicious of abuse. The bruise may be a manifestation of rough handling or an underlying fracture. Smacking (although clearly inappropriate in this case) is not unlawful in the UK (except

unishment of young children in public in Scotland). The
ved to play truant by his parents is at high risk of harm,
issing out on his education. Condoning truancy is illegal, but
ot of itself a child protection matter unless there are wider concerns
about neglect. Many teenagers smoke, with or without their parents'
knowledge. Although injurious to health, it would not be considered
child abuse to permit smoking. Prematurely sexualized behaviour
is often seen in sexually abused children. Exposure to inappropriate
sexual imagery is often used by abusers as a technique of 'grooming'
children to take part in sexual abuse.

7. **(a), (d), (e)**

8. **(a), (d), (e)**

9. **(c), (e)**

   In sickle-cell anaemia, growth is impaired, and puberty delayed.
   Special growth charts are available for children with sickle-cell
   anaemia in the UK. Progressive autoinfarction of the spleen means
   that by the age of 5 years, most children have functional hyposplenism, putting them at increased risk of infection with encapsulated organisms, including *Streptococcus pneumoniae, Haemophilus
   influenzae* and *Salmonella* spp. Nevertheless, the spleen and other
   organs may become massively enlarged in a sequestration crisis
   resulting in circulatory collapse. Recurrent vaso-occlusive crises
   are relatively common, although a small number of individuals
   are affected disproportionately.

10. **(a), (c), (e)**

    The frequent and copious administration of emollients to all
    affected areas is a cornerstone of management. Topical tacroli-
    mus and pimecrolimus may be tried but should only be done so
    under specialist supervision. Antibiotics may be necessary for the
    management of secondary bacterial infection. Their use should
    be restricted to short courses to avoid antibiotic resistance. Cows'
    milk-free diets may be useful for some but the evidence for uni-
    versal recommendation is lacking. Corticosteroids should be used
    carefully and the more potent forms should only be used in short
    courses.

11. **(c), (d)**

    Erythema toxicum is a common newborn skin condition. It pres-
    ents as asymptomatic papules and vesicles surrounded by small
    areas of erythema. It is self-limiting and requires no treatment.
    Milia are similarly common. They present as white papules
    1–2 mm in size, mainly seen on the face.

12. **(a), (c)**

Prophylactic monoclonal antibody therapy is advocated for high-risk infants, such as those with existing respiratory disease. There is no established role for its administration in the acute phase. There is no clear and established link between bronchiolitis and a later diagnosis of asthma, however, half of infants will wheeze with subsequent viruses. There is no evidence that steroids offer clinical benefit.

13. **(b), (c), (d)**

Pertussis immunization is not completely effective in preventing all cases of pertussis, but is associated with a less severe course. Encephalopathy and seizures complicate pertussis in 3–4% of cases and may prove fatal, but the great majority of deaths occur secondary to pneumonia. The lymphocyte count is reliably elevated, and may be a useful indicator of potential pertussis infection, as culture results usually take 7–10 days. Coughing paroxysms with cyanosis are typical of whooping cough, and do not indicate a worse prognosis.

14. **(a), (b), (d), (e)**

Antibiotics, such as flucloxacillin, are used in all young children because of the high risk of staphylococcal pneumonia. When *Pseudomonas* infection occurs, strenuous attempts are made to eradicate it, as persistent carriage is associated with more rapid deterioration of lung function and a worse prognosis. Most, but not all, patients have pancreatic insufficiency. Liver disease in cystic fibrosis affects 40–50% of teenagers. The majority have simple fatty change (steatotic hepatitis), but a minority develop secondary biliary cirrhosis.

15. **All true**.

Diabetes complications are rare in childhood, but poor control will result in the appearance of complications in early adult life. It is vital to continue insulin during illness to avoid the risk of diabetic ketoacidosis. Good diabetes control (HbA1c <7.5%) is associated with an increased risk of severe hypoglycaemia, but a reduced risk of long-term complications. Insulin should normally be reduced (but not omitted) before strenuous exercise, due to the risk of hypoglycaemia. Annual screening for autoimmune thyroid disease is now recommended for children with diabetes.

16. **(a), (c), (e)**

The great majority of children with treated congenital hypothyroidism have normal intelligence, whereas without treatment, severe mental retardation ('cretinism') results. Treatment is with levothyroxine in sufficient doses to restore TSH to normal, as

ssible. The usual cause of congenital hypothyroidism
plasia or ectopia, but up to 15% of cases arise from
hormone dyshormonogenesis, in which the thyroid
and is normally situated, but unable to synthesize thyroxine.
Dyshormonogenesis is associated with deafness in some cases
(Pendred syndrome) and carries a 1:4 recurrence risk. Screening
for hypothyroidism, phenylketonuria and other disorders is normally done in the 2nd week of life.

17. **(b), (c), (d)**

Parathyroid hormone is the main regulator of serum calcium. It
promotes calcium and vitamin D absorption from the gut, mobilizes calcium from bone, reduces renal excretion and activates the
enzyme 1-alpha-hydroxylase which converts vitamin D to its active
form. In the UK, sunlight during the winter months is insufficient
for vitamin D synthesis in skin. Lack of vitamin D results in rickets
and hypocalcaemia. If severe, hypocalcaemia may result in tetany,
seizures and laryngeal spasm, which may be fatal. The best dietary
sources of vitamin D are fish, meat, eggs and dairy products.

18. **(a), (c), (e)**

Intersex is discussed in Chapter 12, p. 153. The sex of rearing
depends on what it is possible to achieve. In practice, the majority
of infants with intersex are reared as girls. Female intersex arises
from antenatal androgen exposure, most commonly from congenital adrenal hyperplasia (CAH). The majority of children presenting
with intersex have CAH and will require hydrocortisone (or other
replacement steroid) therapy. However, it is vital to establish the
underlying diagnosis as early as possible, therefore hydrocortisone
is not commenced until initial investigations have been carried out.
An ultrasound examination may be carried out very quickly, and
may confirm the presence or absence of the uterus and ovaries.
Adrenal hyperplasia may also be visualized.

19. **All true**

20. **(a), (b)**

21. **(a), (c)**

22. **(a)**

23. **(b), (e)**

24. **(a)**

Formal advice was issued by the UK Department of Health in 1990 recommending avoidance of vitamin A supplements and all liver-containing foods. Liver contains high concentrations of vitamin A, which, in large quantities, are teratogenic. Pasteurized dairy products are safe from bacterial contamination, if properly stored, and present no risk to health. Unpasteurized foods such as cheese or milk may contain the organism *Listeria monocytogenes*, which may cause severe infections in newborn infants (listeriosis). Folic acid supplementation reduces the risk of fetal neural tube defects. Ideally, it should be taken prior to conception and throughout pregnancy, particularly in women at high risk, e.g. women with previously affected pregnancies, diabetes or epilepsy. Women who have epilepsy should continue to take anticonvulsants in pregnancy as the risks to the fetus of congenital anticonvulsant syndromes are outweighed by the risk to maternal health from untreated epilepsy. Women who are opiate-addicted are usually managed with methadone in pregnancy, as part of a drug-treatment programme. Unfortunately, the result of this is usually neonatal abstinence syndrome (drug withdrawal), which needs careful management with opiates and sedatives.

25. **(a), (b), (c), (d)**
Breech delivery is associated with a flexed hip posture and increased risk of developmental dysplasia of the hip (see Chapter 6, p. 49). Breech delivery carries a significant risk of fetal compromise due to prolonged labour and cord prolapse. This increases the risk of neonatal encephalopathy. Breech delivery occurs more commonly in Down syndrome (1 in 200) but the reason is unknown.

26. **(b), (c), (d), (e)**
Cleft lip is typically left-sided. Cleft lip is usually repaired at about 3 months of age, whereas cleft palate repair is usually carried out at 6 months. Earlier repair may impair development of the mid-face. The association of micrognathia (small jaw) with cleft palate is called Pierre-Robin sequence. In this condition, the tongue may obstruct the airway. All craniofacial anomalies are associated with an increased likelihood of deafness – sensorineural or conductive. Thus all children with cleft lip and palate must have a hearing test at birth, and regular audiological follow-up. Cardiac anomalies also occur more commonly with cleft lip and palate, particularly in association with chromosomal anomalies, notably Di George syndrome and related disorders associated with the 22q11 deletion (see also Chapter 18, p. 278).

27. 1) (c), (d)
2) (e)
3) (a)
4) (f), (g), (i)
5) (h)
See Chapter 4 for details of normal milestones.

28. 1) (h)
2) (f)
3) (a)
4) (b)
5) (i)
These case histories are typical of the accompanying disorders. Secondary enuresis is distinguished from primary by a period of being dry at night. In primary enuresis, it is important to consider neurological abnormalities, but the great majority are otherwise normal and healthy. The autistic spectrum incorporates traits that represent extremes of normality. In this case, the solitary play and unwillingness to depart from routines is typical. Dyspraxia is commonly associated with speech and motor problems in early life, subsequently manifesting as clumsiness. In contrast to children with global developmental delay, in the great majority, intelligence is normal. Learning difficulties are significantly more common in boys, and may be inherited, the most common diagnosis being fragile X.

29. 1) (j)
2) (d)
3) (a)
4) (h)

30. 1) (e)
2) (j)
3) (i)
4) (b)
5) (h)
Thalassaemia, G6PD deficiency and sickle-cell anaemia are thought to give some protection against malaria, and hence are relatively common in individuals in malarial areas. Unfortunately, chloroquine and other drugs may produce acute intravascular haemolysis in G6PD deficiency. It is inherited as an X-linked trait so girls are not usually affected. Intravascular haemolysis results in the passage of haemoglobin in urine, which usually appears dark red or brown. Thalassaemia trait presents incidentally with hypochromic microcytic anaemia. In children from malarial areas, thalassaemia trait may be the cause, although statistically, iron

deficiency anaemia is still the most common reason for this blood picture. This is excluded by the normal ferritin.

Idiopathic thrombocytopenic purpura is an autoimmune disease, and is not associated with hepatosplenomegaly or other features of illness, except bruising and/or bleeding. These indicate the likely diagnosis of aleukaemic leukaemia in which blasts are absent from the peripheral blood, and indicate the need for a bone marrow examination for confirmation. The marrow would show a high proportion of blasts (>25%). In contrast, in aplastic anaemia, although the presentation with bone marrow failure is similar to leukaemia, the bone marrow is hypocellular.

The presentation of von Willebrand's disease (VWD) is similar to mild haemophilia, with a history of easy bruising/bleeding and a prolonged aPTT, however haemophilia is X-linked and thus occurs almost exclusively in boys, whereas autosomal dominant and recessive forms of VWD may occur. Diagnosis is by measurement of specific clotting factors, depending on the diagnosis in question.

31. 1) (f)
2) (h)
3) (a)
4) (d)

The combination of headache and unsteady gait, coupled with neck stiffness, is suggestive of a posterior fossa tumour such as medulloblastoma, although any large intracranial tumour could produce these symptoms, due to associated hydrocephalus.

Osteosarcoma and Ewing's sarcoma both present with a limp, mass or pain. Osteosarcoma is associated with new bone formation, giving a characteristic 'sunburst' appearance. Elevation of the periosteum is typical, giving the appearance of 'Codman's triangle'.

Haematuria with a flank mass is a typical presentation of Wilm's tumour. Neuroblastoma may present in a similar way, but catecholamine metabolites were negative, and haematuria is unusual.

The combination of multiple pituitary hormone deficiencies and elevated prolactin is seen with hypothalamic lesions, as prolactin secretion by the pituitary is repressed by the hypothalamus (via dopamine secretion), whereas the other anterior pituitary hormones require hypothalamic releasing hormones (see Chapter 12, p. 143). A craniopharyngioma may develop very slowly, without overt signs of raised intracranial pressure.

32. 1) (h)
2) (d)
3) (g)
4) (f)

33. 1) (e)
    2) (b)
    3) (d)
    4) (a)
    5) (g)

Glandular fever may result in massive tonsillar hypertrophy with airway obstruction. Parenteral dexamethasone may relieve the obstruction, followed if necessary by tonsillectomy after a few weeks. Case 2 is a classic presentation of epiglottitis. This condition is now extremely rare following introduction of *Haemophilus influenzae* (Type B) immunization. Similarly, case 4 is a classic case of croup, most often caused by parainfluenza virus. Acute onset of upper airway obstruction in a young child should prompt concern about an inhaled foreign body. Inspiratory stridor alone signifies obstruction to the upper airway in the region of the larynx, but inspiratory and expiratory stridor suggests intrathoracic airway obstruction from tracheitis, or as in this case, a foreign body at the carina. Laryngomalacia or 'floppy larynx' is a benign disorder affecting young infants that characteristically results in mild stridor exacerbated by excitement, crying or intercurrent respiratory infections.

34. 1) (f)
    2) (e)
    3) (a)
    4) (c)

Pneumocystis carinii pneumonia (PCP) is a very severe infection complicating HIV-infected individuals. In children, it augers a poor prognosis with a median survival of 2 months. Case 2 is a typical case of bronchiolitis with over 80% of cases being caused by respiratory syncytial virus. Pneumonia with effusion is nearly always due to *Streptococcus pneumoniae*, whereas atypical pneumonia (which is actually more common) rarely causes an effusion. Newcomers to the UK, particularly from Africa and the Indian subcontinent are at increased risk of tuberculosis.

35. 1) (a)
    2) (c)
    3) (b)
    4) (e)

Case 1 shows symmetrical growth retardation indicating a fetal cause. The presence of severe microcephaly, hepatosplenomegaly and thrombocytopenia is characteristic of congenital cytomegalovirus infection. Case 2 is very large at birth. The most common cause of excessive birth weight is maternal diabetes due to relative hyperglycaemia, but this is excluded by the normal antenatal history. A large tongue is characteristic of Beckwith syndrome, which also presents with macrosomia and neonatal hypoglycaemia, and other congenital abnormalities. Case 3 shows features of Down syndrome with symmetrical growth restriction, hypotonia and a distinctive appearance. Case 4 is a rare presentation of hypopituitarism. Hypoglycaemia is commonly found and may be severe enough to result in neonatal seizures.

36. 1) (a)
2) (c)
3) (h)
4) (i)
5) (g)
6) (j)
7) (g)
8) (f)

Case 1 is typical of constitutional delay in growth and adolescence. The most appropriate investigation is an X-ray for bone age to confirm delay. Disproportionate short stature implies an underlying skeletal dysplasia. A skeletal survey will often be diagnostic. The onset of puberty is normally associated with rapid growth, so short stature in association with early puberty is unusual, except in untreated hypothyroidism. Early menarche is often a feature of precocious puberty due to hypothyroidism. Constitutional illness, particularly inflammatory bowel disease, may affect growth. In case 4, this is indicated by low weight, pallor and mouth ulcers typical of Crohn's disease. A blood count and ESR will nearly always be abnormal in this situation. Tall stature with delayed puberty is very unusual, but occurs in Klinefelter syndrome (Karyotype 47 XXY), in which the testes are typically small and hard – hence being prepubertal in size in a child with features of puberty. Case 6 is a classic presentation of coeliac disease. The presence of buttock-wasting and abdominal distension strongly indicate malabsorption. The combination of a relative decline in height with respect to peers is typical of Turner syndrome (as in this case) or acquired growth hormone deficiency. The dysmorphic features and history of glue ear clinch the diagnosis. Extreme growth failure is seen in congenital growth hormone deficiency, typically due to pituitary hypoplasia. Other midline defects such as cleft lip and palate, or single central incisor tooth, occur more commonly in congenital growth hormone deficiency.

37. 1) (f)
2) (h)
3) (i)
4) (e)
5) (b)

Case 1 is almost certainly meningococcal septicaemia. PCR has become a very good way of confirming the diagnosis, sometimes even when blood cultures are negative (e.g. with samples taken after antibiotics have been given). A throat swab would similarly be useful. Case 2's story is consistent with an atypical pneumonia. Features consistent with mycoplasma are: systemic upset and having worse signs on X-ray when compared to clinical findings. *Mycoplasma* is not sensitive to amoxicillin and must be treated with a macrolide antibiotic (e.g. erythromycin). In case 3, children with urinary tract infections (UTIs) can be entirely asymptomatic although there may be some vomiting. If there is a temperature with no clear focus in an otherwise well child it is essential to actively exclude a UTI. In case 4, meningitis is the main differential diagnosis of febrile convulsions. This child is very young and has no clear focus of infection. Typical meningitic signs are not always present at such a young age. With this story it would be prudent to perform a full septic screen, in particular looking for evidence of meningitis and provide cover with IV antibiotics. Case 5's story is typical for lower lobe pneumonia. Children often describe abdominal pain and can be otherwise asymptomatic on examination.

38. 1) (f)
2) (d)
3) (a)
4) (b)

The causes of jaundice are detailed in Chapter 17, Table 17.5, p. 255). Early-onset jaundice or jaundice persisting after 10–14 days is considered abnormal until proven otherwise. Early-onset jaundice (before 48 hours of age), most commonly occurs with haemolysis, as in case 2. The rhesus groups are the same in infant and mother, but the infant has a different blood group from his mother, making the likely diagnosis ABO incompatibility. Persistent jaundice in a breast-fed infant is nearly always due to breast milk jaundice, as in case 4, which is benign. In contrast, in case 1, the infant is failing to thrive, is deeply jaundiced and has white stools suggesting complete biliary obstruction. Biliary atresia requires urgent surgical treatment to create a bile conduit, otherwise irreversible liver failure ensues. Jaundice starting between 3 to 5 days of age is usually physiological. It may be exacerbated if a baby is not feeding well. Phototherapy is effective.

39. 1) (d)
2) (i)
3) (b)
4) (a)
5) (e)

Glossary: Important paediatric definitions and concepts

Autism Specific developmental communication disorder, usually associated with learning disability. Obsessional behaviour traits and stereotyped, repetitive behaviours are commonly seen. Autistic traits, falling short of autism – *autistic spectrum disorder* – are much more common. *Asperger's syndrome* refers to a subgroup of the autistic spectrum with normal intelligence, but impaired social functioning.

Behavioural problems In children, behavioural problems may stem from wider psychological distress within a family, or may be a consequence of upbringing, illness or inherited traits. The best known behaviour disorder is *attention deficit hyperactivity disorder*. *Conduct disorder* refers to children who show disruptive or difficult behaviour, such as stealing or physical aggression. *Tourette's syndrome* is a distinctive behaviour disorder characterized by vocal and motor tics, hyperactivity and *obsessive compulsive disorder*. Other behavioural problems include *school refusal* and *truancy*.

Cerebral palsy The effects of a neurological insult to the developing brain, on motor function, occurring in fetal life or infancy. A variety of patterns of cerebral palsy are recognized, depending on the type of movement disorder and the affected parts of the body, e.g. spastic diplegia. Cerebral palsy is non-progressive, in contrast to *progressive intellectual and neurological deterioration* in childhood, which may be a consequence of metabolic or infectious causes.

Child health professionals Aside from doctors and nurses, many other professionals are involved in children's healthcare. *Health visitors* support young children and families, which includes performing growth and developmental check-ups. Children with disabilities, chronic illness or psychosocial problems may be further supported by *social workers*. Particular problems or needs are met through the work of specific therapists – *physiotherapists, speech and language therapists, occupational therapists, orthotists* (footwear), *orthoptists* (vision assessment), *psychologists* and *play therapists*. The complexity of health and social care arrangements may require the assistance of a *key worker* to help families through the maze.

Child protection See 'Safeguarding'.

Developmental assessment Maximizing any child's potential requires tools to help recognize abnormal development, and thus to help the child with appropriately targeted interventions. A child's development is signalled by the achievement of developmental milestones. For formal assessment of development, various tools of differing complexity are available. These include the *Schedule of Growing Skills*, the *Denver Score*, the *Bayley Scale*, the *Griffiths Assessment* and, for assessment of intelligence, the *Weschler Intelligence Scale for Children (Revised) – WISC-R*.

Disability Living Allowance   A tax-free, non-means-tested benefit for people with an illness or disability who need help with mobility or personal care; it is available to people resident in the UK. Many children with chronic conditions, such as cerebral palsy, leukaemia or diabetes, are eligible.

Disorders of sexual development   Formerly known as intersex, disorders of sexual development (DSD) is now the preferred term. Most commonly intersex arises from erroneous sexual development – XX or XY DSD. The commonest cause of this is congenital adrenal hyperplasia, leading to virilization of a female infant (XX DSD). Much rarer are true hermaphrodites who have both ovarian and testicular tissue.

Embryonal tumours   A number of the most common childhood tumours arise from primitive embryonal tissues, including neuroblastoma (neural), Wilms' tumour (renal), retinoblastoma (eye) and medulloblastoma (brain). The tumours typically occur in early to mid-childhood, and are often aggressive, rapidly growing tumours.

Enuresis and encopresis   Enuresis refers to the involuntary passage of urine, most commonly at night – *nocturnal enuresis* or *bedwetting*. If the child has never been dry at night, the condition is said to be *primary*. *Secondary nocturnal enuresis*, which occurs after a period of continence, is most often a consequence of intercurrent illness (e.g. urinary tract infection) or psychological distress. *Encopresis* may refer to the involuntary passage of stool – *soiling*, or *overflow incontinence* – commonly associated with constipation, whereas *non-retentive encopresis* refers to passage of stool in inappropriate places, and is a psychological disorder which may be associated with *toilet phobia*.

Faltering growth   Also known as failure-to-thrive. Refers to infants and young children who are failing to put on weight at the expected rate. Faltering growth may arise from underlying ill health, or from inadequate nutrition or neglect.

Growth   The accretion of bone at the *growth plates* of long bones. The growth plate consists of a plate of cartilage separating the *metaphysis* (shaft) and *epiphysis*. The pattern of bone maturation is consistent between individuals, and may be monitored by X-rays – most commonly of the left hand and wrist. The appearance may then be compared with standard radiographs to give a *bone age*.

Growth charts   Charts available in the UK for a range of growth parameters, from birth to adulthood. Aside from height and weight, charts are available for other dimensions such as head circumference, body mass index and waist circumference, body proportions and blood pressure. Special charts are also available for some children with specific growth disorders such as Down syndrome. Conventionally, the charts define the normal range for growth, between the 2nd and 98th *centiles*, average growth being indicated by the 50th centile.

Inborn errors of metabolism   Inherited metabolic disorders usually result in a block to a particular metabolic pathway, resulting in accumulation of toxic metabolites, and deficiency of the intended product.

For example, the condition *phenylketonuria* arises from deficiency of the *enzyme* phenylalanine hydroxylase, leading to accumulation of toxic metabolites with resultant brain injury, if untreated. Hypopigmentation (fair hair, blue eyes) is also due to reduced tyrosine synthesis. Inborn errors of metabolism are rare, and usually of autosomal recessive inheritance.

Intersex   See 'Disorders of sexual development'.

Learning disability   Children with delayed or abnormal intellectual development are said to have learning disability or developmental delay. Terms formerly used include mental handicap and mental retardation.

Legal definitions   The *perinatal period* refers to the first 7 days of life, the *neonatal period* to the first 28 days of life and *infancy* to the first 12 months. Children are defined as such in law until they have reached their 19th birthday, but from the age of 16 years are autonomous for the purposes of consent to treatment and other legal rights. Younger children, if '*Gillick-competent*', may seek treatment without approval of their parents or legal guardian.

Micro-array   A newer genetic screening test, replacing the conventional cytogenetic karyotype test. It is more sensitive, quicker and cheaper than a karyotype, but in the investigation of balanced translocations a karyotype remains the investigation of choice.

Parent and family support groups   A range of charitable bodies that have been established, often by parents of affected children, to provide help, support and advice for parents and professionals for a range of health problems. For example *Scope* supports children and families with cerebral palsy. The organization *Contact a Family* provides an online directory of self-help groups (www.cafamily.org.uk), invaluable for signposting parents and professionals to appropriate groups.

Personal Child Health Record   Also referred to as the 'red book', this is given to every child in the UK. It contains information for parents on normal development, weaning, immunizations, dental care, etc. and contains charts for recording measurements and growth. It serves as a common document for parents to share with all healthcare givers.

Primitive reflexes   The newborn infant has a number of intrinsic motor reflexes – primitive reflexes. These include the palmar and plantar *grasp reflexes*, the *Moro reflex*, the *asymmetric tonic neck reflex* and *stepping* and *crawling reflexes*. Abnormal persistence of these reflexes signals impaired development.

Puberty   The process of achieving sexual maturity, culminating in cessation of growth, is a complex process. The average girl begins puberty at around 11 years of age, signalled by breast development (*thelarche*), followed by the appearance of pubic hair (*pubarche*). The onset of periods (*menarche*) occurs about 2 years later. In boys, the mean age of puberty is 12 years, and is signalled by the appearance of pubic hair and progressive testicular enlargement, associated with enlargement of the penis. Testicular enlargement may be monitored with an *orchidometer* – a string of oval beads of increasing size. Puberty before 8 years in girls and 9 years in boys is described as *precocious puberty*. Normal variants of puberty include isolated breast development (*premature thelarche*) or pubic hair (*premature pubarche*). Premature pubarche occurs most commonly due to premature production of adrenal androgens – *premature adrenarche*. Failure to enter puberty by the age of 13 years in girls and 14 years in boys is referred to as *delayed puberty*, and is most commonly idiopathic – *constitutional delay* in growth and puberty. It is usually associated with short stature.

Safeguarding   The procedures used to protect children who are at risk or who have suffered child abuse or neglect. In England and Wales, the Children Act (1989) lays down the appropriate procedures. Similar legislation applies to Scotland and Northern Ireland. Assessments of suspected child abuse and neglect are led by a social worker. Following an initial assessment a strategy meeting may be convened by social services to consider the immediate next steps. A case conference will later consider the appropriate action needed for the child and family. Children deemed at risk of further harm may be placed in the care of the local authority, or placed on the Child Protection Register. A young child who has suffered physical harm will usually require a skeletal survey – a series of X-rays to look for evidence of other injuries, past or present. Other investigations needed may include CT and/or MRI scans and blood tests.

Seizures   This term describes any abrupt transient change in behaviour, movement or sensaton. The term attach has the same connotation. Seizures associated with an abrupt discharge of abnormal brainwaves should be entitled *'epileptic seizures'*. Patients with a tendency to recurrent unprovoked *epileptic seizures* are said to have *'epilepsy'*. Many other conditions in childhood are characterized by attacks or seizures, e.g. the syncopies. The generic term for these used to be *turns* but *non-epileptic attack* is probably a better term.

Special educational needs   Children with physical, behavioural or intellectual difficulties require support to get the most from education. They are said to have special educational needs. Children requiring high levels of support undergo *a Statement of the Education and Health Care Plan. An educational psychologist* is invaluable in the assessment of children with behavioural problems.

Sudden unexpected death in infancy   Known also as *'cot death'*, this refers to the unexplained death of an infant. Many possible causes have been advanced; however, since the introduction of the *'Back to Sleep'* campaign in the 1990s, in which parents were told to lay babies on their backs, rather than prone, the incidence has reduced dramatically.

Syndrome   The word syndrome refers to the occurrence of a number of characteristics together. The characteristics may be physical (e.g. Down syndrome), behavioural (e.g. Asperger's syndrome), biochemical (e.g. syndrome of inappropriate ADH secretion) or a combination (e.g. Williams' syndrome). *Dysmorphic features*, i.e. distinctive physical characteristics, may indicate an underlying congenital syndrome.

Index

Page numbers ending in 'b', 'f' and 't' refer to Boxes, Figures and Tables respectively